Advances in Esophageal and Gastric Cancers

Advances in Esophageal and Gastric Cancers

Edited by Reginald Kelly

STATES
ACADEMIC PRESS
www.statesacademicpress.com

States Academic Press,
109 South 5th Street,
Brooklyn, NY 11249, USA

Visit us on the World Wide Web at:
www.statesacademicpress.com

ISBN: 978-1-63989-022-4

Cataloging-in-Publication Data

Advances in esophageal and gastric cancers / edited by Reginald Kelly.
p. cm.
Includes bibliographical references and index.
ISBN 978-1-63989-022-4
1. Esophagus--Cancer. 2. Digestive organs--Cancer. 3. Gastrointestinal system--Cancer. I. Kelly, Reginald.
RC280.E8 A28 2022
616.994 32--dc23

Table of Contents

Preface

Gastric cancer is the cancer that usually originates from the cells that line the stomach. The cancer may start as a polyp or an ulcer that initially may not cause any symptom or may cause bleeding or pain. Risk factors for gastric cancer are smoking, bacterial infection and acid reflux. Stomach cancer can also occur in the proximal part of the stomach which is close to esophagus. Esophageal cancer is a cancer that primarily develops in the esophagus. Ways of diagnosing stomach cancer include barium swallow, which examines the esophagus, stomach and duodenum, esophagogastroduodenoscopy, endoscopic ultrasound, computed tomography scan, fecal occult blood test, etc. This book brings forth some of the unexplored aspects of esophageal and gastric cancers. Also included herein is a detailed explanation of the various methods used for the diagnosis and treatment of these cancers. The extensive content of this book provides the readers with a thorough understanding of the subject.

The information contained in this book is the result of intensive hard work done by researchers in this field. All due efforts have been made to make this book serve as a complete guiding source for students and researchers. The topics in this book have been comprehensively explained to help readers understand the growing trends in the field.

I would like to thank the entire group of writers who made sincere efforts in this book and my family who supported me in my efforts of working on this book. I take this opportunity to thank all those who have been a guiding force throughout my life.

Editor

1

Nutritional Management of Esophageal Cancer Patients

Dimitrios Schizas, Irene Lidoriki,
Demetrios Moris and Theodore Liakakos

Abstract

Esophageal cancer is associated with malnutrition in the vast majority of patients. This phenomenon is partly attributed to the disease process itself, the location of the tumor and other factors, such as dysphagia which is often accentuated due to chemotherapy/radiotherapy treatment or surgical intervention. The poor nutritional status of these patients is often related to the presence of cancer cachexia, altered metabolism, and tissue wasting. Malnutrition in this patient population affects quality of life, worsens patient's tolerance to chemotherapy and accounts for lower survival. Nutritional management of these patients includes both proper nutritional assessment and support and might prevent, to a certain extent, the manifestation of malnutrition-related consequences. The purpose of this article is to review the current literature in order to focus on the etiology and diagnosis of malnutrition in esophageal cancer patients, emphasizing also on the optimal nutritional support during multimodality treatment.

Keywords: nutritional assessment, nutritional support, perioperative nutritional care, esophageal cancer

1. Introduction

Esophageal cancer is one of the most fatal cancers worldwide as it was ranked ninth for cancer incidence and sixth for cancer death in 2013. In 2013, there were 442,000 new cases of esophageal cancer and 440,000 deaths [1]. There are two main histologic subtypes of esophageal cancer: squamous cell carcinoma and adenocarcinoma, each one of them is related to several risk factors. Among them, modifiable lifestyle factors, such as alcohol consumption, tobacco use, and nutrition should be considered as key points in order to prevent esophageal cancer.

Excess alcohol consumption and consumption of hot food and beverages increase the risk of esophageal squamous cell carcinoma, whereas many components of Western type diet, such as red and processed meat increase the risk of esophageal adenocarcinoma [2–4]. Moreover, obesity, especially central type, and gastroesophageal reflux disease are risk factors toward developing esophageal adenocarcinoma [5, 6]. On the other hand, healthy dietary habits could be a shield against some types of esophageal cancer [7], while nutritional support could be beneficial for the management of these patients after cancer diagnosis.

Esophageal cancer is commonly associated with malnutrition and impaired nutritional intake. Nutritional management of these patients may differ according to the type of therapy and stage of disease, in order to alleviate symptoms, ameliorate nutritional status, and improve quality of life. Furthermore, cancer cachexia affects a great percentage of esophageal cancer patients emerging as a significant factor the multidisciplinary team should deal with [8]. Regarding the perioperative care, the proper type of feeding (i.e. enteral/parenteral nutrition (EN/PN), immunonutrition, oral supplements, etc.) as well as the right time of feeding is a matter of controversy due to lack of consistent evidence for patients undergoing esophagectomy [9]. Special nutritional needs in the long run are also of great significance for patients with both resectable and unresectble disease, bearing in mind that the majority of these patients strive to meet their caloric and protein needs. Considering the treatment approach, nutritional screening and assessment leads to early detection of malnourished patients in need of nutritional support. Taking into account patient's specific needs helps to choose the most suitable routes of delivering nutritional support (nutritional counseling and artificial nutrition). Personalized nutritional support could modify poor nutritional status resulting in reduced postoperative complications and improved survival. Moreover, the implementation of nutritional protocols could reduce toxicity of treatment regimens and in conjunction with nutritional monitoring could have impact on patients' daily living [10]. Therefore, nutritional therapy should be an essential part of a multidisciplinary approach in the clinical setting, in order to improve short- and long-term outcomes.

The aim of the current review is to focus on the etiology of malnutrition, review the various methods of nutritional assessment, and analyze the aspects of nutritional management of esophageal cancer patients as a fundamental part of multimodality therapy.

2. Nutritional status

2.1. Malnutrition rates and weight loss

Esophageal cancer patients often suffer from malnutrition, the manifestation of which is strongly linked to the stage of the disease and therapeutic regimens. Excessive weight loss is partly attributed to the disease process itself and is often deteriorated due to chemotherapy/radiotherapy treatment [11]. Malnutrition occurs in 60–85% of esophageal cancer patients, which is one of the highest reported rates when compared to other malignancies, such as lung, head and neck, stomach, and pancreatic cancers [12]. According to recent publications, 32% of patients who underwent esophagectomy experienced more than 10% weight loss preoperatively [13], while 90% of patients had a 5% weight loss at 3 months postoperatively [14]. It is noteworthy that in many patients weight loss persists for at least 3 years after surgical intervention [15]. Another study revealed that 43.8% of patients with esophageal cancer were underweight based on BMI values, 29.7% of patients were undernourished as indicated from anthropometric measurements and 69% had weight loss within 2 weeks before hospital admission [16]. Chemotherapy and radiotherapy affect nutritional status by promoting weight loss and muscle wasting. More specifically, malnutrition developed in 83.8% of patients after the end of radiotherapy [17] and the number of patients requiring nutritional intervention increased from 56 to 75% during induction chemotherapy [10]. These facts highlight the need of nutritional assessment at several time points in order to identify patients who are candidates for nutritional support.

2.2. Methods of nutritional assessment and impact on clinical outcome

There are various methods of nutritional assessment in the clinical setting providing clinicians with tools for the evaluation of the nutritional status and the estimation of nutritional needs of esophageal cancer patients. One commonly used criterion of malnutrition is the percentage of weight loss in a certain period of time. A weight loss of more than 5% in the previous month or more than 10% in the last 3–6 months is considered significant malnutrition [18]. One retrospective study concluded that weight loss <10% and BMI>18 kg/m^2 were significantly correlated with a better response to chemoradiotherapy, while BMI>18 kg/m^2 was predictive of survival at both univariate and multivariate analysis [19]. Other anthropometric measurements, such as mid-arm circumference and mid upper-arm muscle area can give information about the nutritional status and body composition of these patients.

Biochemical markers, such as plasma proteins are often used as nutritional markers. For instance, albumin is commonly used for the assessment of protein status, but given its long half-life (14–20 days), it has a slow response to dietary interventions and cannot detect subtle changes in nutritional status. Furthermore, albumin reflects an acute phase response and is not always a reliable marker of malnutrition [20]. However, albumin is an independent risk factor for complications after esophagectomy, since patients with hypoalbuminemia have twice the risk of postoperative infection and increased incidence of acute respiratory distress syndrome [21]. A recent review examined the association of serum albumin with postoperative complications in patients undergoing esophagectomy, suggesting that low serum albumin does increase the risk of postoperative complications, but there is still conflicting evidence regarding the prognostic value of this biomarker [22].

Other methods of nutritional assessment include questionnaires that incorporate many factors that impede adequate nutritional intake, as well as laboratory parameters, and unintentional weight loss. For example, Subjective Global Assessment (SGA), a questionnaire based on four parameters of patient's history (percentage of weight loss, changes in habitual diet, presence of significant gastrointestinal symptoms, and changes in patient's functional capacity) and three elements of their physical examination (loss of subcutaneous fat, muscle wasting, and presence of edema or ascites) is one the most commonly used tool for nutritional screening in malnourished hospital patients with cancer. SGA is strongly correlated with performance status in esophageal cancer patients [16] as well as with The Glasgow prognostic score and with complications during cancer treatment [23]. Other tools that have been studied in cancer patients is the Prognostic Nutritional Index (PNI), the Nutritional Risk Screening 2002 (NRS 2002), the Controlling Nutritional Status (CONUT) and the Nutritional Risk Index (NRI). Esophagectomized patients with a high Prognostic Nutritional Index—a tool which includes serum albumin and absolute peripheral lymphocyte count—had a higher prevalence of postoperative complications [24]. These results are in accordance with later studies, indicating that nutritional status preoperatively, expressed as PNI, was significantly related with the occurrence of severe complications and was a predictive factor for long-term survival [25, 26]. Nevertheless, Han-Geurts et al. showed that PNI was not associated with postoperative infectious complications in patients who underwent esophageal resection for malignancy [27]. NRS-2002 is recommended by the European Society for Clinical Nutrition and Metabolism as a standard tool for the assessment of surgical patients [28], but it is not tailored to esophageal cancer patients, thus limiting its prognostic value in this population. The CONUT score, which is calculated by serum albumin concentration, total peripheral lymphocyte count, and total cholesterol concentration, was developed as a screening tool for early detection of patients at risk of malnutrition [29]. Patients classified preoperatively as moderate or severe malnourished had a higher incidence of pulmonary and other severe morbidities, surgical site infections, and reoperation. Consequently, the duration of hospital stay in patients with moderate or severe malnutrition was significantly longer compared to well-nourished or slightly malnourished patients [30]. Similarly, Hirahara et al. [31] and Toyokawa et al. [32] demonstrated that CONUT was significantly associated with cancer death and poorer disease-free survival in patients with resectable esophageal squamous cell carcinoma. NRI is another tool used for the assessment of malnutrition based on serum albumin concentration and weight loss. Increased nutritional risk, derived from NRI, is associated with reduced survival in esophageal cancer patients treated with definitive chemoradiotherapy [10, 33], but is not associated with postoperative infectious complications in patients treated with esophagectomy [27]. The Geriatric Nutritional Risk Index (GNRI) is a new index recently introduced for the assessment of nutritional status of elderly patients. Patients diagnosed with poor nutritional status according to GNRI had significantly higher rate of respiratory complications after esophagectomy and gastric tube reconstruction [34]. In conclusion, there are several nutrition assessment tools for esophageal cancer patients, but since many of the studies mentioned above are of retrospective nature, the gold standard for the evaluation of nutritional status in this cancer subpopulation is yet to be determined (**Table 1**).

Percentage of unintentional weight loss	*Biochemical markers* (albumin, prealbumin, total peripheral lymphocyte count)	*Questionnaires and indices:* SGA, NRS2002, CONUT, NRI, PNI, Glasgow Prognostic Score

Table 1. Nutritional assessment of esophageal cancer patients.

2.3. Sarcopenia and cancer cachexia

Patients with esophageal cancer often witness loss of muscle mass and/or muscle strength, a condition described as sarcopenia. Although there are many different definitions of the term sarcopenia, all of them place emphasis on the impaired physical function following decreased muscle mass [35–37]. Sarcopenia is a component of cancer cachexia, especially in advanced stage cancer patients. Cancer cachexia is a complex syndrome which combines anorexia, early satiety, weakness, anemia, inflammation, weight loss, and loss of muscle mass with or without loss of fat mass [38]. A recent study pointed out that the prevalence of cancer cachexia in advanced esophageal cancer patients was 52.9% [39]. There is lack of consensus on the definition, diagnostic criteria, and classification of cancer cachexia, but the most commonly used definition includes one of the following: Weight loss >5% over past 6 months (in absence of simple starvation); or BMI <20 and any degree of weight loss >2%; or appendicular skeletal muscle index consistent with sarcopenia (males <7.26 kg/m^2; females <5.45 kg/m^2),and any degree of weight loss >2% [40]. Furthermore, assessment of sarcopenia plays an emerging role in cancer patients owing to the fact that CT scanning is a gold standard imaging method of body composition analysis at the tissue-organ level [41]. CT scans can identify reduced muscle mass and predict negative cancer outcomes in people with abdominal malignancies, where traditional methods of assessment are less effective [42]. Handgrip strength is another method used to measure muscle strength, which is directly related to the physiologic status of the individual and reflects patient's nutritional status. It could be easily used in patient's nutritional assessment due to the fact that it is an inexpensive and not time-consuming method.

Sarcopenia and cachexia are prognostic factors for surgical complications, decreased survival, and poor response to chemotherapy. More specifically, patients with weak handgrip strength had higher risk of complications and mortality after elective esophagectomy [43]. Decreased muscle mass, assessed by preoperative computed tomography scans, seems to be an independent predictor of both overall survival (**Figure 1**) [44] and disease-free survival, as significant as tumor stage, in patients following esophagectomy [45, 46]. In addition, sarcopenic patients who underwent esophagectomy had significantly higher rate of respiratory complications compared to nonsarcopenic subjects, but there was no difference in the incidence of overall complications between the two groups [47–49]. Sarcopenia has also impact on chemotherapy outcome since decreased muscle mass is associated with dose-limiting toxicity and pathological chemotherapy response in patients receiving neoadjuvant chemotherapy [50–52]. Therefore, it is imperative to estimate patients' muscle mass not only preoperatively but also before the onset of chemotherapy, bearing in mind that sarcopenia is frequently masqued by obesity making it more difficult to define patients' needs for intervention.

2.4. Mechanisms of malnutrition

Malnutrition, as mentioned above, affects a great percentage of esophageal cancer patients. Most patients are not able to achieve a positive energy balance and in many cases, initial body weight cannot even be maintained. This is ascribed mainly to impaired metabolism and side effects caused by esophagectomy or chemotherapy/radiation treatment. Dysphagia is a very common mechanical cause of malnutrition and is accompanied by dietary changes in order to

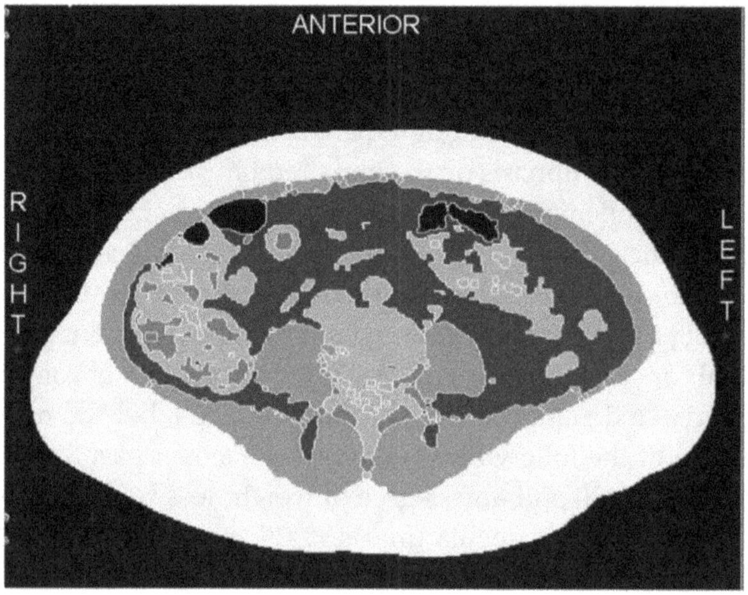

Figure 1. Example of CT scan analysis by the Slice-O-Matic software. Lumbar vertebrae 3 slice with Hounsfield units used to measure area of skeletal muscle, subcutaneous fat and visceral fat. White outer ring, subcutaneous fat; Light grey inner ring, muscle; Dark grey central area, visceral fat. Reproduced from Gibson et al. [42].

avoid foods that worsen symptoms leading to inadequate intake of calories. The surgical procedure often causes deficiencies in macronutrients and micronutrients, with the most prevailing side effects being postprandial dumping syndrome, dysphagia, anorexia, reflux, and early satiety [53–55]. Furthermore, chemotherapy affects rapidly proliferating cells preferentially and, consequently, affects the cells of the gastrointestinal tract. Chemotherapy-related causes of reduced food intake include nausea, vomiting, diarrhea, mucositis, and decreased appetite. Radiotherapy also contributes to malnutrition, and combined with chemotherapy exacerbates patients' nutritional status. Common side effects of radiotherapy include mucositis, esophagitis, odynophagia, mouth and throat soreness, and hypogeusia [56]. Tumor-related causes of malnutrition are also of great significance, but the mechanisms involved are still under investigation. Cancer-induced anorexia may result from circulating factors produced by the tumor or by the host in response to the tumor. For instance, cytokines, such as interleukins (IL) and tumor necrosis factor-alpha (TNF-α) cause anorexia [57], whereas other tumor-secreted factors promote central- and peripheral-mediated cancer cachexia. Tumor growth results in the secretion of pro-inflammatory factors that promote cachexia by signaling anorexia, muscle wasting, and white adipose tissue atrophy. Tumors also secrete both the proteolysis-inducing factor and activin, which promote skeletal muscle degradation and sarcopenia [58, 59].

Even though the mechanisms behind muscle wasting have been widely studied, less is known about the factors implicated in adipose tissue loss in cancer cachectic patients, such as lipid-mobilizing factor, as well as about the derangement in the neuroendocrine regulation of food intake and anorexia [60]. Additionally, changes in carbohydrate, lipid, and protein metabolism account for altered substrate metabolism. Changes in resting energy expenditure (REE) are considered one of the causes of nutritional depletion in cancer. In particular, measured REE by indirect calorimetry (IC) was elevated in patients with newly detected esophageal cancer, compared to healthy individuals [61]. A cross-sectional study involved 30 patients admitted with a diagnosis of squamous cell carcinoma who underwent IC before starting cancer therapy. The basal energy expenditure (BEE) was evaluated using IC and was also estimated using the Harris-Benedict Equation (HBE). The results showed that BEE of patients with squamous cell carcinoma was underestimated when using the HBE [62]. However, current evidence is inconsistent, since some studies suggest that REE is normal and is not affected by stage of disease [63–65]. Consequently, more research should be conducted in order to shed light on this controversial field.

3. Perioperative nutritional care

3.1. Enteral versus parenteral nutrition

Esophagectomy is one of the most invasive and time-consuming operations among gastrointestinal surgical procedures. It induces a strong stress response in the human body [66]. Consequently, patients' nutritional status is deteriorated after surgery, making postoperative nutritional care very important. The use of enteral nutrition (EN) postoperatively is a matter of debate, while scientific research attempts to define the role of enteral and parenteral nutrition (PN) on the clinical outcome of patients undergoing esophagectomy. Enteral feeding is considered the method of choice for the nutritional support of cancer patients with functioning gastrointestinal tract. Enteral nutrition is advantageous over parenteral nutrition for the following reasons: it provides all the necessary micro- and macronutrients in a more intact form, maintains gut mucosal integrity, inhibits the cytokine response, reduces the secretion of stress hormones, inhibits bacterial translocation, has a decreased risk of complications, and is less expensive [67]. Nevertheless, enteral nutrition is often avoided in order to minimize strain to the anastomoses, and reduce the risk of postoperatively impaired gastrointestinal motility. Another concern involves the return of gut motility or peristalsis and the ability of the gut to absorb nutrients. Surgical advances have increased the integrity of all anastomoses, making early oral enteral feeding after surgery a feasible option.

A randomized control trial investigated the outcomes of PN or EN after thoracoscopic esophagectomy. The rate of weight loss at postoperative day (POD) 14 was significantly lower in the EN group than in the PN group. Prealbumin levels at POD 10 showed no differences between the two groups. However, the incidence of postoperative pneumonia was higher in the PN group than in the EN group [68]. The results of another randomized clinical trial showed that there was no significant difference between EN and PN groups in terms of postoperative serum albumin, prealbumin, or transferrin. However, complement component 3 (C3) and 4 (C4) levels were significantly higher in the EN group compared with the PN group, while C-reactive protein level was significantly lower in the enteral feeding group. Bowel movements were restored sooner and costs of treatment were lower in the EN group. Postoperative complications did not differ significantly between the two groups [69]. Results from a recent meta-analysis of 10 randomized controlled trials concerning cancer patients following esophagectomy indicated that early postoperative enteral nutrition could significantly decrease pulmonary complications and anastomotic leakage compared with parenteral nutrition. On the eighth postoperative day, the EN group had higher levels of albumin and prealbumin compared with the PN group, suggesting that postoperative EN support is more effective in maintaining patients' nutritional status than PN support. No difference was observed in digestive complications between these two approaches. However, this meta-analysis is characterized by heterogeneity issues, especially regarding the postoperative nutritional status [70]. Furthermore, others suggest that combination of enteral and parenteral feeding is more beneficial, since total parenteral nutrition (TPN) could lead to hyperglycemia in stressed patients. A combination of EN and TPN might have some benefits when compared to TPN alone, such as improvement of intestinal integrity and stimulation of incretin production contributing to improved glucose control in patients undergoing esophagectomy [71]. Moreover, supplemental parenteral nutrition after esophagectomy contributes to better coverage of patients' calorie requirements, since large amounts of enteral nutrition are not usually tolerated in the first postoperative days [72].

The European Society for Parenteral and Enteral Nutrition (ESPEN) guidelines for nutritional support recommend that interruption of nutritional intake is unnecessary after surgery in most patients and in patients who require postoperative artificial nutrition, enteral feeding, or a combination of enteral and supplementary parenteral feeding is the first choice. Also this combination should be considered in patients in whom more than 60% of energy needs cannot be met via the enteral route. Postoperative parenteral nutrition is beneficial in undernourished patients in whom enteral nutrition is not feasible or not tolerated. In addition, postoperative parenteral nutrition is beneficial in patients with postoperative complications impairing gastrointestinal function that are unable to receive and absorb adequate amounts of oral/enteral feeding for at least 7 days [28]. Moreover, the American Society for Parenteral and Enteral Nutrition (ASPEN) guidelines for critically ill patients recommends that patients who have undergone major upper gastrointestinal tract surgery and EN is not feasible, PN should be initiated (only if the duration of therapy is anticipated to be more than 7 days). Unless the patient is at high nutrition risk, PN should not be started in the immediate postoperative period, but should be delayed for 5–7 days [73]. In conclusion, although enteral nutrition seems to be a safe and feasible option postoperatively in terms of immunological parameters and postoperative complications, no firm conclusion can be drawn regarding postoperative nutritional markers that reflect patients' nutritional status.

3.2. Time of feeding

3.2.1. Early enteral nutrition

The initiation of enteral feeding after esophagectomy remains a controversial topic and many studies examine whether or not early enteral feeding affects negatively or positively the postoperative outcome. One study that investigated early enteral feeding after esophagectomy included 208 patients who received enteral nutrition postoperatively and were divided into three groups (Group 1, 2, and 3) based on whether they received EN within 48 h, 48–72 h or more than 72 h, respectively. The postoperative complications, length of hospital (LOH) stay, days for first fecal passage, cost of hospitalization, and the difference in serum albumin values pre- and postoperatively were all recorded. Group 1 had the lowest thoracic drainage volume, the earliest first fecal passage, and the lowest LOH and hospitalization expenses of all the three groups. The incidence of pneumonia was higher in Group 3. Finally, all postoperative outcomes of nutritional status were worst in Group 3 [74]. Similarly, one systematic review demonstrated that early oral EN was associated with reduced length of stay and did not increase complication rates [75]. More randomized clinical trials are required to confirm the results from retrospective studies that indicated that early EN promotes early recovery of intestinal movement and better recovery from systemic inflammation [66]. In addition, current literature is inconclusive with respect to the right time of EN administration postoperatively, that is, EN initiation within 24 h versus EN initiation during 24–72 h [76, 77].

3.2.2. *Enhanced recovery after surgery (ERAS)*

Early enteral nutrition is an essential part of fast-track surgery protocols in order to maximize the effects of enhanced recovery. Fast-track programs incorporate new methods regarding anesthesia, nutritional care, pain control, and surgical techniques in the preoperative, intraoperative, and postoperative period, aiming to promote postoperative rehabilitation of patients [78]. ESPEN guidelines recommend that all cancer patients undergoing either curative or palliative surgery should be managed within an enhanced recovery program postoperatively; within this program every patient should be screened for malnutrition and if deemed at risk, given additional nutritional support [79]. Nutritional aspects of ERAS could be summarized as follows: limitation of preoperative fasting, preoperative fluid and carbohydrate loading, and initiation of oral diet on the first postoperative day [80]. A recently published review demonstrated that utilization of enhanced recovery programs in esophageal cancer patients was associated with a reduction in the incidence of anastomotic leak, pulmonary complications, and length of hospital stay, but no significant change was observed in postoperative mortality or readmission rate. Nevertheless, there was significant heterogeneity between the studies in terms of enhanced recovery protocols, surgical approach, and utilization of neoadjuvant therapies that should be taken into account [81]. Results from a randomized controlled clinical study showed that the implementation of a fast-track protocol improved postoperative clinical recovery and cellular and humoral immunity of patients undergoing esophagectomy for esophageal cancer (**Table 2**) [82]. In this context, the implementation of fast-track programs in esophagectomy patients is promising, but the majority of patients included in the studies are relatively healthy patients. More randomized controlled studies and evidence-based research are required in order to justify the routine use of fast-track protocols in esophageal cancer patients [83].

3.3. Perioperative immunonutrition

Immunonutrition is one of the most debated topics in nutritional support of esophageal cancer patients. The term immunonutrition includes formulas that contain immune-modulating substances, such as arginine, glutamine, ribose nucleic acid, and omega-3-fatty acids. A recent review concluded that postoperative enteral immunonutrition could be promising in improving humoral immunity in patients undergoing esophagogastric resection, but this improvement is not related to a reduced hospital stay, nor does it reduce the rate of infections. The authors reported that there is heterogeneity regarding the types of operations undertaken (two studies included patients undergoing esophagectomy, three studied patients undergoing gastrectomy,

Day	FTS pathway
POD1	Jejunostomy tube feeding 500 ml (starting at 20 ml/h)
	Early postoperative mobilization program
	(>2 h out of bed)
	Physical therapy and nebulizers
	Remove urine catheter
	Head of bed put at 30°
	Supply albumin
	Chest tube to suction
	Promoted to lung recruitment
POD2	Jejunostomy tube feeding 1000 ml (40 ml/h)
	Chest tube to suction
	Expand mobilization (>4 h out of bed)
	Continue physical therapy and nebulizers
	Continue supply albumin
POD3	Jejunostomy tube feeding 1500 ml (60–80 ml/h)
	Remove chest tube
	Remove epidural catheter
	Expand mobilization (>6 h out of bed)
	Continue physical therapy and nebulizers
	Continue supply albumin
POD4	Gastrograffin opacification of upper gastrointestine
	If swallow shows no leak, advance patient to oral drink
	Jejunostomy tube feeding 1500 ml (60–80 ml/h)
	Continue physical therapy and nebulizers
	Education on aspiration precaution
	Education on chewing and swallowing
POD5	Jejunostomy tube feeding 1500 ml (60–80 ml/h)
	Advance patient to a full liquid diet
	Continue aspiration precautions
	Continue physical therapy and nebulizers
POD6	Increase liquid diet
	Decrease jejunostomy tube feeding
	(500 or 1000 ml)
	Continue aspiration precautions
	Continue physical therapy and nebulizers
POD7	Remove jejunostomy tube
	Full liquid diet
	Discharge home on soft diet and liquid diet
	Continue aspiration precautions

Note: FTS: Fast track surgery. Adapted from Chen et al. [82].

Table 2. Daily guideline of postoperative care of patients with fast-track surgery pathway.

and one had patients undergoing both operations). Additionally, the included randomized clinical trials used different formulations of enteral immunonutrition and standard enteral nutrition, further limiting the accuracy of the results. Moreover, not all studies reported the same outcomes as far as inflammatory and immunological markers are concerned. Therefore, the authors suggest that there is no convincing evidence in terms of routine immunonutrition in patients undergoing esophageal resection for cancer [84].

On the other hand, preoperative nutritional supplementation with immune-enhancing formulas was associated with reduced infectious complications, duration of hospitalization, improved short-term survival and less mortality in patients with esophageal cancer. These results highlight the possible need to provide immunonutrients before surgery to obtain sufficient levels at the time of surgical stress when there is an increased need for stimulation of the immune system [85]. One meta-analysis that included studies with patients that underwent esophagectomy, gastrectomy and pancreatectomy, demonstrated that patients who received immunonutrition postoperatively, had a significantly lower risk of wound infection and shorter length of hospital stay. No significant effect of immunonutrition on other postoperative morbidities and mortality was noticed [86]. The reduction in hospital stay and/or in postoperative complications seems to compensate for the higher cost of immunonutrition compared to standard enteral feeding in a cost-effectiveness analysis [87]. According to ESPEN guidelines on nutrition in cancer patients, upper gastrointestinal tract cancer patients undergoing surgical resection should receive oral/enteral immunonutrition in the context of traditional perioperative care [79]. Furthermore, ASPEN guidelines suggest the routine use of an immunemodulating formula (containing both arginine and fish oils) in the surgical intensive care unit for the postoperative patient who requires enteral nutrition therapy [73].

Synbiotics, which are a combination of prebiotics and probiotics, are speculated to have beneficial effects on human health, but little is known about their clinical value in patients who have undergone esophagectomy. Administration of synbiotics prevented postoperative deterioration of the intestinal microfloral environment and suppressed excessive inflammatory response, possibly by exerting immunomodulatory effects and by inhibiting bacterial translocation [88, 89]. Additionally, synbiotics led to decreased incidence of severe diarrhea and lower interruption or reduction of enteral nutrition. Passage of flatus postoperatively occurred significantly earlier in patients who received synbiotics than in the control group, suggesting that synbiotics maintain intestinal motility [88]. Taking all the aforementioned things into consideration, larger scale studies are needed in order to define whether or not immunonutrition has beneficial effects on the postoperative outcome of esophageal cancer patients. Future research should focus on the optimal dose of specific immunonutrients, on the timing (preoperatively and/or postoperatively) and duration of immunonutrition delivery and clarify which is the target group the intervention should be addressed to.

3.4. Type of feeding

Enteral feeding postoperatively seems to be the method of choice for uncomplicated esophageal cancer patients. Enteral feeding options after surgery include mainly nasoenteric tubes and jejunostomy catheters, in order to bypass recently constructed anastomoses. However there is no general agreement regarding the best method for postoperative feeding, and the optimal access route remains questionable. Tube-related complications include occlusion, catheter displacement and local cellulitis at the site of insertion. More severe complications include leakage into the peritoneal cavity resulting in peritonitis, volvulus at the point of fixation to the anterior abdominal wall, aspiration pneumonia, necrotizing fasciitis or jejunal necrosis at the site of catheter insertion and septicemia [90, 91].

A retrospective analysis of 90 patients who underwent esophagectomy demonstrated that early enteral nutrition can be administered using three different routes (nasojejunal tube, jejunostomy tube, and pharyngostomy tube) with similar results regarding tube-related complications, length of stay, and 30-day morbidity [92]. Another study of esophageal cancer patients with dysphagia examined the effects of jejunostomy feeding on weight loss and treatment outcomes. The palliative group of patients was able to maintain a stable weight despite the presence of cancer cachexia. This was also evident in the esophagectomy group of patients despite the catabolic effect of the operation, indicating the effectiveness of the jejunostomy feeding catheter as a means of nutritional support. The feeding catheter was well tolerated by the majority of patients (86.8%) and the most frequently occurred complications included catheter clogging (10.1% of the study population) and catheter dislodgement (3.1% of the study population) [93]. A randomized clinical study that compared nasoenteric tubes to jejunostomy feeding in upper gastrointestinal tract cancer patients showed that the length of enteral feeding use was less in the nasoenteric group and parenteral feeding was required more frequently than in jejunostomy feeding group. Complications related to the different feeding routes were similar between the two groups [94]. A recent review investigated the best route for enteral nutrition following esophagectomy (oral intake, jejunostomy, or nasojejunal tube feeding) in terms of postoperative complication rates, percentage of patients meeting their nutritional needs, weight loss, tube feeding complications, mortality, patient satisfaction, and length of hospital stay. Complications and catheter efficacy did not differ between postoperative nasojejunal tube feeding and jejunostomy tube feeding. Moreover, jejunostomy feeding patients were able to meet their short-term nutritional requirements, but data concerning long-term outcomes and patients satisfaction were scarce. This review concluded that the best route for the delivery of early enteral nutrition postoperatively is still unclear [75].

ESPEN guidelines on enteral nutrition in surgical patients recommends that tube feeding should be applied in patients who cannot start early oral nutrition, including those undergoing gastrointestinal surgery for cancer and patients with obvious undernutrition at the time of surgery, in whom oral intake will be inadequate (<60%) for more than 10 days. Initiation of tube feeding should start within 24 h after surgery with a low flow rate (i.e. 10–20 ml/h) due to limited intestinal tolerance. Placement of a needle catheter jejunostomy or nasojejunal tube is recommended for all candidates for tube feeding undergoing major abdominal surgery. When anastomoses of the proximal gastrointestinal tract have been performed, enteral nutrition should be delivered via a tube placed distally to the anastomosis [95].

Postoperative nutritional management of esophageal cancer patients can be summarized as in **Figure 2**.

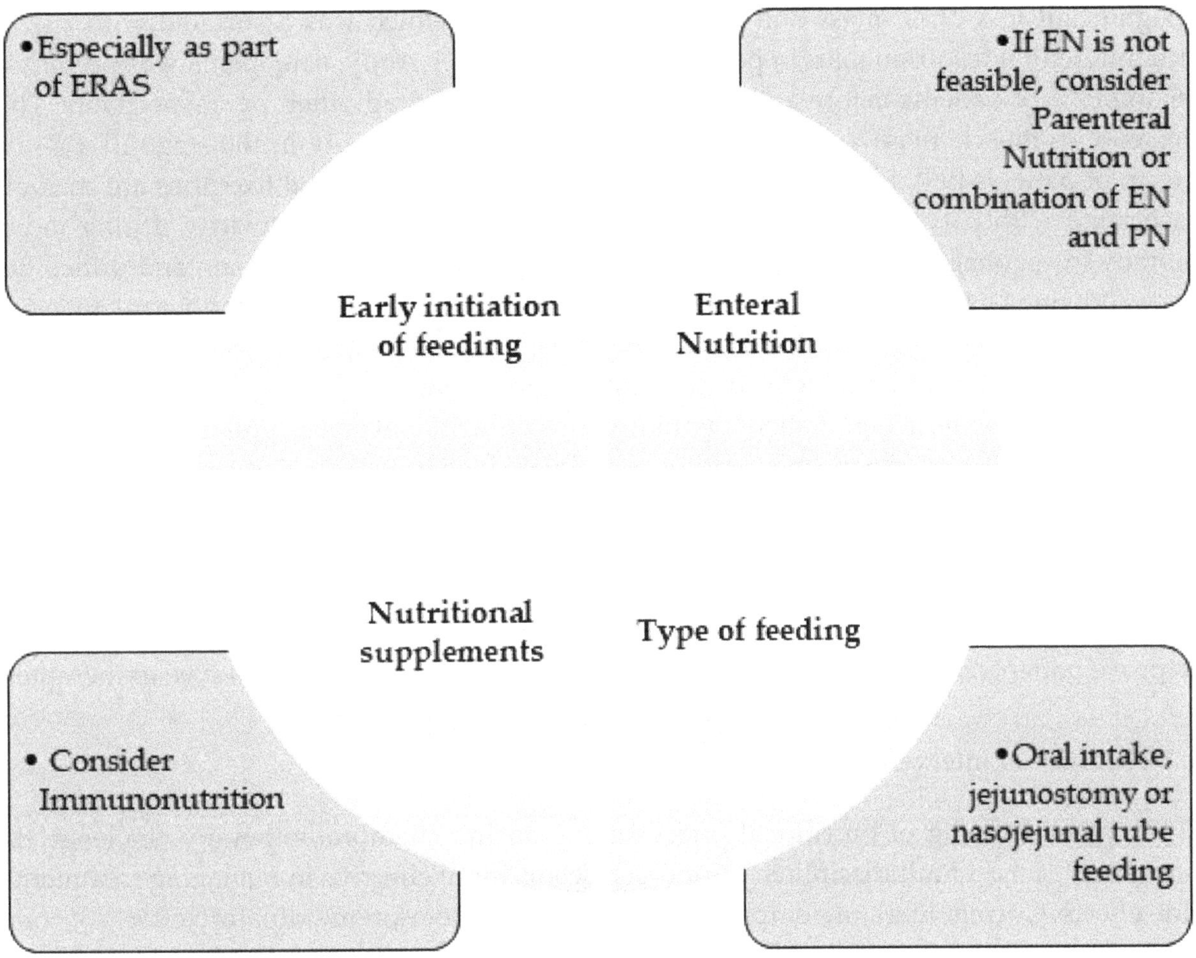

Figure 2. Postoperative nutritional management of esophageal cancer patients.

4. Nutritional care during chemoradiotherapy

4.1. Nutrition issues during chemotherapy and radiotherapy

Currently, perioperative chemotherapy is frequently administered for the treatment of resectable advanced esophageal cancer. The neoadjuvant administration of chemotherapy or chemoradiotherapy preoperatively results in reduced tumor size before surgery. Perioperative chemotherapy improves significantly disease-free survival and overall survival rates compared to surgery alone. However, a great percentage of these patients are not able to complete the planned postoperative chemotherapeutic regimens. This is mainly caused because of postoperative complications and impaired nutritional and physical status [96–98]. Gastrointestinal disorders caused by chemotherapy itself, including nausea, vomiting, diarrhea, and anorexia, negatively affect patients' quality of life and make completion of chemotherapy difficult. Neoadjuvant chemotherapy induces changes in body composition which, in turn have negative impact on clinical outcomes. Results from a small cohort of esophageal cancer patients showed that 26% of patients were sarcopenic before the initiation of neoadjuvant chemotherapy and this percentage increased to 43% after its completion. There was a significant loss of fat mass and skeletal muscle mass which was associated with risk of circumferential resection margin positivity [50]. In another study, sarcopenia was present in 56 and 67% of patients before and after neoadjuvant chemoradiotherapy, respectively. This decrease in muscle mass was predictive of postoperative mortality in the stage III–IV subgroup of patients [99]. Furthermore, most of the radiotherapy-related toxicities are strongly associated with patient's nutritional status. Esophagitis is the main toxicity during radiotherapy in esophageal cancer patients. These patients often suffer from pain and difficulties in swallowing [100]. One study in patients receiving concurrent chemoradiotherapy revealed that malnutrition was observed in 83.8% of patients, while 68.8% of patients developed severe dysphagia. Malnourished patients developed more treatment-related toxicities compared to those without malnutrition. Patients with impaired nutritional status presented severe dysphagia, anorexia, severe nausea/vomiting, and severe hematologic toxicities more frequently than those in a good nutrition status [17]. Although nutritionally related side effects occur frequently, nutritional assessment of patients with cancer receiving chemoradiotherapy is often omitted in the clinical setting. Scientific research has to focus on nutritional interventions during neoadjuvant chemoradiotherapy or postoperative adjuvant therapy that seems to improve patients' nutritional status, alleviate symptoms and increase tolerance to therapies.

4.2. Nutritional interventions during chemoradiotherapy

The type and timing of nutritional interventions during chemoradiotherapy challenge the caregivers, since a multidisciplinary approach seems more effective in managing treatment's side effects. Current literature emphasizes mainly on the immunomodulatory effects of some nutrients, on the impact of oral/tube administration of high-energy, and/or high protein supplements on the clinical outcome and on patients education about selecting an enriched diet. In cancer patients, it has been shown that the use of supplemental formulas and *n*-3 fatty acids, such as eicosapentaenoic acid (EPA) and docosahexaenoic acid (DHA), can improve body composition, preserve muscle mass, and possibly reverse or stop the development of cancer cachexia [101]. A controlled, randomized prospective, double-blind, multicenter study investigated the impact of enteral nutrition (via percutaneous endoscopic gastrostomy (PEG)) enriched with EPA and DHA on body composition, nutritional and functional status of esophageal and head and neck cancer patients undergoing concurrent chemoradiotherapy. There was a tendency toward improvement regarding loss of body cell mass and body weight following chemoradiotherapy, but did not reach statistical significance. However, Karnofsky score and subjective parameters, such as the NRS 2002 and the SGA score were significantly improved in the experimental group compared with the control group, indicating improved nutritional and functional status [102]. Similar results reported by another randomized double-blind clinical trial showed that administration of immunonutrition during chemoradiotherapy in head and neck and esophageal cancer patients was advantageous over standard enteral nutrition in terms of body weight, lean body mass, serum albumin levels, NRI assessment, plasma antioxidant capacity, and functional capacity [103].

Moreover, immunonutrition can modulate the immunological and inflammatory systems, thus reducing the risks of concurrent chemoradiotherapy. One randomized clinical trial examined the effects of immunonutrition on serum cytokine and inflammatory markers, and cellular immunity in locally advanced esophageal cancer patients undergoing chemoradiotherapy. The levels of C-Reactive Protein (CRP) and TNF increased more during treatment in the control group (standard enteral nutrition) than in the treatment group, whereas all other markers did not differ significantly between the two groups [104]. In addition, the impact of immunonutrients on immune system of head and neck and esophageal cancer patients during chemoradiotherapy was examined in another randomized clinical trial. Immune cells metabolism and functions were assessed at the initiation and at the completion of treatment. The experimental group had better adaptation to the systematic inflammation and oxidative stress, as indicated by $CD4^+/CD8^+$ T-lymphocyte counts ratio, CD3 membrane expression, polymorphonuclear cells CD62L and CD15 densities, reactive oxygen species (ROS) production, and peripheral blood mononuclear cells production of pro-inflammatory prostaglandin-E2 [105].

Another role of immunonutrition is the potential protection against chemotherapy-induced toxicities. Miyata et al. compared the effects between enteral nutrition rich in *n*-3 fatty acids (900 mg/d) and enteral nutrition poor in *n*-3 fatty acids (250 mg/d) on chemotherapy-related adverse events and inflammatory markers during neoadjuvant chemotherapy in esophageal cancer patients. This randomized control trial showed no significant difference in the incidence of grade 3/4 leukopenia and neutropenia, but stomatitis was observed less frequently in the *n*-3-rich group, than in the *n*-3-poor group. Grade 3/4 diarrhea was also observed less frequently in the *n*-3-rich group than in the *n*-3-poor group, but this was not statistically significant. Moreover, *n*-3-rich enteral nutrition seems to have hepatoprotective properties by preventing an increase of aspartate aminotransferase and alanine aminotransferase values [106].

Synbiotics seem also to mitigate chemotherapy-related side effects through adjustments to the intestinal microbiota. A randomized clinical trial investigated the effects of synbiotics in esophageal cancer patients undergoing neoadjuvant chemotherapy, on the intestinal microbiota, and the adverse events of treatment. Severe lymphopenia and diarrhea were less frequent in patients who received synbiotics than in the control group. Furthermore, febrile neutropenia occurred less in the synbiotics group compared to the control group [107]. Chemotherapy may disturb the intestinal microbiota, leading to reduced production of organic acids in the bowel, impaired mucosal integrity, and increased harmful bacteria. These, in turn, may induce chemotherapy-related toxicities, such as diarrhea and infectious complications [108]. Administration of synbiotics results in increased concentrations of short-chain fatty acids, such as acetate and propionate. These fatty acids are an important energy source of enterocytes, maintain intestinal environment acidity and intestinal motility. Synbiotics also maintain the number of beneficial bacteria and inhibit the overgrowth of possible diarrheal pathogens, thus reducing the incidence of diarrhea [109].

ESPEN guidelines on nutrition in cancer patients recommend the supplementation with long-chain *n*-3 fatty acids or fish oil to stabilize or improve appetite, food intake, lean body mass, and body weight in patients with advanced cancer undergoing chemotherapy and at risk of weight loss or malnourished [79]. It is therefore evident that immunonutrition enhances immune system and exerts anti-inflammatory properties, but the promising effects on clinical outcome during chemoradiotherapy in esophageal cancer are still under investigation. Additional clinical trials are needed to determine the preferred type, timing and duration of immunonutrition required to reduce inflammation and chemotherapy-induced toxicities, and maintain muscle mass.

Nutritional interventions, other than that examining the impact of specific immunonutrients on chemoradiotherapy-related outcomes, include nutritional counseling and/or enteral supplements in order to maintain stable body weight and cope with feeding difficulties (**Table 3**). A recent randomized controlled trial compared the effects of a walk-and-eat intervention versus conventional medical care for patients with esophageal cancer undergoing neoadjuvant chemoradiotherapy. This intervention consisted of a structured walking protocol and weekly nutritional advice including weight and intake evaluation, counseling to overcome feeding difficulties, supplementation, if necessary, with enteral formulas, and patient's education concerning food texture modification and oral care before and after eating. During chemoradiotherapy, the group that received the walk-and-eat intervention had 100-m less decline than controls in walk distance, 3 kg less decrease in handgrip strength, and 2.7 kg less reduction in body weight. Moreover, the experimental group had significantly reduced rates of intravenous nutritional support and wheel chair use [110]. Another randomized trial tested the effects of an interdisciplinary nutrition support team on clinical and hospitalized outcomes of esophageal cancer patients receiving concurrent chemoradiotherapy. Nutritional support included dietary counseling, oral nutritional supplements, enteral nutrition, and parenteral nutrition according to patient's needs. At the completion of treatment, nutritional status of patients in the interventional group was better compared to control group, as demonstrated by prealbumin, transferrin, and albumin levels. Bone marrow suppression and complications related to infections were significantly lower in the nutritional support group. Nutritional intervention was also associated with a lower average length of hospital stay and in-patient cost [111]. Furthermore, nutritional intervention improved survival of esophageal cancer patients treated with definitive chemoradiotherapy. It is noticeable that this effect was observed only if nutritional support was provided at baseline (dietary advice, oral supplementation, or major intervention), and not if provided later in the treatment course [10].

According to ESPEN, in patients receiving radiotherapy, especially radiotherapy of the head and neck, thorax, and gastrointestinal tract, an adequate nutritional intake should be ensured primarily by individualized nutritional counseling and/or with use of oral nutritional

Nutritional counseling
Oral supplementation
Immunonutrition
Synbiotics
Parenteral nutrition support

Table 3. Nutritional interventions during chemoradiotherapy.

supplements, in order to avoid nutritional deterioration, maintain intake, and avoid radiotherapy interruptions. In addition, for patients undergoing curative anticancer drug treatment who cannot meet their nutritional requirements despite counseling and oral nutritional supplements, ESPEN recommends supplemental enteral nutrition or, if this is not sufficient or possible, parenteral nutrition [79]. Therefore, assessment and maintenance of good nutritional status at baseline may be a simple and cost-effective intervention that improves clinical outcomes in esophageal cancer patients during chemoradiotherapy treatment.

4.3. Stent insertion

There are various types of stents available, such as self-expandable metallic stents, self-expandable plastic stents, and biodegradable stents. Esophageal stenting can be implemented to relieve dysphagia during preoperative chemotherapy and/or radiotherapy. A systematic review investigated the impact of stent insertion during neoadjuvant treatment on dysphagia improvement. Placement of an esophageal stent significantly improved overall dysphagia scores in all 12 studies reviewed. However, no consistent improvement in nutritional status was observed, defined by body weight and albumin levels. Moreover, stent insertion was associated with complications, such as migration and chest pain, frequently resulting in stent removal or replacement [112]. The European Society of Gastrointestinal Endoscopy (ESGE) does not recommend self-expandable metal stents placement as a bridge to surgery or prior to preoperative chemoradiotherapy, since it is associated with a high incidence of adverse events. Other options, such as feeding tube placement are preferable and should be considered in dysphagic or malnourished patients in the neoadjuvant setting [113].

5. Palliative care

Management of patients undergoing noncurative treatments due to advanced disease is difficult, since the goals are not to cure patients but to improve length and quality of remaining life. Nutritional support is a crucial part in the palliative care as long as its benefits outweigh its costs. Patients with metastatic disease present for the clinician not only clinical but ethical issues as well. Dysphagia is the main symptom in patients with unresectable disease which aggravates malnutrition and requires nutritional intervention [114]. Nutritional support of these patients includes intravenous fluids for hydration, feeding tubes, parenteral nutrition, and stent placement in order to supplement dietary and caloric intake. Various techniques have been proposed to manage dysphagia, such as brachytherapy, self-expanding metal stents, thermal laser therapy, and photodynamic therapy. Each one of them has specific advantages and risks that should be taken into consideration. The authors of a recent meta-analysis of 53 randomized controlled trials concluded that self-expanding metal stent insertion is safe, effective, and improves dysphagia faster compared to other modalities. High-dose intraluminal brachytherapy is a satisfactory alternative and might provide additional survival benefit with a better quality of life. Combinations of brachytherapy with self-expanding metal stent insertion or radiotherapy seem to be the preferable option addressed to inoperative patients [115]. ESGE recommends placement of partially or fully covered self-expandable metal stents for palliative treatment of malignant dysphagia over laser therapy, photodynamic therapy, and esophageal bypass [113].

Moreover, in esophageal cancer patients with short life expectancy unsuitable for esophageal stenting, percutaneous endoscopic gastrostomy (PEG) may be a suitable means in order to achieve nutritional support, while allowing patients to be at home [116]. Endoscopically assisted nasogastric tube feeding is also a feasible palliative option for nutritional support, with a low complication rate. Tube-feeding patients had significantly higher enteral calorie intake, higher serum albumin, shorter hospital stay, and longer median survival compared to those who received *nil per os*, according to a retrospective study of patients with malignant esophageal obstruction [117]. Palliative care in the terminal phase should be followed in an individualized manner. ESPEN recommends that in dying patients, artificial hydration and nutrition are unlikely to benefit patients. Nevertheless, in acute confusional states, patients might receive a short and limited hydration to rule out dehydration as precipitating cause [79].

6. Conclusion

Esophageal cancer patients suffer from malnutrition and cannot easily meet their nutritional needs. Nutritional assessment, in the perioperative phase, but also in patients undergoing chemoradiotherapy should be performed regularly, in order to identify undernourished patients. Regarding the perioperative management of these patients, early enteral nutrition support seems to be the method of choice in uncomplicated patients, especially as a part of ERAS programs. However, the impact of immunonutrition on clinical outcome is still under investigation. During chemoradiotherapy, prevention of weight loss is of great significance and might be achieved through close nutritional monitoring. Nutritional support mainly encompasses dietary counseling, oral supplementation, tube feeding, and combination of them and has promising results in ameliorating nutritional status and affecting the oncologic outcome. Moreover, patients with terminal-stage esophageal cancer might benefit from early stent insertion in order to reduce dysphagia. Individualized nutritional support should be addressed to every patient who is in need of nutritional intervention.

Author details

Dimitrios Schizas[1*], Irene Lidoriki[1], Demetrios Moris[2] and Theodore Liakakos[1]

*Address all correspondence to: schizasad@gmail.com

1 First Department of Surgery, Laikon General Hospital, National and Kapodistrian University of Athens, Athens, Greece

2 Department of Surgery, Division of Surgical Oncology, The Ohio State University Wexner Medical Center and James Cancer Hospital and Solove Research Institute, Columbus, OH, USA

References

[1] Global Burden of Disease Cancer Collaboration. The global burden of cancer 2013. JAMA Oncology. 2015;**1**(4):505-527. DOI: 10.1001/jamaoncol.2015.0735

[2] Yang CS, Chen X, Tu S. Etiology and prevention of esophageal cancer. Gastrointestinal Tumors. 2016;**3**(1):3-16. DOI: 10.1159/000443155

[3] Choi Y, Song S, Song Y, Lee JE. Consumption of red and processed meat and esophageal cancer risk: Meta-analysis. World Journal of Gastroenterology. 2013;**19**(7):1020-1029. DOI: 10.3748/wjg.v19.i7.1020

[4] Andrici J, Eslick G. Hot food and beverage consumption and the risk of esophageal cancer. American Journal of Preventive Medicine. 2015;**49**(6):952-960. DOI: 10.1016/j.amepre.2015.07.023

[5] Corley DA, Kubo A, Zhao W. Abdominal obesity and the risk of esophageal and gastric cardia carcinomas. Cancer Epidemiology, Biomarkers & Prevention: A Publication of the American Association for Cancer Research, Cosponsored by the American Society of Preventive Oncology. 2008;**17**(2):352-358. DOI: 10.1158/1055-9965.EPI-07-0748

[6] Cook MB, Corley DA, Murray LJ, et al. Gastroesophageal reflux in relation to adenocarcinomas of the esophagus: A pooled analysis from the Barrett's and Esophageal Adenocarcinoma Consortium (BEACON). Suzuki H, ed. PLoS One. 2014;**9**(7):e103508. DOI: 10.1371/journal.pone.0103508

[7] Kubo A, Block G, Quesenberry CP, et al. Effects of dietary fiber, fats, and meat intakes on the risk of Barrett's esophagus. Nutrition and Cancer. 2009;**61**(5):607-616. DOI: 10.1080/01635580902846585

[8] Anandavadivelan P, Lagergren P. Cachexia in patients with oesophageal cancer. Nature Reviews Clinical Oncology. 2016;**13**(3):185-198. DOI: 10.1038/nrclinonc.2015.200

[9] Llop-Talaveron JM, Farran-Teixidor L, Badia-Tahull MB, et al. Artificial nutritional support in cancer patients after esophagectomy: 11 years of experience. Nutrition and Cancer. 2014;**66**(6):1038-1046. DOI: 10.1080/01635581.2014.939292.

[10] Cox S, Powell C, Carter B, et al. Role of nutritional status and intervention in oesophageal cancer treated with definitive chemoradiotherapy: Outcomes from SCOPE1. British Journal of Cancer. 2016;**115**(2):172-177. DOI: 10.1038/bjc.2016.129

[11] Deans DAC, Tan BH, Wigmore SJ, et al. The influence of systemic inflammation, dietary intake and stage of disease on rate of weight loss in patients with gastro-oesophageal cancer. British Journal of Cancer. 2009;**100**(1):63-69. DOI: 10.1038/sj.bjc.6604828

[12] Riccardi D, Allen K. Nutritional management of patients with esophageal and esophagogastric junction cancer. Cancer Control. 1999;**6**(1):64-72

[13] Bailey SH, Bull DA, Harpole DH, et al. Outcomes after esophagectomy: A ten-year prospective cohort. The Annals of Thoracic Surgery. 2003;**75**(1):217-222

[14] Bower MR, Martin RC. Nutritional management during neoadjuvant therapy for esophageal cancer. Journal of Surgical Oncology. 2009;**100**(1):82-87. DOI: 10.1002/jso.21289

[15] Martin L, Lagergren P. Long-term weight change after oesophageal cancer surgery. British Journal of Surgery. 2009;**96**(11):1308-1314. DOI: 10.1002/bjs.6723

[16] Quyen TC, Angkatavanich J, Thuan TV, et al. Nutrition assessment and its relationship with performance and Glasgow prognostic scores in Vietnamese patients with esophageal cancer. Asia Pacific Journal of Clinical Nutrition. 2017;**26**(1):49-58. DOI: 10.6133/apjcn.122015.02

[17] Pan P, Tao G, Sun X. Subjective global assessment and prealbumin levels of esophageal cancer patients undergoing concurrent chemoradiotherapy. Nutricion Hospitalaria. 2015;**31**(5):2167-2173. DOI: 10.3305/nh.2015.31.5.8596

[18] Nitenberg G, Raynard B. Nutritional support of the cancer patient: Issues and dilemmas. Critical Reviews in Oncology/Hematology. 2000;**34**(3):137-168

[19] DiFiore F, Lecleire S, Pop D, et al. Baseline nutritional status is predictive of response to treatment and survival in patients treated by definitive chemoradiotherapy for a locally advanced esophageal cancer. American Journl of Gastroenterology. 2007;**102**(11):2557-2563. DOI: 10.1111/j.1572-0241.2007.01437.x

[20] National Collaborating Centre for Acute Care. Nutrition Support for Adults Oral Nutrition Support, Enteral Tube Feeding and Parenteral Nutrition Methods, Evidence and Guidance; 1e176. 2006. London: National Collaborating Centre for Acute Care at The Royal College of Surgeons of England; 2011

[21] Ryan AM, Hearty A, Prichard RS, et al. Association of hypoalbuminemia on the first postoperative day and complications following esophagectomy. Journal of Gastrointestinal Surgery. 2007;**11**(10):1355-1360

[22] Goh SL, De Silva RP, Dhital K, et al. Is low serum albumin associated with postoperative complications in patients undergoing oesophagectomy for oesophageal malignancies? Interactive CardioVascular and Thoracic Surgery. 2015;**20**(1):107-113. DOI: 10.1093/icvts/ivu324

[23] da Silva JB, Maurício SF, Bering T, Correia MI. The relationship between nutritional status and the Glasgow prognostic score in patients with cancer of the esophagus and stomach. Nutrition and Cancer. 2013;**65**(1):25-33. DOI: 10.1080/01635581.2013.741755

[24] Nozoe T, Kimura Y, Ishida M, et al. Correlation of pre-operative nutritional condition with post-operative complications in surgical treatment for oesophageal carcinoma. European Journal of Surgical Oncology. 2002;**28**(4):396-400. DOI: 10.1053/ejso.2002.1257

[25] Feng J-F, Chen Q-X. Significance of the prognostic nutritional index in patients with esophageal squamous cell carcinoma. Therapeutics and Clinical Risk Management. 2014;**10**:1-7. DOI: 10.2147/TCRM.S56159

[26] Filip B, Scarpa M, Cavallin F, et al. Postoperative outcome after oesophagectomy for cancer: Nutritional status is the missing ring in the current prognostic scores. European Journal of Surgical Oncology. 2015;**41**(6):787-794. DOI: 10.1016/j.ejso.2015.02.014

[27] Han-Geurts IJ, Hop WC, Tran TC, Tilanus HW. Nutritional status as a risk factor in esophageal surgery. Digestive Surgery. 2006;**23**(3):159-163. DOI: 10.1159/000093756

[28] Braga M, Ljungqvist O, Soeters P, et al. ESPEN guidelines on parenteral nutrition: Surgery. Clinical Nutrition. 2009;**28**(4):378-386. DOI: 10.1016/j.clnu.2009.04.002

[29] Ignacio de Ulibarri J, Gonzalez-Madrono A, de Villar NG, et al. CONUT: A tool for controlling nutritional status. First validation in a hospital population. Nutricion Hospitalaria. 2005;**20**(1):38-45

[30] Yoshida N, Baba Y, Shigaki H, et al. Preoperative nutritional assessment by controlling nutritional status (CONUT) is useful to estimate postoperative morbidity after esophagectomy for esophageal cancer. World Journal of Surgery. 2016;**40**(8):1910-1917. DOI: 10.1007/s00268-016-3549-3

[31] Hirahara N, Matsubara T, Hayashi H, et al. Prognostic importance of controlling nutritional status in patients undergoing curative thoracoscopic esophagectomy for esophageal cancer. American Journal of Therapeutics. 2016;**0**(0):1-9. DOI: 10.1097/MJT.0000000000000414

[32] Toyokawa T, Kubo N, Tamura T, et al. The pretreatment controlling nutritional status (CONUT) score is an independent prognostic factor in patients with resectable thoracic esophageal squamous cell carcinoma: Results from a retrospective study. BMC Cancer. 2016;**16**(1):722. DOI: 10.1186/s12885-016-2696-0

[33] Clavier JB, Antoni D, Atlani D, et al. Baseline nutritional status is prognostic factor after definitive radiochemotherapy for esophageal cancer. Diseases of the Esophagus. 2014;**27**(6):560-567. DOI: 10.1111/j.1442-2050.2012.01441.x

[34] Yamana I, Takeno S, Shibata R, et al. Is the geriatric nutritional risk index a significant predictor of postoperative complications in patients with esophageal cancer undergoing esophagectomy? European Surgical Research. 2015;**55**(1-2):35-42. DOI: 10.1159/000376610

[35] Cruz-Jentoft AJ, Baeyens JP, Bauer JM, et al. Sarcopenia: European consensus on definition and diagnosis—Report of the European Working Group on Sarcopenia in Older People. Age Ageing. 2010;**39**(4):412-423. DOI: 10.1093/ageing/afq034

[36] Muscaritoli M, Anker SD, Argiles J, et al. Consensus definition of sarcopenia, cachexia and pre-cachexia: Joint document elaborated by special interest groups (SIG) "cachexia-anorexia in chronic wasting diseases" and "nutrition in geriatrics". Clinical Nutrition. 2010;**29**(2):154-159. DOI: 10.1016/j.clnu.2009.12.004

[37] Fielding RA, Vellas B, Evans WJ, et al. Sarcopenia: An undiagnosed condition in older adults—Current consensus definition: Prevalence, etiology, and consequences. International working group on Sarcopenia. Journal of the American Medical Directors Association. 2011;**12**(4):249-256. DOI: 10.1016/j.jamda.2011.01.003

[38] Argilés JM, Olivan M, Busquets S, López-Soriano FJ. Optimal management of cancer anorexia–cachexia syndrome. Cancer Management and Research. 2010;**2**:27-38

[39] Sun L, Quan XQ, Yu S. An epidemiological survey of cachexia in advanced cancer patients and analysis on its diagnostic and treatment status. Nutrition and Cancer. 2015;**67**(7):1056-1062. DOI: 10.1080/01635581.2015.1073753

[40] Fearon K, Strasser F, Anker SD, et al. Definition and classification of cancer cachexia: An international consensus. Lancet Oncology. 2011;**12**(5):489-495. DOI: 10.1016/S1470-2045(10)70218-7

[41] Prado CM, Birdsell LA, Baracos VE. The emerging role of computerized tomography in assessing cancer cachexia. Current Opinion in Supportive and Palliative Care. 2009;**3**(4):269-275. DOI: 10.1097/SPC.0b013e328331124a

[42] Gibson DJ, Burden ST, Strauss BJ, et al. The role of computed tomography in evaluating body composition and the influence of reduced muscle mass on clinical outcome in abdominal malignancy: A systematic review. European Journal of Clinical Nutrition. 2015;**69**(10):1079-1086. DOI: 10.1038/ejcn.2015.32

[43] Chen CH, Ho-Chang, Huang YZ, Hung TT. Hand-grip strength is a simple and effective outcome predictor in esophageal cancer following esophagectomy with reconstruction: A prospective study. Journal of Cardiothoracic Surgery. 2011;**6**:98. DOI: 10.1186/1749-8090-6-98

[44] Levolger S, van Vugt JL, de Bruin RW, IJzermans JN. Systematic review of sarcopenia in patients operated on for gastrointestinal and hepatopancreatobiliary malignancies. British Journal of Surgery. 2015;**102**(12):1448-1458. DOI: 10.1002/bjs.9893

[45] Sheetz KH, Zhao L, Holcombe SA, et al. Decreased core muscle size is associated with worse patient survival following esophagectomy for cancer. Diseases of the Esophagus. 2013;**26**(7):716-722. DOI: 10.1111/dote.12020

[46] Tamandl D, Paireder M, Asari R, et al. Markers of sarcopenia quantified by computed tomography predict adverse long-term outcome in patients with resected oesophageal or gastro-oesophageal junction cancer. European Radiology. 2016;**26**(5):1359-1367. DOI: 10.1007/s00330-015-3963-1

[47] Ida S, Watanabe M, Yoshida N, et al. Sarcopenia is a predictor of postoperative respiratory complications in patients with esophageal cancer. Annals of Surgical Oncology. 2015;**22**(13):4432-4437. DOI: 10.1245/s10434-015-4559-3

[48] Nishigori T, Okabe H, Tanaka E, et al. Sarcopenia as a predictor of pulmonary complications after esophagectomy for thoracic esophageal cancer. Journal of Surgical Oncology. 2016;**113**(6):678-684. DOI: 10.1002/jso.24214

[49] Makiura D, Ono R, Inoue J, et al. Preoperative sarcopenia is a predictor of postoperative pulmonary complications in esophageal cancer following esophagectomy: A retrospective cohort study. Journal of Geriatric Oncology. 2016;**7**(6):430-436. DOI: 10.1016/j.jgo.2016.07.003

[50] Yip C, Goh V, Davies A, et al. Assessment of sarcopenia and changes in body composition after neoadjuvant chemotherapy and associations with clinical outcomes in oesophageal cancer. European Radiology. 2014;**24**(5):998-1005. DOI: 10.1007/s00330-014-3110-4

[51] Tan BH, Brammer K, Randhawa N, et al. Sarcopenia is associated with toxicity in patients undergoing neo-adjuvant chemotherapy for oesophago-gastric cancer. European Journal of Surgical Oncology. 2015;**41**(3):333-338. DOI: 10.1016/j.ejso.2014.11.040

[52] Anandavadivelan P, Brismar TB, Nilsson M, et al. Sarcopenic obesity: A probable risk factor for dose limiting toxicity during neo-adjuvant chemotherapy in oesophageal cancer patients. Clinical Nutrition. 2016;**35**(3):724-730. DOI: 10.1016/j.clnu.2015.05.011

[53] Aghajanzadeh M, Safarpour F, Koohsari MR, et al. Functional outcome of gastrointestinal tract and quality of life after esophageal reconstruction of esophagus cancer. Saudi Journal of Gastroenterology. 2008;**15**(1):24e8. DOI: 10.4103/1319-3767.45050

[54] Ginex P, Thom B, Jingeleski M, et al. Patterns of symptoms following surgery for esophageal cancer. Oncology Nursing Forum. 2013;**40**(3):E101-E107. DOI: 10.1188/13.ONF.E101-E107

[55] Greene CL, DeMeester SR, Worrell SG, et al. Alimentary satisfaction, gastrointestinal symptoms, and quality of life 10 or more years after esophagectomy with gastric pull-up. Journal of Thoracic and Cardiovascular Surgery. 2014;**147**(3):909-914. DOI: 10.1016/j.jtcvs.2013.11.004

[56] Mak RH, Mamon HJ, Ryan DP, et al. Toxicity and outcomes after chemoradiation for esophageal cancer in patients age 75 or older. Diseases of the Esophagus. 2010;**23**(4):316-323. DOI: 10.1111/j.1442-2050.2009.01014.x

[57] Sonti G, Ilyin SE, Plata-Salaman CR. Anorexia induced by cytokine interactions at pathophysiological concentrations. American Journal of Physiology. 1996;**270**(6 Pt 2): R1394-R402

[58] Zhou X, Wang JL, Lu J, et al. Reversal of cancer cachexia and muscle wasting by ActRIIB antagonism leads to prolonged survival. Cell. 2010;**142**(4):531-543. DOI: 10.1016/j.cell.2010.07.011

[59] Johns N, Stephens NA, Fearon KC. Muscle wasting in cancer. The International Journal of Biochemistry & Cell Biology. 2013;**45**(10):2215-2229. DOI: 10.1016/j.biocel.2013.05.032

[60] Mendes MC, Pimentel GD, Costa FO, Carvalheira JB. Molecular and neuroendocrine mechanisms of cancer cachexia. Journal of Endocrinology. 2015;**226**(3):R29-R43. DOI: 10.1530/JOE-15-0170

[61] Wu J, Huang C, Xiao H, et al. Weight loss and resting energy expenditure in male patients with newly diagnosed esophageal cancer. Nutrition. 2013;**29**(11-12):1310-1314. DOI: 10.1016/j.nut.2013.04.010

[62] Becker Veronese CB, Guerra LT, Souza Grigolleti S, et al. Basal energy expenditure measured by indirect calorimetry in patients with squamous cell carcinoma of the esophagus. Nutricion Hospitalaria. 2013;**28**(1):142-147. DOI: 10.3305/nh.2013.28.1.6152

[63] Cao DX, Wu GH, Zhang B, et al. Resting energy expenditure and body composition in patients with newly detected cancer. Clinical Nutrition. 2010;**29**(1):72-77. DOI: 10.1016/j.clnu.2009.07.001

[64] Dempsey DT, Feurer ID, Knox LS, et al. Energy expenditure in malnourished gastrointestinal cancer patients. Cancer. 1984;**53**(6):1265-1273

[65] Okamoto H, Sasaki M, Johtatsu T, et al. Resting energy expenditure and nutritional status in patients undergoing transthoracic esophagectomy for esophageal cancer. Journal of Clinical Biochemistry and Nutrition. 2011;**49**(3):169-173. DOI: 10.3164/jcbn.11-13

[66] Kobayashi K, Koyama Y, Kosugi S, et al. Is early enteral nutrition better for postoperative course in esophageal cancer patients? Nutrients. 2013;**5**(9):3461-3469. DOI: 10.3390/nu5093461

[67] Demeyer I, Bataillie K, Baute L. Long-term sedation in the ICU: Enteral versus parenteral feeding. Clinical Intensive Care. 1994;**5**(5 Suppl):13-16

[68] Takesue T, Takeuchi H, Ogura M, et al. A prospective randomized trial of enteral nutrition after thoracoscopic esophagectomy for esophageal cancer. Annals of Surgical Oncology. 2015;**22**(Suppl 3):S802-S809. DOI: 10.1245/s10434-015-4767-x

[69] Rajabi Mashhadi MT, Bagheri R, Ghayour-Mobarhan M, et al. Early postoperative enteral versus parenteral feeding after esophageal cancer surgery. Iranian Journal of Otorhinolaryngology. 2015;**27**(82):331-336

[70] Peng J, Cai J, Niu ZX, Chen LQ. Early enteral nutrition compared with parenteral nutrition for esophageal cancer patients after esophagectomy: A meta-analysis. Diseases of the Esophagus. 2016;**29**(4):333-341. DOI: 10.1111/dote.12337

[71] Lidder P, Flanagan D, Fleming S, et al. Combining enteral with parenteral nutrition to improve postoperative glucose control. British Journal of Nutrition. 2010;**103**(11):1635-1641. DOI: 10.1017/S0007114509993631

[72] Wu W, Zhong M, Zhu DM, et al. Effect of early Full-Calorie nutrition support following esophagectomy: A randomized controlled trial. Journal of Parenteral and Enteral Nutrition. 2016. pii: 0148607116651509. [Epub ahead of print]

[73] McClave SA, Taylor BE, Martindale RG, et al. Guidelines for the provision and assessment of nutrition support therapy in the adult critically ill patient: Society of Critical Care Medicine (SCCM) and American Society for Parenteral and Enteral Nutrition (A.S.P.E.N.). Journal of Parenteral and Enteral Nutrition. 2016;**40**(2):159-211. DOI: 10.1177/0148607115621863

[74] Wang G, Chen H, Liu J, et al. A comparison of postoperative early enteral nutrition with delayed enteral nutrition in patients with esophageal cancer. Nutrients. 2015;**7**(6):4308-4317. DOI: 10.3390/nu7064308

[75] Weijs TJ, Berkelmans GH, Nieuwenhuijzen GA, et al. Routes for early enteral nutrition after esophagectomy. A systematic review. Clinical Nutrition. 2015;**34**(1):1-6. DOI: 10.1016/j.clnu.2014.07.011

[76] Fujita T, Daiko H, Nishimura M. Early enteral nutrition reduces the rate of life-threatening complications after thoracic esophagectomy in patients with esophageal cancer. European Surgical Research. 2012;**48**(2):79-84. DOI: 10.1159/000336574

[77] Manba N, Koyama Y, Kosugi S, et al. Is early enteral nutrition initiated within 24 hours better for the postoperative course in esophageal cancer surgery? Journal of Clinical Medicine Research. 2014;**6**(1):53-58. DOI: 10.4021/jocmr1665w

[78] Langelotz C, Spies C, Müller JM, Schwenk W. "Fast-track"-rehabilitation in surgery, a multimodal concept. Acta Chirurgica Belgica. 2005;**105**:555-559

[79] Arends J, Bachmann P, Baracos V, et al. ESPEN guidelines on nutrition in cancer patients. Clinical Nutrition. 2017; **36**(1):11-48. DOI: 10.1016/j.clnu.2016.07.015

[80] Gustafsson UO and Ljungqvist O. Perioperative nutritional management in digestive tract surgery. Current Opinion in Clinical Nutrition and Metabolic Care. 2011;**14**(5):504-509. DOI: 10.1097/MCO.0b013e3283499ae1

[81] Markar SR, Karthikesalingam A, Low DE. Enhanced recovery pathways lead to an improvement in postoperative outcomes following esophagectomy: systematic review and pooled analysis. Diseases of the Esophagus. 2015;**28**(5):468-475. DOI: 10.1111/dote.12214

[82] Chen L, Sun L, Lang Y, et al. Fast-track surgery improves postoperative clinical recovery and cellular and humoral immunity after esophagectomy for esophageal cancer. BMC Cancer. 2016;**16**:449. DOI: 10.1186/s12885-016-2506-8

[83] Wang JY, Hong X, Chen GH, et al. Clinical application of the fast track surgery model based on preoperative nutritional risk screening in patients with esophageal cancer. Asia Pacific Journal of Clinical Nutrition. 2015;**24**(2):206-211. DOI: 10.6133/apjcn.2015.24.2.18

[84] Mabvuure NT, Roman A, Khan OA. Enteral immunonutrition versus standard enteral nutrition for patients undergoing oesophagogastric resection for cancer. International Journal of Surgery. 2013;**11**(2):122-127. DOI: 10.1016/j.ijsu.2012.12.012

[85] Kubota K, Kuroda J, Yoshida M, et al. Preoperative oral supplementation support in patients with esophageal cancer. The Journal of Nutrition Health and Aging. 2014;**18**(4):437-440. DOI: 10.1007/s12603-014-0018-2

[86] Wong CS, Aly EH. The effects of enteral immunonutrition in upper gastrointestinal surgery: A systematic review and meta-analysis. International Journal of Surgery. 2016;**29**:137-150. DOI: 10.1016/j.ijsu.2016.03.043

[87] dos Reis AM, Kabke GB, Fruchtenicht AVG, et al. Cost-effectiveness of perioperative immunonutrition in gastrointestinal oncologic surgery: A systematic review. Arquivos Brasileiros de Cirurgia Digestiva. 2016;**29**(2):121-125. DOI: 10.1590/0102-6720201600020014

[88] Tanaka K, Yano M, Motoori M, et al. Impact of perioperative administration of synbiotics in patients with esophageal cancer undergoing esophagectomy: A prospective randomized controlled trial. Surgery. 2012;**152**(5):832-842. DOI: 10.1016/j.surg.2012.02.021

[89] Yokoyama Y, Nishigaki E, Abe T, et al. Randomized clinical trial of the effect of perioperative synbiotics versus no synbiotics on bacterial translocation after oesophagectomy. British Journal of Surgery. 2014;**101**(3):189-199. DOI: 10.1002/bjs.9385

[90] Han-Geurts IJ, Hop WC, Verhoef C, et al. Randomized clinical trial comparing feeding jejunostomy with nasoduodenal tube placement in patients undergoing oesophagectomy. British Journal of Surgery. 2007;**94**(1):31-35. Doi: 10.1002/bjs.5283

[91] Wani ML, Ahangar AG, Lone GN, et al. Feeding jejunostomy: does the benefit overweight the risk (a retrospective study from a single centre). International Journal of Surgery. 2010;**8**(5):387-390. DOI: 10.1016/j.ijsu.2010.05.009

[92] Elshaer M, Gravante G, White J, et al. Routes of early enteral nutrition following oesophagectomy. Annals of the Royal College of Surgeons of England. 2016;**98**(7):461-467. DOI: 10.1308/rcsann.2016.0198

[93] Abdelgadir MA, Mahadi SE, Nasr AO, Ahmed ME. Role of jejunostomy feeding catheter as a model for nutritional support. International Journal of Surgery. 2010;**8**(6):439-443. DOI: 10.1016/j.ijsu.2010.05.006

[94] Torres Júnior LG, de Vasconcellos Santos FA, Correia MI. Randomized clinical trial: Nasoenteric tube or jejunostomy as a route for nutrition after major upper gastrointestinal operations. World Journal of Surgery. 2014;**38**(9):2241-2246. DOI: 10.1007/s00268-014-2589-9

[95] Weimann A, Braga M, Harsanyi L, et al. ESPEN Guidelines on Enteral Nutrition: Surgery including organ transplantation. Clinical Nutrition. 2006;**25**(2):224-244. DOI: 10.1016/j.clnu.2006.01.015

[96] Cunningham D, Allum WH, Stenning SP, et al. Perioperative chemotherapy versus surgery alone for resectable gastroesophageal cancer. New England Journal of Medicine. 2006;**355**(1):11-20. DOI: 10.1056/NEJMoa055531

[97] Ychou M, Boige V, Pignon JP, et al. Perioperative chemotherapy compared with surgery alone for resectable gastroesophageal adenocarcinoma: An FNCLCC and FFCD multicenter phase III trial. Journal of Clinical Oncology. 2011;**29**(13):1715-1721. DOI: 10.1200/JCO.2010.33.0597

[98] Sjoquist KM, Burmeister BH, Smithers BM, et al. Survival after neoadjuvant chemotherapy or chemoradiotherapy for resectable oesophageal carcinoma: an updated meta-analysis. Lancet Oncology. 2011;**12**(7):681-692. DOI: 10.1016/S1470-2045(11)70142-5

[99] Reisinger KW, Bosmans JW, Uittenbogaart M, et al. Loss of skeletal muscle mass during neoadjuvant chemoradiotherapy predicts postoperative mortality in esophageal cancer surgery. Annals of Surgical Oncology. 2015;**22**(13):4445-4452. DOI: 10.1245/s10434-015-4558-4

[100] Jiang N, Zhao JZ, Chen XC, et al. Clinical determinants of weight loss in patients with esophageal carcinoma during radiotherapy: A prospective longitudinal view. Asian Pacific Journal of Cancer Prevention. 2014;**15**(5):1943-1948

[101] Hardman WE. (n-3) fatty acids and cancer therapy. Journal of Nutrition. 2004;**134**(12): 3427S-3430S

[102] Fietkau R, Lewitzki V, Kuhnt T, et al. A disease-specific enteral nutrition formula improves nutritional status and functional performance in patients with head and neck and esophageal cancer undergoing chemoradiotherapy: results of a randomized, controlled, multicenter trial. Cancer. 2013;**119**(18):3343-3353. DOI: 10.1002/cncr.28197

[103] Vasson MP, Talvas J, Perche O, et al. Immunonutrition improves functional capacities in head and neck and esophageal cancer patients undergoing radiochemotherapy: A randomized clinical trial. Clinical Nutrition. 2014;**33**(2):204-210. DOI: 10.1016/j.clnu.2013.06.008

[104] Sunpaweravong S, Puttawibul P, Ruangsin S, et al. Randomized study of antiinflammatory and immune-modulatory effects of enteral immunonutrition during concurrent chemoradiotherapy for esophageal cancer. Nutrition and Cancer. 2014;**66**(1):1-5. DOI: 10.1080/01635581.2014.847473

[105] Talvas J, Garrait G, Goncalves-Mendes N, et al. Immunonutrition stimulates immune functions and antioxidant defense capacities of leukocytes in radiochemotherapy-treated head & neck and esophageal cancer patients: A double-blind randomized clinical trial. Clinical Nutrition. 2015;**34**(5):810-817. DOI: 10.1016/j.clnu.2014.12.002

[106] Miyata H, Yano M, Yasuda T, et al. Randomized study of the clinical effects of ω-3 fatty acid-containing enteral nutrition support during neoadjuvant chemotherapy on chemotherapy-related toxicity in patients with esophageal cancer. Nutrition. 2017;**33**:204-210. DOI: 10.1016/j.nut.2016.07.004

[107] Motoori M, Yano M, Miyata H, et al. Randomized study of the effect of synbiotics during neoadjuvant chemotherapy on adverse events in esophageal cancer patients. Clinical Nutrition. 2017; **36**(1):93-99. DOI: 10.1016/j.clnu.2015.11.008

[108] van Vliet MJ, Harmsen HJ, de Bont ES, Tissing WJ. The role of intestinal microbiota in the development and severity of chemotherapy-induced mucositis. PLoS Pathogens. 2010;**6**(5):e1000879. DOI: 10.1371/journal.ppat.1000879

[109] Bowen JM, Stringer AM, Gibson RJ, et al. VSL#3 probiotic treatment reduces chemotherapy-induced diarrhea and weight loss. Cancer Biology & Therapy. 2007;**6**(9):1449e54

[110] Xu Y-J, Cheng JC-H, Lee J-M, et al. A Walk-and-Eat intervention improves outcomes for patients with esophageal cancer undergoing neoadjuvant chemoradiotherapy. Oncologist. 2015;**20**(10):1216-1222. DOI: 10.1634/theoncologist.2015-0178

[111] Cong M-H, Li S-L, Cheng G-W, et al. An interdisciplinary nutrition support team improves clinical and hospitalized outcomes of esophageal cancer patients with concurrent chemoradiotherapy. Chinese Medical Journal (England). 2015;**128**(22):3003-3007. DOI: 10.4103/0366-6999.168963

[112] Jones CM, Griffiths EA. Should oesophageal stents be used before neo-adjuvant therapy to treat dysphagia in patients awaiting oesophagectomy? Best evidence topic (BET). International Journal of Surgery. 2014;**12**(11):1172-1180. DOI: 10.1016/j.ijsu.2014.09.008

[113] Spaander MC, Baron TH, Siersema PD, et al. Esophageal stenting for benign and malignant disease: European Society of Gastrointestinal Endoscopy (ESGE) Clinical Guideline. Endoscopy. 2016;**48**(10):939-948. DOI: 10.1055/s-0042-114210

[114] Gray RT, O'donnell ME, Scott RD, et al. Impact of nutritional factors on survival in patients with inoperable oesophageal cancer undergoing self-expanding metal stent insertion. European Journal of Gastroenterology & Hepatology. 2011;**23**(6):455-460. DOI: 10.1097/MEG.0b013e3283469761

[115] Dai Y, Li C, Xie Y, et al. Interventions for dysphagia in oesophageal cancer. The Cochrane Database of Systematic Reviews. 2014;(10):CD005048. DOI: 10.1002/14651858.CD005048.pub4

[116] Grilo A, Santos CA, Fonseca J. Percutaneous endoscopic gastrostomy for nutritional palliation of upper esophageal cancer unsuitable foresophageal stenting. Arquivos de Gastroenterologia. 2012;**49**(3):227-231

[117] Yang C, Lin H, Hsieh T, Chang W. Palliative enteral feeding for patients with malignant esophageal obstruction: A retrospective study. BMC Palliative Care. 2015;**14**:58. DOI: 10.1186/s12904-015-0056-5

2

Immunotherapy for Esophageal Cancer

Tian Wang and Yi Zhang

Abstract

As the third most common cancer of the gastrointestinal tract, esophageal cancer has a rather worse prognosis treated with current therapy strategies, and a poor 5-year survival rate lower than 15%. Recent years, emerging immunotherapy has showed a gratifying effect in treating other solid tumors which illuminates its usage for esophageal cancers. Immunotherapy for esophageal cancer basically includes adoptive-cell-therapy-based, antibody-based and vaccine-based therapies, and all of which have shown preliminary favorable results in treating esophageal cancer. However, due to the rather lower mutation rate and a tough microenvironment inside the cancer, promising immunotherapies like immune checkpoint blockade drugs, gene-modified-T cell therapies are hindered by the immunosuppressive factors from microenvironment. Future endeavors will be focusing on targeting immunosuppressive factors, combining immunotherapies with classical treatments to create a satisfying effect.

Keywords: esophageal cancer, tumor microenvironment, immunotherapy, immune checkpoint blockade drugs, CAR-T cell therapy

1. Introduction

Esophageal cancer is one of the leading culprits of mortality worldwide and is responsible for a total number of 746,000 [1] new cases and 439,000 [2] deaths every year. A large number of these cancers are diagnosed at an advanced stage and the metastasis causes bad outcomes. Endoscopic surgery, cytotoxic chemotherapy and radiotherapy remain to be the active and essential clinical treatment but only provide modest benefits, with median overall survival (OS) only in the range of 8–10 months [3]. After nearly 20 years of fast development, immunotherapy turned to be a promising method for treating esophageal cancer. Recent advances have brought some therapeutic regimens to be approved by Food and Drug Administration (FDA) then coming to clinical practice in first- and second-line settings (**Table 1**). The future

Treatment	Cancer type	Treating method	Phase	Study number
ACT				
	EC	CIK	II	NCT02490735
	Multiple cancer types (including EC)	CTL	I	NCT00004178
	EC	NY-ESO-1-TCR T cells	II	NCT01795976
Tumor vaccine				
Cell vaccine	Multiple cancer types (including EC)	Tumor cell vaccine	I	NCT01258868
	Multiple cancer types (including EC)	H1299 lysate vaccine	I/II	NCT02054104
	Multiple cancer types (including EC)	Allogeneic tumor vaccine	I	NCT01143545
Peptide vaccine	EC	IMF-001	I	NCT01003808
	EC	LY6K, VEGFR1, VEGFR2	I	NCT00561275
	EC	URLC10, TTK, KOC1, VEGFR1, VEGFR2, cisplatin, fluorouracil	I	NCT00632333
	EC	URLC10	I	NCT00753844
	EC, GC	G17DT, cisplatin, fluorouracil	III	NCT00020787
Immune checkpoints therapies	EC + GEJC + GC	Nivolumab/placebo	III	NCT02743494
	EC + GEJC Siewert I	Pembrolizumab vs. investigator's choice	III	NCT02564263
	EC	Pembrolizumab + brachytherapy	I	NCT02642809
	EC	Nivolumab vs. paclitaxel/docetaxel	III	NCT02569242
	EC + GEJC Siewert I	Pembrolizumab	II	NCT02971956
	EC + GC	Pembrolizumab + trastuzumab	II	NCT02318901
	EC	Durvalumab (anti-PD-L1) + chemoradiotherapy	I/II	NCT02735239
	Solid tumors (including ESCC)	LAG525 (anti-LAG3) + PD001 (anti-PD-1)	I/II	NCT02460224
	Solid tumors (including ESCC)	Nivolumab + ipilimumab	I	NCT02834013

ACT: adoptive cell therapy; CIK: cytokine-induced killer cells; CTL: cytotoxic T-cells; VEGFR: vascular endothelial growth factor receptors; PD: programmed cell death receptor; EC: esophageal cancer; ESCC: esophageal squamous cell carcinoma; GEJC: gastroesophageal junction carcinoma.

Table 1. Recent or completed clinical trials of potential therapeutic approaches for immunotherapy of esophageal cancer.

of immunotherapy is promising in treating solid tumors, yet still there is a desperate need for more effective and less toxic treatment options for patients with advanced esophageal cancer.

In recent years, emergence of immunotherapy towards cancer has improved the management of several malignancies dramatically, especially melanoma, renal cell carcinoma, non-small cell lung cancer and so on, shedding light on its usage on esophageal cancer as well. Identification of more suppressive factors in tumor microenvironment and insights into the biology of T cell functioning yielded a large number of diverse and novel anti-tumor regimens. Global efforts continue to explore how and when to integrate these agents in treatment of esophageal cancer. Immune checkpoint inhibition through antibodies that block cytotoxic T-lymphocyte antigen 4 (CTLA-4) and programmed cell death protein 1 (PD-1) has led to meaningful improvements in survival [4]. Vaccine adjuvant administration has also reduced tumor recurrence to some degree. CAR-T (chimeric antigen receptor T-cell) immunotherapy is a typical example of recent advances in synthetic biology, genome engineering, and cell manufacturing that has made it possible to develop highly specific and potent tumor-reactive T cells and offer many opportunities for experimentation and broader clinical translation. Combined regimens of immunotherapy with other classical esophageal treating procedures will illuminate the future of clinical oncotherapy. Recent achievements, which are illustrated below, including finished or ongoing clinical trials and laboratory findings of immunotherapy for esophageal cancer, bringing optimism for meaningful changes in treatment algorithms and for better outcomes in this fatal disease.

2. Immunotherapy regimens for esophageal cancer

2.1. History of immunotherapy

A few decades ago, several rare clinical regression of advanced cancer in response to immune stimulation aroused interests in the area of cancer treatment. A passionate handful of immunologists, oncologists and surgeons carried out forward-looking researches into the relations between tumor progress and body immune system. Their respectable efforts turned the seemingly insignificant clinical phenomenon into reproducible concrete success by revealing the hidden mechanisms of tumor response.

At the earliest period of cancer immunotherapies, the exact mechanism remained unknown and the anti-tumor growth effect was limited yet providing impetus for in-depth study. The first effective immunotherapies aiming at directly modulating cell function using well-characterized recombinant cytokines including interleukin-2 (IL-2) and interferon alpha (IFNα), yet the safety was lowered associated with substantial toxicity. Other cytokines, including IFNγ, IL-4, IL-7, IL-10, IL-12, IL-15, IL-18, IL-25, etc., failed to provide substantive benefit. The following breakthrough was the emerging conception of monoclonal antibodies (mAbs) targeting tumor cell surface receptor proteins (human epidermal growth factor receptor 2 (HER2)/Neu, epidermal growth factor receptor (EGFR), etc.) and were integrated into cancer care. Vaccination therapies using the modified peptide, whole tumor, recombinant proteins, dendritic cells (DCs), and adjuvants were only modestly successful. With researching deeper into the cross-talk happening in the tumor microenvironment between tumor cells and immune cells, the modern era of immunotherapy launched with the extraordinary novel efficacy (and toxicities) of mAbs targeting immune checkpoints in patients with various cancer types in order to decrease the suppressive potential that would prevent immune cells from functioning. Current alternative approach to overcoming the suppressive tumor microenvironment was the administration of genetically modified autologous T cells targeting specific cancer-related antigens [5]. This could be done in the form of T cells in which modified specific T cell receptors (TCR) were inserted for a shared tumor antigen or a tumor-specific neoantigen accompanied by co-transduction of stimulatory cytokines such as IL-12 or could co-administrate with PD-1 pathway blockers to sustain the capability before being expanded in large numbers *in vitro* following lymphodepleting chemotherapy. These approaches have produced dramatic responses in a few patients with a variety of individual tumor types, especially hematological malignancies [6]. Further improvement of adoptive cell transfer therapy came from the modified T cells expressing chimeric antigen receptors (CAR) targeting tumor-specific binding domains. After several generations of amelioration, CAR-T therapy showed extraordinary effect in treating hematological malignancies yet treatment of patients with solid tumors using CAR-T cells had been less fruitful and had troubled clinicians much through the off-tumor/on-target toxicity. Given the virtually limitless possibility of *ex vivo* engineering of T cells, many of these potential hurdles will likely be resolved by the additional modification of T cell products prior to treatment.

Immunotherapy showed great potential in the treatment of esophageal cancer. Modern treatments of patients with esophageal cancer integrated immunotherapy with conventional surgical, chemotherapeutic, and radiation oncologic strategies. In spite of the seemingly gratifying results, the 5-year survival rate of patients with esophageal cancer in the middle and late stages is still lower than 15%, the 5-year survival rate of patients with locally advanced surgery alone is only 20–25% [7]. Postoperative chemotherapy or neoadjuvant chemoradiation only turns the 5-year survival rate up to only 30–35% [8]. One of the causes to blame of the rather poor prognosis of esophageal cancer is the rapid disease progression. More than 50% of patients already have visible metastases at the time of diagnosis [7]. Therefore, further investigation of esophageal cancer microenvironment and its impact on disease progression will lay a solid theoretical foundation for early diagnosis and treatment improvement of esophageal cancer.

In this chapter, we tried to converge concepts relevant to the complicated relationship between the host and the neoplastic tissue.

2.2. Immune microenvironment and molecular correlations in esophageal cancer

As early as 100 years ago, Paget [9] had put forward the hypothesis of "seeds and soil", which laid the foundation for the concept of tumor microenvironment. Numerous data indicate that many immune-related cells, factors and immune-related signaling pathways in the tumor microenvironment play an important role in the occurrence, metastasis, recurrence, angiogenesis, and drug resistance of tumors. The in-depth study of the tumor immune microenvironment is to search for molecular pathogenesis and new therapeutic models of esophageal cancer.

Tumor microenvironment is constituted by various immune cells, endothelial cells, adipocytes, paravascular cells, nerve cells, fibroblasts, and extracellular matrix components around the cancer cells [10]. Some stromal cells in the tumor microenvironment have immunosuppressive potential to inhibit the function of immune effector cells and promote tumor progression. Thus inhibiting cancer cell apoptosis and promoting mechanisms such as proliferation, angiogenesis, drug resistance, and immune escape to promote tumorigenesis [11]. Chemokines CCL17 and CCL22 secreted by tumor cells or tumor-associated macrophages (TAMs) recruit CCR4+ regulatory T cells (Treg), which then inhibit immune effector cells by contacting directly or secretion of cytokines (IL-10 and IL-35). Th17 cells can be transformed into Treg cells stimulated by IL-6 and transforming growth factor-β (TGF-β). Inflammation and tumor-derived factors stimulate the activation of myeloid-derived suppressor cells (MDSCs). Activated MDSCs can directly inhibit the expression of CD8 + T cells. Activation and induction of Treg cells and other mechanisms contribute to immune escape of cancer cells. TAM cells and CAF cells promote the growth, invasion, metastasis, and angiogenesis of tumor cells through the secretion of cytokines, chemokines, and various growth factors. In addition, tumor cells and TAM cells can express programmed cell death ligand (PD)-L1/2 inhibiting T cell activation after binding to PD-1.

MDSCs have been shown to play an important role in promoting tumor immune escape, activating CAF cells and angiogenesis [12]. The presence of proinflammatory cytokines such as IL-1, IL-6 and prostaglandins in esophageal cancer microenvironment can activate MDSC [13]. MDSC inhibits activation of T cells by direct inhibition [14], cytotoxicity of natural killer cells (NK) [15], depletion of arginine and cysteine, induction of Treg cells, etc. to achieve immune escape [16]. Another group of immunosuppressive cells that exert similar functions are Treg cells. Under physiological conditions, Treg cells can regulate the activation and proliferation of T cells, B cells, and cytotoxicity of NK cells. But in tumor microenvironment, Treg cells can promote the occurrence and progression of tumor cells by secreting immunosuppressive related factors, secreting tumor-associated antigens (TAAs), and suppressing the cellular adverse reactions of immune effector cells and the release of granzymes [17]. Studies have shown that tumor cells and TAMs can recruit CCR4+ Treg cells to tumor sites by secreting CCL17 and CCL22 and other chemokines [18]. Treg cells are highly aggregated in tumor cites, promoting tumor invasion and metastasis, and are associated with disease severity, survival after chemotherapy, and prognosis [17]. Additionally, Th17 cells can secrete IL-17 and IL-22 and activate STAT3 related signaling pathways to promote angiogenesis and tumor growth [23]. However, the role of Th17 cells is still controversial. What factors affect the function of Th17 have not yet been well defined [18]. Therefore, we still have to know more about Th17 cells in esophageal cancer to explore potential therapeutic targets.

The tumorigenic mechanisms of TAMs are varied. Phenotype spectrum of macrophage ranges from M1 to M2: M1 macrophages represent the classical activated macrophages, with functions of cytokines secretion, antigen presentation, resistance to infection and anti-tumor ability, etc., while M2 macrophages secrete type II cytokines and induce activation of COX2/prostaglandin E and other mechanisms that cause tumorigenesis [19]. The presence of cancer associated fibroblasts (CAFs) in patients with esophageal cancer is associated with microvessel density, and can also promote tumor progression and metastasis through epithelial mesenchymal transition (EMT). CAFs are also associated with 3-year survival rates and disease recurrence after radiotherapy and chemotherapy [20].

PD-1 is a member of the CD28 superfamily and is an important immunosuppressive molecule that inhibits the activation of T cells after binding to its ligand PD-L1/PD-L2 [4]. Multiple experiments confirmed that PD-L1 and PD-L2 are highly expressed in esophageal cancer [21], in which PD-L1 expression is closely related to tumor invasion depth and poor prognosis, whereas PD-L2 expression is associated with decreased CD8+ T cell infiltration [21]. The increasing PD-L2 expression can promote the secretion of Th2 cytokines such as IL-4/IL-13 [22]. These pieces of evidence suggest that blockers targeting PD-1 are of great significance in the treatment of esophageal cancer [23].

In the early stages of esophageal cancer, TGF-β signaling suppresses tumor growth by down-regulating the expression of Smad4 and c-Myc genes, while promoting growth and EMT in advanced esophageal cancer [24]. This "switching" effect is thought to be caused by the loss of adaptor proteins. For instance, an important adaptor protein, β2-spectrin, plays an important part in cell–cell interactions and maintenance of epithelial cell polarity. In esophageal adenocarcinoma, decreasing β2-spectrin in tumor cells results in increased expression of SOX9 and c-Myc, but it also reduces other TGF-β targets such as E-cadherin and cell cycle-regulated p21 and p27 genes [25]. In summary, these changes make TGF-β promote the progression and metastasis of the tumor by inducing EMT, especially in epithelial tumors like esophageal cancer.

In addition to growth factors, chemokines in the tumor microenvironment also play an important role in the development of tumors. Mainly, there is stromal cell derived factor-1 (CXCL12/SDF-1) secreted by fibroblasts [26], binding to its corresponding receptor CXCR4 or CXCR7 thus inducing tumor growth, promoting angiogenesis, stimulating tumor movement, invasion and metastasis [26]. SDF-1/CXCR4/CXCR7 axis is closely related to tumor invasion, metastasis and survival. However, the use of these separate components as indicators of prognostic analysis has yielded inconsistent results [27]. Nonetheless, CXCL12 has been shown to regulate the migration of CXCR4-positive tumor cells in esophageal adenocarcinoma *in vitro* and *in vivo*. Knockout of CXCR4 expression in KYSE-150 and TE-13 esophageal cancer cells by small interfering RNA can inhibit the proliferation, invasion and metastasis of tumor cells. Local CCL5 and CXCL10 in esophageal squamous cell carcinoma can recruit CD8+ T cells to the tumor site [28].

Further researches showed that remodeling body immune state by various means in esophageal cancer patients will be the main research direction of immunotherapy for esophageal cancer.

2.3. Checkpoint inhibitor regimens

Immune system has sophisticated regulatory mechanisms. Several checkpoints are involved to maintain the balance between effective immune-responses fighting against infection or cancer state yet won't activate excessively to prevent damaging healthy cells. Cytotoxic T lymphocyte antigen-4 (CTLA-4) and PD-1 are among the major inhibitory receptors expressed by Tregs which downregulate immune responses [29]. Inhibitory antibodies modulating these immune checkpoints have been most frequently used in immune-oncology trials in esophageal cancers.

PD-1/PD-L1 blockers have achieved encouraging clinical results in treating melanoma, lung cancer and other cancer types [30, 31]. The potential role of PD-1 blockers in treatment of esophageal cancer can be predicted by genomic map of the tumor immune microenvironment. The expression of PD-L1 on MDSCs isolated from esophageal cancer tissue was higher obviously, and PD-1 expression was detected in approximately 60% of the tumor infiltrating lymphocytes (TILs) from esophageal cancer tissues [32]. Therefore, inhibition of the PD-1/PD-L1 pathway for esophageal cancer treatment cannot be ignored.

Preliminary results of ongoing studies indicated that PD-1 blocker Pembrolizumab had acceptable safety in PD-L1 positive esophageal cancer patients. The objective response rate for mid-term analysis was approximately 30% with a sustained response period of up to 40 weeks [33]. These results laid the foundation for the continued completion of checkpoint inhibitor regimens pivotal study in esophageal cancer patients.

CTLA-4, also known as CD152, belongs to the immunoglobulin superfamily and serves as an immunological checkpoint. When activated CD4+ helper T cells express CTLA-4, this kind of cells sends inhibitory signals to T cells [34]. High CTLA-4 expressing CD4+ Treg cells block T cells by reducing IL-2 secretion and downregulating IL-2 receptor expression then retard T cells in G1 phase of the cell cycle [35]. Ipilimumab and tremelimumab have two fully humanized monoclonal anti-CTLA-4 antibodies that have already received FDA approval for the treatment of melanoma and mesothelioma [36, 37]. A survey of tremelimumab has been completed in phase II clinical trials for treating advanced gastric and esophageal cancer (n = 18). Although only a 5% response rate was observed, four patients were controlled and one patient was observed with partial remission (25.4 Mo) after treatment and continued for several months [38]. The results of ongoing clinical trials are expected to further highlight the clinical value of monoclonal anti-CTLA-4 antibodies in esophageal cancer.

2.4. Vaccine regimens

Tumor vaccine treatment involves the administration of TAAs into patients thus triggering specific anti-tumor immune responses. Rosenberg et al. [39, 40] conducted a comprehensive review of 1306 cancer vaccine usage studies conducted before 2004 and found that the overall target response rate was only 3.3%. The explanation may be that these immune cells have low affinity or are inhibited by endogenous factors like the checkpoints mentioned above.

For the treatment of esophageal cancer, some vaccine-based clinical trial reports have been published. A Phase I clinical trial of 10 patients with refractory stage III or IV esophageal squamous cell carcinoma treated with peptide vaccine found that 9 patients developed antigen-specific T cell immune response. One of the patients with liver metastases showed complete remission for 7 months, another had partial remission within all metastatic lung lesions, and 3 patients had progression-free survival lasting 2.5 months. The peptide vaccine used was derived from three HLA-A24-restricted cancer testis antigens (TTK protein kinase, lymphocyte antigen 6 complex locus K, and insulin-like growth factor-II mRNA binding protein 3) [41]. The multicenter, phase II clinical trial of the vaccine evaluated the OS, PFS, and immune response after vaccinations in patients with HLA-A*2402 positive and negative esophageal squamous cell carcinoma, and immune response was observed in HLA-A*2402 positive patients (n = 35), but there was no statistical difference in OS compared to HLA-A*2402-negative patients (n = 25) (4.6 mo vs. 2.6 mo, P > 0.05), yet there is a significant difference in PFS (P = 0.032) [42]. In a tumor vaccine trial hosted by Saito et al. [43] (n = 20), 4 patients with high levels of MAGE-A4 or MHC class I antigen in autologous tumor cells not only showed MAGE-A4 specific immune responses after vaccination, but compared with patients without using antibodies, their OS was also significantly prolonged. Wada et al. [44] used NY-ESO-1 as a cancer vaccine in 8 patients with esophageal cancer. The results showed that 7 patients had an immune response. Of the 6 patients evaluated for efficacy, 1 patient experienced partial remission, 2 patients continued to maintain progression-free status, and 2 patients had mixed clinical responses. Given the preliminary results of these peptide vaccines in clinical trials, safety inspections and the related researches combined with radiotherapy and chemotherapy are also being carried out gradually in treating multiple cancer types including esophageal cancer.

2.5. Adoptive cell therapy regimens

The concept of ACT (adoptive cell therapy) was first proposed by Dietrich et al. [45]. It refers to the treatment of utilizing autologous or allogeneic immune cells by infusing them back into the patients after being amplified *in vitro* by certain means. Currently effector cells can be divided into two categories: the first type is non-specific immune cells, including autologous lymphokine-activated killer cells (LAK), cytokine-induced killer cells (CIK) and NK cells. Cells are isolated from peripheral blood cells and are stimulated by lymphokines or cytokines; another type of effector cells is antigen-specific T cells, including TILs, cytotoxic T cells (CTL) and genetically engineered T cells including T cell receptor transferred T-cells (TCR-T) and CAR-T [46].

The first ACT trial in human improved the survival of patients with metastatic cancer by reintroduction of CIK and recombinant IL-2 to their body, which has been successfully applied to the treatment of refractory metastatic melanoma, and for other types of cancer such as glioma, renal cell carcinoma, non-small cell lung cancer, etc. The objective response rate varies from 20 to 72% [47], encouraging its further usage in esophageal cancer, too.

So far, ACT treatment of esophageal cancer has been evaluated in several clinical trials. In the first published study by Besser et al. [48] and Toh et al. [49], mononuclear cells were isolated from peripheral blood of esophageal squamous cell carcinoma patients and were given autologous tumor cell stimulation *in vitro*. Latter results showed that half of the patients had an objective response, and 36% of the subjects achieved complete remission or partial remission. CTL and TIL cells are now hot spots for carrying out immunotherapy for solid tumors as the mechanism of killing tumor is rather clear.

TCR-T cells transduce the α and β chains of the antigen-specific high-affinity TCR into T cells and express them on the cell surface, thereby effectively identifying and killing the tumor cells expressing the antigen. Currently, the most common TAAs found in esophageal cancer are cancer testis MAGE-A3/4 and NY-ESO-1. Several studies [50, 51] showed that the expression ratio of MAGE-A3 in esophageal cancer was about 90%, and the expression rate of NYESO-1 in esophageal cancer was up to 40–90%. A preliminary phase 1 clinical trial of genetically engineered T cells was carried out by Kageyama et al. [52], TCR-T cells were readopted to patients with MAGE-A4-positive recurrent esophageal cancer, and administered the MAGE-A4 peptide vaccine subsequently, the level of TCR-T cells in the peripheral blood of 10 subjects was monitored for 5 months, and 5 of them were able to detect specific T cells continuously. Seven subjects appeared tumor progress after 2 months of treatment, but another 3 subjects survived more than 27 months.

CAR-T is another type of genetically engineered T cells. CAR-T was obtained by translocating chimeric antigen receptor such as CARs into T cells. Gross et al. [53] successfully constructed the structure of CARs into T cells for the first time to exert their specific killing function. Up to now, tens of clinical trial data of CAR-T treatment on malignant hematological malignancies have been published. The Novartis' tisagenlecleucel, a synthetic bioimmune product of anti-CD19 CAR-T cells has been approved by FDA on treating relapsed/refractory B-cell acute lymphoblastic leukemia (B-ALL) in 2017 [54]. The early generation of CAR-T therapy for solid tumors did not appear ideal outcomes during clinical use [55]. The reasonable explanation might be lack of unique TAAs in solid tumors, less efficiency and persistency of T cell homing to tumor sites, and the intratumoral immunosuppressive environment strongly inhibited CAR-T cell function. Clinical trials targeting solid tumors using second or third-generation CAR techniques had been limited, but some of the more significant clinical trials are carrying out good results. Patients with metastatic or recurrent HER2-positive medulloblastoma treated with HER2-CAR-T had came out with stable conditions [56]. Feng et al. [57] showed the results of a clinical trial of an EGFR-CAR-T treatment for EGFR-positive relapsed/refractory NSCLC patients revealed partial remission in 2 of the 11 patients involved in the evaluation and 5 patients had a stable condition ranging from 2 to 8 months. There were no obvious adverse reactions in the entire clinical trial. In the treatment of esophageal cancer, no CAR-T therapy-related studies have been conducted yet. However, anti-tumor targets are now erupting in esophageal cancer. Points such as HER2 can also provide references for future steps in the development of research.

3. Combined treatment

Currently, comprehensive therapy shed light on tumor treatment to a large degree. Clinical practice has proven that it is difficult to achieve the best results with any single treatment method. Therefore, the principle of treatment for most tumors depends on comprehensive treatment. Recent research results showed that the combined usage of immunotherapy and chemotherapy in a variety of cancer treatment achieved better results than a single therapy, it can not only reverse the immunosuppression effects caused by the late stage of the tumor, increase the cross-presentation of tumor antigens, promote the proliferation of killer T cells and make it more easy to kill tumor cells, but can also reduce the incidence of adverse reactions from chemotherapy and reduce drug resistance of tumor cells to some extent. Combination of chemotherapy and immunotherapy has been a common available method in some cancer types. Neoadjuvant chemotherapy regimens together with HER2-targeted therapy achieved pathologic complete response in relapse-free survival among patients with breast cancer [58].

New treatment targeting specific mutant genes illustrated clinical success in a phase II study of metastatic melanoma combined with interleukin-2 aldesleukin and BRAF inhibitor vemurafenib [59]. The effectiveness of combined therapy can even cover the metastatic areas, in melanoma brain metastases, complete intracranial response was observed after using dual checkpoint-inhibition of talimogene laherparepvec (T-Vec), pembrolizumab and whole brain radiotherapy. Additionally, immunotherapy also showed potential augmented effect plus cryotherapy [60], focused ultrasound therapy [61] and photothermal therapy [62], etc. Tumor vaccine also took another leap when combined with other immunotherapies, clinical results showed that nivolumab in combination with talimogene laherparepvec (T-Vec) in resected melanoma carried out better outcomes [63]. The clinical value of immunotherapy and radiotherapy showed even more outstanding clinical effects, anti-tumor immune response was enhanced by anti-PD-1 immunotherapy in recurrent nasopharyngeal carcinoma, showing a bright prospect of further combination [64]. In treating esophageal cancer, there are also many creative comprehensive treatment methods that are constantly developing. In patients with drug-resistant esophageal cancer, a phase Ib/II study of low-dose decitabine-primed chemoimmunotherapy showed undeniable safety and efficacy [65]. A combination therapy of multi-peptide vaccine with chemoradiation therapy performed satisfying safety thus can be an effective treatment for patients with unresectable ESCC [66]. Novel multitarget tyrosine kinase inhibitor anlotinib in a third-line treatment of refractory advanced non-small-cell lung cancer (RA-NSCLC) provided significant PFS benefits compared with placebo, and accompanied with acceptable toxicity [67]. Though has a guaranteed future, there need to be more rational and effective trials of combinations to be excavated in the field of treating esophageal cancer together with other solid tumors.

4. Conclusions and future directions

The success of immunotherapy in some tumors came from years of research deep into the immune system and tumor itself and brought hope of healing cancer. It is worth mentioning that several immune checkpoint blockers have been or are being approved by the FDA, and it is expected that the next step will be to accelerate the pace of application of single drug or other treatment modes in combination within clinical usage. However, opportunities and challenges coexist, and there are still some key questions that have not been answered in immunotherapy. First of all, many targeted cancer drugs that treat cancer need to be explored to determine the biological dose that achieves the greatest clinical benefit with minimal toxicity. Second, given that most of the current immunotherapy is mainly to activate anti-tumor effects by activating the immune system, this kind of treatment requires patient to have some degree of immunity before receiving the initial immunotherapy. Therefore, it is imperative to fully evaluate patient's immune status and find biomarkers that predict the effectiveness of immunotherapy. In addition, there is abundant evidence that exposure to radiation and chemotherapy drugs may affect the rate of DNA mutations in tumor cells, prompting the formation of some new antigens. As the current immunotherapy is always combined with radiotherapy and chemotherapy, determining the proper dose for each regimen is the prerequisite for maximum benefit of combined therapy.

Immunotherapy has a broad application prospect in the treatment of malignant tumors. The high frequency of esophageal cancer mutations and the effective results of immunotherapy highlighted in other gastrointestinal cancers provide strong evidence for the study of esophageal cancer immunotherapy. Treatment strategies combined with existing or new treatment modes will be the direction of future esophageal cancer treatment.

Author details

Tian Wang and Yi Zhang*

*Address all correspondence to: yizhang@zzu.edu.cn

Biotherapy Center, The First Affiliated Hospital of Zhengzhou University, Zhengzhou, Henan, China

References

[1] GBD 2015 Disease and Injury Incidence and Prevalence, Collaborators. Lancet. 2016; **388**(10053):1545-1602. DOI: 10.1016/S0140-6736(16)31678-6. PMC: 5055577 PMID: 277-33282

[2] GBD 2015 Mortality and Causes of Death, Collaborators. Lancet. 2016;**388**(10053): 1459-1544. DOI: 10.1016/s0140-6736(16)31012-1. PMC: 5388903 PMID: 27733281

[3] Chang S, Kohrt H, Maecker HT. Monitoring the immune competence of cancer patients to predict outcome. Cancer Immunology, Immunotherapy. 2014;**63**:713-719. DOI: 10. 1007/s00262-014-1521-3. PMID: 24487923

[4] Smyth E, Thuss-Patience PC. Immune checkpoint inhibition in gastro-oesophageal cancer. Oncology Research and Treatment. 2018;**41**(5):272-280. DOI: 10.1159/000489099. PMID: 29705787

[5] Li F, Zhang T, Cao L, Zhang Y. Chimeric antigen receptor T cell based immunotherapy for cancer. Current Stem Cell Research & Therapy. 2018 Apr 19. DOI: 10.2174/1574888X 13666180420110239. PMID: 29676233

[6] Kueberuwa G, Kalaitsidou M, Cheadle E, Hawkins RE, Gilham DE. CD19 CAR T cells expressing IL-12 eradicate lymphoma in fully lymphoreplete mice through induction of host immunity. Molecular Therapy—Oncolytics. 2017 Dec 19;**8**:41-51. DOI: 10.1016/j. omto.2017.12.003 eCollection 2018 Mar 30. PMID: 29367945

[7] Enzinger PC, Mayer RJ. Esophageal cancer. The New England Journal of Medicine. 2003;**349**:2241-2252. DOI: 10.1056/NEJMra035010 PMID: 14657432

[8] Rubenstein JH, Shaheen NJ. Epidemiology, diagnosis, and management of esophageal adenocarcinoma. Gastroenterology. 2015;**149**:302-17.e1. DOI: 10.1053/j.gastro.2015.04.053 PMID: 25957861

[9] Paget S. The distribution of secondary growths in cancer of the breast. 1889. Cancer Metastasis Reviews. 1989;**8**:98-101 PMID: 2673568

[10] Karakasheva TA, Dominguez GA, Hashimoto A, Lin EW, Chiu C, Sasser K, Lee JW, Beatty GL, Gabrilovich DI, Rustgi AK. CD38+ M-MDSC expansion characterizes a subset of advanced colorectal cancer patients. JCI Insight. 2018 Mar 22;**3**(6):pii-97022. DOI: 10.1172/jci.insight.97022 PMID: 29563330

[11] Whiteside TL. The tumor microenvironment and its role in promoting tumor growth. Oncogene. 2008;**27**:5904-5912. DOI: 10.1038/onc.2008.271 PMID: 18836471

[12] Zhu Y, Zhang L, Zha H, Yang F, Hu C, Chen L, Guo B, Zhu B. Stroma-derived fibrinogen-like protein 2 activates cancer-associated fibroblasts to promote tumor growth in lung cancer. International Journal of Biological Sciences. 2017 Jun 1;**13**(6):804-814. DOI: 10.7150/ijbs.19398 eCollection 2017. PMID: 28656005

[13] Okano S, Abu-Elmagd K, Kish DD, Keslar K, Baldwin WM 3rd, Fairchild RL, Fujiki M, Khanna A, Osman M, Costa G, Fung J, Miller C, Kayashima H, Hashimoto K. Myeloid-derived suppressor cells increase and inhibit donor-reactive T cell responses to graft intestinal epithelium in intestinal transplant patients. American Journal of Transplantation. 2018 Mar 6. DOI: 10.1111/ajt.14718. PMID: 29509288

[14] Parker KH, Beury DW, Ostrand-Rosenberg S. Myeloid-derived suppressor cells: Critical cells driving immune suppression in the tumor microenvironment. Advances in Cancer Research. 2015;**128**:95-139. DOI: 10.1016/bs.acr.2015.04.002

[15] Spallanzani RG1, Dalotto-Moreno T, Raffo Iraolagoitia XL, Ziblat A, Domaica CI, Avila DE, Rossi LE, Fuertes MB, Battistone MA, Rabinovich GA, Salatino M, Zwirner NW. Expansion of CD11b(+)Ly6G (+)Ly6C (int) cells driven by medroxyprogesterone acetate in mice bearing breast tumors restrains NK cell effector functions. Cancer Immunology, Immunotherapy. 2013 Dec;**62**(12):1781-1795. DOI: 10.1007/s00262-013-1483-x. PMID: 24114144

[16] Fleming V, Hu X, Weber R, Nagibin V, Groth C, Altevogt P, Utikal J, Umansky V. Targeting myeloid-derived suppressor cells to bypass tumor-induced Immunosuppression. Frontiers in Immunology. 2018 Mar 2;**9**:398. DOI: 10.3389/fimmu.2018.00398 eCollection 2018. PMID: 29552012

[17] Ahrends T, Borst J. The opposing roles of CD4+ T cells in anti-tumor immunity. Immunology. 2018 Apr 27. DOI: 10.1111/imm.12941. PMID: 29700809

[18] Yang G, Li H, Yao Y, Xu F, Bao Z, Zhou J. Treg/Th17 imbalance in malignant pleural effusion partially predicts poor prognosis. Oncology Reports. 2015 Jan;**33**(1):478-484. DOI: 10.3892/or.2014.3576

[19] Wang Y, Xu G, Wang J, Li XH, Sun P, Zhang W, Li JX, Wu CY. Relationship of Th17/Treg cells and radiation pneumonia in locally advanced esophageal carcinoma. Anticancer Research. 2017 Aug;**37**(8):4643-4647

[20] Qiao Y, Zhang C, Li A, Wang D, Luo Z, Ping Y, Zhou B, Liu S, Li H, Yue D, Zhang Z, Chen X, Shen Z, Lian J, Li Y, Wang S, Li F, Huang L, Wang L, Zhang B, Yu J, Qin Z, Zhang Y. IL6 derived from cancer-associated fibroblasts promotes chemoresistance via CXCR7 in esophageal squamous cell carcinoma. Oncogene. 2018 Feb 15;**37**(7):873-883. DOI: 10.1038/onc.2017.387

[21] Guo W, Wang P, Li N, Shao F, Zhang H, Yang Z, Li R, Gao Y, He J. Prognostic value of PD-L1 in esophageal squamous cell carcinoma: A meta-analysis. Oncotarget. 2017 Dec 27;**9**(17):13920-13933. DOI: 10.18632/oncotarget.23810. PMID: 29568405

[22] Freeman GJ, Long AJ, Iwai Y, Bourque K, Chernova T, Nishimura H, Fitz LJ, Malenkovich N, Okazaki T, Byrne MC, Horton HF, Fouser L, Carter L, Ling V, Bowman MR, Carreno BM, Collins M, Wood CR, Honjo T. Engagement of the PD-1 immunoinhibitory receptor by a novel B7 family member leads to negative regulation of lymphocyte activation. The Journal of Experimental Medicine. 2000;**192**:1027-1034. DOI: 10.1084/jem.192.7.1027. PMID: 11015443

[23] Walsh EM, Kelly RJ. Single agent anti PD-1 inhibitors in esophageal cancer—A first step in a new therapeutic direction. Journal of Thoracic Disease. 2018 Mar;**10**(3):1308-1313. DOI: 10.21037/jtd.2018.03.43

[24] Caja L, Dituri F, Mancarella S, Caballero-Diaz D, Moustakas A, Giannelli G, Fabregat I. TGF-β and the tissue microenvironment: Relevance in fibrosis and cancer. International Journal of Molecular Sciences. 2018 Apr 26;**19**(5). DOI: 10.3390/ijms19051294

[25] Song S, Maru DM, Ajani JA, Chan CH, Honjo S, Lin HK, Correa A, Hofstetter WL, Davila M, Stroehlein J, Mishra L. Loss of TGF-β adaptor 2SP activates notch signaling and SOX9 expression in esophageal adenocarcinoma. Cancer Research. 2013;**73**:2159-2169. DOI: 10.1158/0008-5472.CAN-12-1962

[26] Givel AM, Kieffer Y, Scholer-Dahirel A, Sirven P, Cardon M, Pelon F, Magagna I, Gentric G, Costa A, Bonneau C, Mieulet V, Vincent-Salomon A, Mechta-Grigoriou F. miR200-regulated CXCL12β promotes fibroblast heterogeneity and immunosuppression in ovarian cancers. Nature Communications. 2018 Mar 13;**9**(1):1056. DOI: 10.1038/s41467-018-03348-z

[27] Nazari A, Khorramdelazad H, Hassanshahi G. Biological/pathological functions of the CXCL12/CXCR4/CXCR7 axes in the pathogenesis of bladder cancer. International Journal of Clinical Oncology. 2017 Dec;**22**(6):991-1000. DOI: 10.1007/s10147-017-1187-x. PMID: 29022185

[28] Liu J, Li F, Ping Y, Wang L, Chen X, Wang D, Cao L, Zhao S, Li B, Kalinski P, Thorne SH, Zhang B, Zhang Y. Local production of the chemokines CCL5 and CXCL10 attracts CD8+ T lymphocytes into esophageal squamous cell carcinoma. Oncotarget. 2015;**6**: 24978-24989. DOI: 10.18632/oncotarget.4617

[29] Liu Z, McMichael EL, Shayan G, Li J, Chen K, Srivastava RM, Kane LP, Lu B, Ferris RL. Novel effector phenotype of Tim-3+ regulatory T cells leads to enhanced suppressive

function in head and neck cancer patients. Clinical Cancer Research. 2018 Apr 30. DOI: 10.1158/1078-0432.CCR-17-1350. PMID: 29712685

[30] Borghaei H, Paz-Ares L, Horn L, Spigel DR, Steins M, Ready NE, Chow LQ, Vokes EE, Felip E, Holgado E, Barlesi F, Kohlhäufl M, Arrieta O, Burgio MA, Fayette J, Lena H, Poddubskaya E, Gerber DE, Gettinger SN, Rudin CM, Rizvi N, Crinò L, Blumenschein GR, Antonia SJ, Dorange C, Harbison CT, Graf Finckenstein F, Brahmer JR. Nivolumab versus docetaxel in advanced nonsquamous non-small-cell lung cancer. The New England Journal of Medicine. 2015;**373**:1627-1639. DOI: 10.1056/NEJMoa1507643. PMID: 26412456

[31] Long GV, Atkinson V, Lo S, Sandhu S, Guminski AD, Brown MP, Wilmott JS, Edwards J, Gonzalez M, Scolyer RA, Menzies AM, McArthur GA. Combination nivolumab and ipilimumab or nivolumab alone in melanoma brain metastases: A multicentre randomised phase 2 study. The Lancet Oncology. 2018 Mar 27. DOI: 10.1016/S1470-2045(18)30139-6. PMID: 29602646

[32] Huang H, Zhang G, Li G, Ma H, Zhang X. Circulating CD14(+)HLA-DR(−/low) myeloid-derived suppressor cell is an indicator of poor prognosis in patients with ESCC. Tumour Biology. 2015;**36**:7987-7996. DOI: 10.1007/s13277-015-3426-y. PMID: 25967454

[33] Doi T, Piha-Paul SA, Jalal SI, Saraf S, Lunceford J, Koshiji M, Bennouna J. Safety and antitumor activity of the anti-programmed death-1 antibody pembrolizumab in patients with advanced esophageal carcinoma. Journal of Clinical Oncology. 2018 Jan 1;**36**(1): 61-67. DOI: 10.1200/JCO.2017.74.9846

[34] Santoni G, Amantini C, Morelli MB, Tomassoni D, Santoni M, Marinelli O, Nabissi M, Cardinali C, Paolucci V, Torniai M, Rinaldi S, Morgese F, Bernardini G, Berardi R. High CTLA-4 expression correlates with poor prognosis in thymoma patients. Oncotarget. 2018 Mar 30;**9**(24):16665-16677. DOI: 10.18632/oncotarget.24645. eCollection 2018 Mar 30

[35] Liu D, Badell IR, Ford ML. Selective CD28 blockade attenuates CTLA-4-dependent CD8+ memory T cell effector function and prolongs graft survival. JCI Insight. 2018 Jan 11;**3**(1). DOI: 10.1172/jci.insight.96378 PMID: 29321374

[36] Diao K, Bian SX, Routman DM, Yu C, Ye JC, Wagle NA, Wong MK, Zada G, Chang EL. Stereotactic radiosurgery and ipilimumab for patients with melanoma brain metastases: Clinical outcomes and toxicity. Journal of Neuro-Oncology. 2018 Apr 25. DOI: 10.1007/s11060-018-2880-y. PMID: 29696531

[37] Maio M, Scherpereel A, Calabrò L, Aerts J, Cedres Perez S, Bearz A, Nackaerts K, Fennell DA, Kowalski D, Tsao AS, Taylor P, Grosso F, Antonia SJ, Nowak AK, Taboada M, Puglisi M, Stockman PK, Kindler HL. Tremelimumab as second-line or third-line treatment in relapsed malignant mesothelioma (DETERMINE): A multicentre, international, randomised, double-blind, placebo-controlled phase 2b trial. The Lancet Oncology. 2017 Sep;**18**(9):1261-1273. DOI: 10.1016/S1470-2045(17)30446-1 Epub 2017 Jul 17. PMID: 28729154

[38] Ralph C, Elkord E, Burt DJ, O'Dwyer JF, Austin EB, Stern PL, Hawkins RE, Thistlethwaite FC. Modulation of lymphocyte regulation for cancer therapy: A phase II trial of tremelimumab in advanced gastric and esophageal adenocarcinoma. Clinical Cancer Research. 2010;**16**:1662-1672. DOI: 10.1158/1078-0432.CCR-09-2870. PMID: 20179239

[39] Rosenberg SA, Yang JC, Restifo NP. Cancer immunotherapy: Moving beyond current vaccines. Nature Medicine. 2004;**10**:909-915. DOI: 10.1038/nm1100. PMID: 15340416

[40] Rosenberg SA, Sherry RM, Morton KE, Scharfman WJ, Yang JC, Topalian SL, Royal RE, Kammula U, Restifo NP, Hughes MS, Schwartzentruber D, Berman DM, Schwarz SL, Ngo LT, Mavroukakis SA, White DE, Steinberg SM. Tumor progression can occur despite the induction of very high levels of self/tumor antigen-specific CD8+ T cells in patients with melanoma. Journal of Immunology. 2005;**175**:6169-6176. DOI: 10.4049/jimmunol.175.9.6169. PMID: 16237114

[41] Kono K, Mizukami Y, Daigo Y, Takano A, Masuda K, Yoshida K, Tsunoda T, Kawaguchi Y, Nakamura Y, Fujii H. Vaccination with multiple peptides derived from novel cancer-testis antigens can induce specific T-cell responses and clinical responses in advanced esophageal cancer. Cancer Science. 2009;**100**:1502-1509. DOI: 10.1111/j.1349-7006.2009.01200.x. PMID: 19459850

[42] Kono K, Iinuma H, Akutsu Y, Tanaka H, Hayashi N, Uchikado Y, Noguchi T, Fujii H, Okinaka K, Fukushima R, Matsubara H, Ohira M, Baba H, Natsugoe S, Kitano S, Takeda K, Yoshida K, Tsunoda T, Nakamura Y. Multicenter, phase II clinical trial of cancer vaccination for advanced esophageal cancer with three peptides derived from novel cancer-testis antigens. Journal of Translational Medicine. 2012;**10**:141. DOI: 10.1186/1479-5876-10-141. PMID: 22776426

[43] Saito T, Wada H, Yamasaki M, Miyata H, Nishikawa H, Sato E, Kageyama S, Shiku H, Mori M, Doki Y. High expression of MAGE-A4 and MHC class I antigens in tumor cells and inductionof MAGE-A4 immune responses are prognostic markers of CHP-MAGE-A4 cancer vaccine. Vaccine. 2014;**32**:5901-5907. DOI: 10.1016/j.vaccine.2014.09.002. PMID: 25218300

[44] Wada H, Sato E, Uenaka A, Isobe M, Kawabata R, Nakamura Y, Iwae S, Yonezawa K, Yamasaki M, Miyata H, Doki Y, Shiku H, Jungbluth AA, Ritter G, Murphy R, Hoffman EW, Old LJ, Monden M, Nakayama E. Analysis of peripheral and local anti-tumor immune response in esophageal cancer patients after NY-ESO-1 protein vaccination. International Journal of Cancer. 2008;**123**:2362-2369. DOI: 10.1002/ijc.23810. PMID: 18729190

[45] Dietrich A, Mitchison NA, Rajnavölgyi E, Schneider SC. Primed lymphocytes are boosted by type II collagen of their hosts after adoptive transfer. Journal of Autoimmunity. 1994;**7**:601-609. DOI: 10.1006/jaut.1994.1044. PMID: 7840853

[46] Alsina M, Moehler M, Lorenzen S. Immunotherapy of esophageal cancer: Current status, many trials and innovative strategies. Oncology Research and Treatment. 2018;**41**(5): 266-271. DOI: 10.1159/000488120. Epub 2018 Apr 20

[47] Rosenberg SA, Lotze MT, Muul LM, Leitman S, Chang AE, Ettinghausen SE, Matory YL, Skibber JM, Shiloni E, Vetto JT. Observations on the Systemic Administration of Autologous Lymphokine-Activated Killer Cells and Recombinant Interleukin-2 to Patients with Metastatic Cancer

[48] Besser MJ, Shapira-Frommer R, Schachter J. Tumor-infiltrating lymphocytes: Clinical experience. Cancer Journal. 2015;**21**:465-469 PMID: 26588677. DOI: 10.1097/PPO.0000-000000000154

[49] Toh U, Yamana H, Sueyoshi S, Tanaka T, Niiya F, Katagiri K, Fujita H, Shirozou K, Itoh K. Locoregional cellular immunotherapy for patients with advanced esophageal cancer. Clinical Cancer Research. 2000;**6**:4663-4673. PMID: 11156218

[50] Chen X, Wang L, Yue D, Liu J, Huang L, Yang L, Cao L, Qin G, Li A, Wang D, Wang M, Qi Y, Zhang B, van der Bruggen P, Zhang Y. Correlation between the high expression levels of cancer-germline genes with clinical characteristics in esophageal squamous cell carcinoma. Histology and Histopathology. 2017 Aug;**32**(8):793-803. DOI: 10.14670/HH-11-847. Epub 2016 Nov 21

[51] Bujas T, Marusic Z, Peric Balja M, Mijic A, Kruslin B, Tomas D. MAGE-A3/4 and NY-ESO-1 antigens expression in metastatic esophageal squamous cell carcinoma. European Journal of Histochemistry. 2011;**55**:e7. DOI: 10.4081/ejh. 2011.e7. PMID: 21556122

[52] Kageyama S, Wada H, Muro K, Niwa Y, Ueda S, Miyata H, Takiguchi S, Sugino SH, Miyahara Y, Ikeda H, Imai N, Sato E, Yamada T, Osako M, Ohnishi M, Harada N, Hishida T, Doki Y, Shiku H. Dose-dependent effects of NY-ESO-1 protein vaccine complexed with cholesteryl pullulan (CHP-NY-ESO-1) on immune responses and survival benefits of esophageal cancer patients. Journal of Translational Medicine. 2013;**11**:246. DOI: 10.1186/1479-5876-11-246. PMID: 24093426

[53] Gross G, Waks T, Eshhar Z. Expression of immunoglobulin-T-cell receptor chimeric molecules as functional receptors with antibodytype specificity. Proceedings of the National Academy of Sciences of the United States of America. 1989;**86**:10024-10028. DOI: 10.1073/pnas.86.24.10024. PMID: 2513569

[54] Liu Y, Chen X, Han W, Zhang Y. Tisagenlecleucel, an approved anti-CD19 chimeric antigen receptor T-cell therapy for the treatment of leukemia. Drugs Today (Barc). 2017 Nov;**53**(11):597-608. DOI: 10.1358/dot.2017.53.11.2725754. PMID: 29451276

[55] Kershaw MH, Westwood JA, Parker LL, Wang G, Eshhar Z, Mavroukakis SA, White DE, Wunderlich JR, Canevari S, Rogers-Freezer L, Chen CC, Yang JC, Rosenberg SA, Hwu P. A phase I study on adoptive immunotherapy using gene-modified T cells for ovarian cancer. Clinical Cancer Research. 2006;**12**:6106-6115. DOI: 10.1158/1078-0432.CCR-06-1183. PMID: 17062687

[56] Nellan A, Rota C, Majzner R, Lester-McCully CM, Griesinger AM, Mulcahy Levy JM, Foreman NK, Warren KE, Lee DW. Durable regression of Medulloblastoma after regional

and intravenous delivery of anti-HER2 chimeric antigen receptor T cells. Journal for Immunotherapy of Cancer. 2018 Apr 30;**6**(1):30. DOI: 10.1186/s40425-018-0340-z

[57] Feng K, Guo Y, Dai H, Wang Y, Li X, Jia H, Han W. Chimeric antigen receptor-modified T cells for the immunotherapy of patients with EGFR expressing advanced relapsed/refractory nonsmall cell lung cancer. Science China. Life Sciences. 2016;**59**:468-479. DOI: 10.1007/s11427-016-5023-8. PMID: 26968708

[58] Weiss A, Bashour SI, Hess K, Thompson AM, Ibrahim NK. Effect of neoadjuvant chemotherapy regimen on relapse-free survival among patients with breast cancer achieving a pathologic complete response: An early step in the de-escalation of neoadjuvant chemotherapy. Breast Cancer Research. 2018;**20**:27. DOI: 10.1186/s13058-018-0945-7

[59] Mooradian MJ, Reuben A, Prieto PA, Hazar-Rethinam M, Frederick DT, Nadres B, Piris A, Juneja V, Cooper ZA, Sharpe AH, Corcoran RB, Flaherty KT, Lawrence DP, Wargo JA, Sullivan RJ. A phase II study of combined therapy with a BRAF inhibitor (vemurafenib) and interleukin-2 (aldesleukin) in patients with metastatic melanoma. Oncoimmunology. 2018 Feb 1;**7**(5):e1423172. DOI: 10.1080/2162402X.2017.1423172. eCollection 2018

[60] Abdo J, Cornell DL, Mittal SK, Agrawal DK. Immunotherapy plus cryotherapy: Potential augmented abscopal effect for advanced cancers. Frontiers in Oncology. 2018 Mar 28;**8**:85. DOI: 10.3389/fonc.2018.00085. eCollection 2018

[61] Mauri G, Nicosia L, Xu Z, Di Pietro S, Monfardini L, Bonomo G, Varano GM, Prada F, Della Vigna P, Orsi F. Focused ultrasound: Tumour ablation and its potential to enhance immunological therapy to cancer. The British Journal of Radiology. 2018 Feb;**91**(1083):20170641. DOI: 10.1259/bjr.20170641

[62] Mi FL, Burnouf T, Lu SY, Lu YJ, Lu KY, Ho YC, Kuo CY, Chuang EY. Self-targeting, immune transparent plasma protein coated nanocomplex for noninvasive photothermal anticancer therapy. Advanced Healthcare Materials. 2017 Jul;**6**(14). DOI: 10.1002/adhm.201700181

[63] Blake Z, Marks DK, Gartrell RD, Hart T, Horton P, Cheng SK, Taback B, Horst BA, Saenger YM. Complete intracranial response to talimogene laherparepvec (T-Vec), pembrolizumab and whole brain radiotherapy in a patient with melanoma brain metastases refractory to dual checkpoint-inhibition. Journal for Immunotherapy of Cancer. 2018 Apr 6;**6**(1):25. DOI: 10.1186/s40425-018-0338-6

[64] Finazzi T, Rordorf T, Ikenberg K, Huber GF, Guckenberger M, Schueler G, HI. Radiotherapy-induced anti-tumor immune response and immune-related adverse events in a case of recurrent nasopharyngeal carcinoma undergoing anti-PD-1 immunotherapy. BMC Cancer. 2018 Apr 6;**18**(1):395. DOI: 10.1186/s12885-018-4295-8

[65] Chen M, Nie J, Liu Y, Li X, Zhang Y, Brock MV, Feng K, Wu Z, Li X, Shi L, Li S, Guo M, Mei Q, Han W. Phase Ib/II study of safety and efficacy of low-dose decitabine-primed chemoimmunotherapy in patients with drug-resistant relapsed/refractory alimentary tract cancer. International Journal of Cancer. 2018 Apr 16. DOI: 10.1002/ijc.31531

[66] Iinuma H, Fukushima R, Inaba T, Tamura J, Inoue T, Ogawa E, Horikawa M, Ikeda Y, Matsutani N, Takeda K, Yoshida K, Tsunoda T, Ikeda T, Nakamura Y, Okinaga K. Phase I clinical study of multiple epitope peptide vaccine combined with chemoradiation therapy in esophageal cancer patients. Journal of Translational Medicine. 2014 Apr 3;**12**:84. DOI: 10.1186/1479-5876-12-84

[67] Han B, Li K, Zhao Y, Li B, Cheng Y, Zhou J, Lu Y, Shi Y, Wang Z, Jiang L, Luo Y, Zhang Y, Huang C, Li Q, Wu G. Anlotinib as a third-line therapy in patients with refractory advanced non-small-cell lung cancer: A multicentre, randomised phase II trial (ALTER0302). British Journal of Cancer. 2018 Mar 6;**118**(5):654-661. DOI: 10.1038/bjc.2017.478

3

Laparoscopic Surgery for Gastric Cancer

Talha Sarigoz, Inanc Samil Sarici, Ozgul Duzgun and Mustafa Uygar Kalayci

Abstract

In patients with gastric cancer, surgical resection is the only treatment that can offer cure or increase long-term survival. With the accumulation of experience in laparoscopic radical gastrectomy and the progress in surgical instruments, laparoscopic surgery for gastric cancer has gained popularity despite initial concerns regarding safety and oncological adequacy. As a result, laparoscopic technique has been widely applied in gastric cancer. Different meta-analyses showed that laparoscopic procedures are associated with less blood loss but longer operation time. Many studies have reported outcomes of laparoscopic surgery for early gastric cancer, but several authors also have shown that a laparoscopic approach can also be used in cases of advanced gastric cancer. We therefore conducted this study to expand our experience and to evaluate laparoscopic gastrectomy step by step in the light of recent reports while defining key points and surgical technique.

Keywords: laparoscopic surgery, gastric cancer, gastrectomy, lymphadenectomy, advanced, early gastric cancer, laparoscopic gastrectomy

1. Introduction

Gastric cancer (GC) is the fifth most common malignancy and the third most common cause of cancer-related deaths worldwide in both sexes combined [1]. Surgery with either total or subtotal gastrectomy and lymphadenectomy is the initial treatment [2]. The first example of gastrectomy for cancer was described by Theodor Billroth and the first laparoscopy-assisted gastrectomy was performed by Kitano et al. in 1991 for a patient with early GC [3, 4]. In the last two decades, in parallel to advances in surgical devices and technical expertise, minimally invasive surgery has become the new trend and the laparoscopy has increasingly started being applied for GC as an alternative to open surgery. However, due to complexity of the lymph node structure and contiguity of stomach to gross vascular structures, it is technically demanding. During the procedure, it is equally important to ensure adequate resection and pay attention to some precautions [5]. In this chapter, we will clarify pre-operative approach, technical considerations as well as clinical outcomes of laparoscopic surgery (LS) for GC based on the recent reports in the literature.

2. Preoperative approach

2.1. Indications for laparoscopic surgery

Most of the reports evaluated early GC population and common consensus is that laparoscopic gastrectomy is appropriate for early-stage GC with benefits of reduced need for painkillers, early discharge, rapid recovery of bowel movement, less pulmonary function disorders, and better cosmetic results [5, 6]. There is agreement about performing laparoscopic total gastrectomy for proximal GC with T1 N0 disease and laparoscopic distal gastrectomy for distal GC with T1–2 N0 disease [5]. Regarding advanced stage cancers, there is still debate over appropriateness of laparoscopy concerning oncologic adequacy of lymphadenectomy with tumor-free margins. Recent meta-analysis and cohorts demonstrated favorable short- and long-term outcomes of laparoscopic gastrectomy for advanced stage GC; but in order to recommend it as an alternative to open surgery, there is still room for prospective clinical trials and longer-follow-up studies [7–9].

2.2. Determination of resection margin

Lack of tactile feedback limits assessment of the tumor during laparoscopic surgery. Since laparoscopic gastrectomy has been performed mostly for early GC and achieving tumor-free margins is important in terms of oncological principles, different methods have been proposed for safe determination of resection line in tumors without serosal surface invasion. Reported various procedures include preoperative or intraoperative endoscopic dye injection, preoperative endoscopic clipping along with intraoperative endoscopy, intraoperative radiography or ultrasonography [10–14]. None of these methods has wide acceptance and choice of technique vary with institution.

2.3. Nutritional status of patients

As gastric cancer is a serious malignancy of the upper intestinal tract, patients are at risk for malnutrition due to maldigestion and malabsorption. On the other hand, surgery itself imposes protein and energy requirements and it can aggravate pre-existing nutritional disorders [15]. There is a lack of clinical evidence about role of laparoscopic gastrectomy in malnourished patients with GC. A recent retrospective study reported significantly less postoperative complications and faster recovery for laparoscopic gastrectomy compared to open surgery [16]. But, prospective clinical trials to analyze short- and long-term effects of preoperative nutritional support, chemotherapy and dissection type are required to recommend laparoscopic gastrectomy for malnourished patients.

2.4. Presence of enlarged lymph nodes in preoperative imaging

There are controversies on the extent of lymphadenectomy for GC. Nevertheless, lymph node dissection is recommended for staging and prevention of local recurrence. Most of the patients with GC are diagnosed at a later stage of the disease, often with enlarged lymph nodes. Since lymphadenectomy is a challenging procedure, especially in laparoscopic setting, enlarged nodes interfere with anatomical structures and disrupt the course of the dissection. In a late retrospective study, performing laparoscopic gastrectomy for GC with pre-operative enlarged lymph nodes was found to be safe and effective [17]. Yet, these results should be supported with prospective research to make recommendation.

2.5. Obese patients

Obese patients carry high risk for comorbid diseases and they are directly associated with intra- and post-operative complications [18]. Obesity was considered as a relative contraindication for laparoscopy, but with the advances in laparoscopic equipment and growing experience, initial studies with laparoscopic surgery in obese patients have shown promise [19]. According to the reports in the literature, due to abundant visceral fat content and difficult manipulation of tissue, operation times in laparoscopic gastrectomy were longer compared to open surgery [20, 21]. Not only obesity, but also high body mass index (BMI ≥ 25 kg/m^2) was shown to affect operation time and retrieved lymph node number negatively [22]. On the other hand, the 5-year survival rates of patients who underwent laparoscopic gastrectomy and open gastrectomy were similar [23]. But regarding early post-operative outcomes, we cannot mention that there is an agreement [20, 21, 23]. Despite negative findings, laparoscopic gastrectomy is likely to be the choice of surgery in obese patients with growing experience.

2.6. Elderly patients

In parallel to increasing age, functional capacity decreases at some point and this situation creates risk for surgery. Considering advantages, elderly may benefit from laparoscopic surgery. In an updated pooled meta-analysis, laparoscopic gastrectomy was found to reduce surgery-related cardiopulmonary disease and also better cognitive outcomes were observed compared to open surgery [24]. But, lack of randomized controlled studies in the literature prevent from making precise conclusions.

3. Technical considerations

3.1. The importance of lymphadenectomy in gastric cancer

Lymph node metastasis (LNM) is the most common pattern of metastatic spread in gastric cancer [25]. The reported frequency of LNM in gastric cancer can be seen up to 80%. Lymphatic networks are plenty in the layer of the gastric wall, particularly in the submucosa and serosa, which simplify metastasis. Oncological outcomes will not be reached if gastrectomy alone is performed for gastric cancer. Therefore, lymphatic flow of the stomach and characteristics of metastasis have been continuously examined by researchers. In the Japanese gastric cancer treatment guidelines based on the third English edition of the Japanese Classification of Gastric Carcinoma and the Japanese Gastric Cancer Association defined the extent of systematic lymphadenectomy according to the type of gastrectomy indicated [26]. Lymph node metastasis in gastric cancer is usually associated with the location of the tumor, and metastasis follows the lymphatic drainage routes from the superficial to the profoundus. For this reason, lymph nodes are numbered and dissection for functional lymph node resection was defined. Laparoscopic gastrectomy, which begins with D1 dissection in early gastric cancer treatment, can now be done easily with the aid of technology (laparoscopy, robotic surgery) and D2 dissection technique is routinely performed in the treatment of advanced GC [27] (**Tables 1** and **2**).

3.2. Surgical technique of laparoscopic gastrectomy with D2 lymphadenectomy

3.2.1. Patient's position and location of trocars

The patient is placed in the modified lithotomy position. The surgical table is adjusted 20–30° into the reverse Trendelenburg position. The surgeon stands on the patient's leg, the assistant is on the right side, and the camera operator is between the patient's left side. Besides routine laparoscopic devices, advance vessel sealing systems, all types of intestinal Endo-GIA and circular staplers must be available on the operating table. The intervention generally performed by using five ports. Additionally, subxiphoid sixth port can be required during the splenic hilar lymph node dissection. 10-mm optic port is placed 1 cm above the umbilicus. 15-mm trocar left preaxillary and 5 mm trocar right preaxillary is inserted in the line 2 cm below the costal margin. Two 5-mm ports are placed bilaterally in each hypochondrium for assisting and dissection purposes (**Figure 1**).

3.2.2. Surgical procedure

Laparoscopic exploration is used for preoperative staging, liver and peritoneal metastasis which can reduce unnecessary laparotomies. Once it is determined that it is suitable for surgery, the procedure continues in four steps as left part region, right part region, cardiac region, and reconstruction (**Table 3**).

3.2.2.1. Left part region (4sa, 4sv, 10, 11d)

The approach for removing the greater omentum begins from the superior border of the transverse colon. After that, the division is extended toward the flexura of left and the right colon. In the continuation of the dissection, splenic ligaments must be separated due to prevent of iatrogenic splenic injury which may be caused by traction. Gastrosplenic, splenocolic, splenorenal, and splenophrenic ligaments need to be separated in this stage. The omentectomy helps to achieve a lymphadenectomy corresponding to lymph node stations 4sa and 4sv according to the Japanese classification. The left gastro-omental vessels are perfectly identified clipped and divided. After this dissection, the short gastric vessels will be divided using the sealing

Regional lymph nodes of stomach

1. Right cardia lymph nodes
2. Left cardia lymph nodes
3. Lymph nodes along the lesser curvature
4. Lymph nodes along the greater curvature
   - Station **4sa:** lymph nodes along the short gastric vessels
   - Station **4sb:** lymph nodes along the left gastroepiploic vessels
   - Station **4d:** lymph nodes along the right gastroepiploic vessel
5. Suprapyloric group of lymph nodes or nodes along the right gastric artery
6. Infrapyloric groups of lymph nodes
7. Lymph nodes along the left gastric artery
8. Lymph nodes along the common hepatic artery
   - Station **8a:** anterosuperior group
   - Station **8b:** posterior group
9. Lymph nodes around the celiac artery
10. Lymph nodes at the splenic hilum
11. Lymph nodes along the splenic artery
    - Station **11p:** along the proximal splenic artery
    - Station **11d:** along the distal splenic artery
12. Lymph nodes in the hepatoduodenal ligament
    - Station **12a:** along the hepatic artery
    - Station **12b:** along the bile duct
    - Station **12p**: behind the portal vein
13. Lymph nodes behind the pancreatic head
14. Lymph nodes at the root of the mesentery or the SMA
15. Lymph nodes along the middle colic artery
16. Para-aortic group of lymph nodes
    - Station **16a1:** lymph node in the aortic hiatus
    - Station **16a2:** lymph node around the abdominal aorta (from the upper margin of the celiac trunk to the lower margin of the left renal vein)
    - Station **16b1:** lymph node around the abdominal aorta (from the lower margin of the left renal vein to the upper margin of the inferior mesenteric artery)
    - Station **16b2:** lymph node around the abdominal aorta (from the upper margin of the inferior mesenteric artery to the aortic bifurcation)

Table 1. Numbering lymph nodes according to the Japanese Research Society for Gastric Cancer.

D0	No dissection or incomplete dissection of the Group 1 nodes
D1	Dissection of all the Group 1 nodes (No.1–6 lymph nodes)
D2	Dissection of all the Group 1 and Group 2 nodes (D1 station + No.7–11 lymph nodes)
D3	Dissection of all the Group 1, Group 2 and Group 3 nodes (D2+ No. 12–16 lymph nodes)

Table 2. Definitions of lymphadenectomy in gastric cancer.

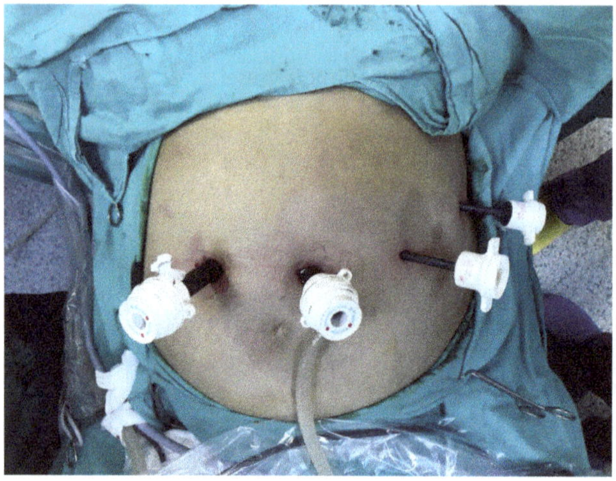

Figure 1. Patient's position and location of trocars.

1	Left part region (4sa, 4sv, 10, 11d)
2	Right part region (4d, 5, 6, 7, 8a, 8p, 9, 11p, 12a, 12b, 12p)
3	Cardiac region [1–3]
4	Gastric resection and reconstruction

Table 3. Steps of laparoscopic gastrectomy for gastric cancer.

systems. This dissection should be continued until the left crus of the diaphragm clearly seen. At this time, the lymph node 10 and 11d in the splenic hilus is gently excised (**Figures 2** and **3**).

3.2.2.2. *Right part region (4d, 5, 6, 7, 8a, 8p, 9, 11p, 12a, 12b, 12p)*

The dissection is then continued toward the right part of the abdomen. Dissection of the gastro-omental ligament is pursued in this area. This dissection allows to drop the right colon and to access the duodenum. This maneuver also allows to expose the anterior aspect of the pancreatic head and to access the right gastro-omental pedicle, where a lymphadenectomy should be performed in order to control lymph node station 6 (**Figure 4**).

Right gastro-omental vessels are dissected, isolated, and divided. Once this first mobilization and 6-station of lymphadenectomy step has been performed, the first portion of the duodenum will be dissected and isolated, prior to moving on to the supragastric compartment. The common bile duct, hepatic artery, and portal vein, which form the hepatoduodenal ligament,

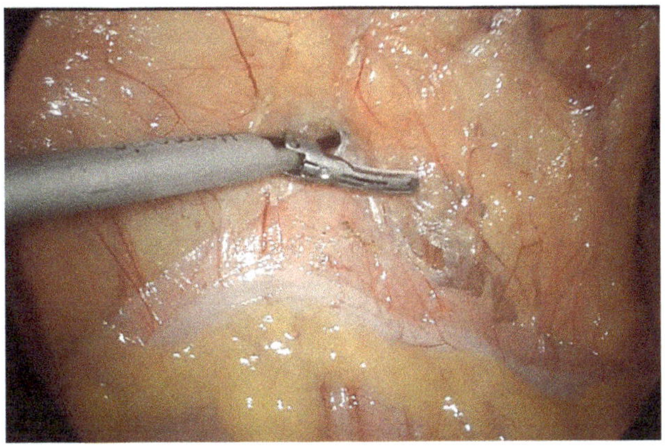

Figure 2. Lift of transvers colon and dissection of anterior transvers mesocolon fascia.

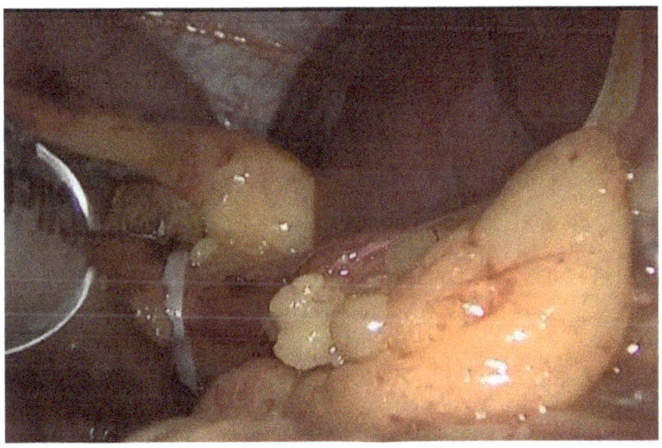

Figure 3. The left gastro-omental vessel is clipped and divided.

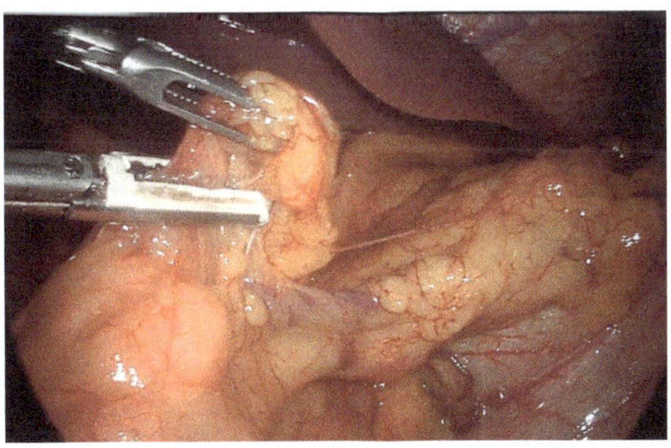

Figure 4. Dissection of number 6 lymphatic area.

are identified. The right gastric artery will also be identified and divided along with lymph node dissection at the level of lymph node station 5. The 12a, 12b, and 12p lymph node stations in the hepatoduodenal ligament are excised with vessel sealing devices (**Figure 5**).

Duodenal division is then performed approximately 2 cm distally from the pylorus by Endo-GIA blue cartridge. After dissection of the hepatic proper artery, resection will be carried on at the superior border of the pancreas at the level of the common hepatic artery, namely lymph node

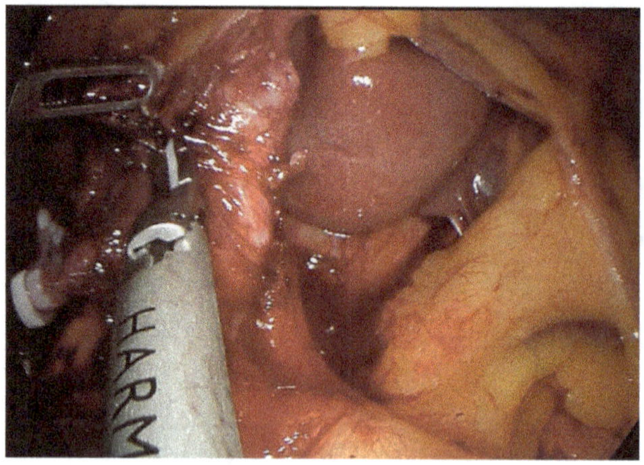

Figure 5. Dissection of hepatoduodenal lymphatic area.

stations 8 and 9. The left coronary vein is also identified, clipped, and divided. Dissection is pursued toward the coeliac trunk with lymph node dissection of stations 9. Dissection of the left gastric artery is begun along with lymph node dissection of station 7. The left gastric artery is clipped and divided. After that 11p lymph node stations along the splenic artery are excised. Care should be taken during dissection due to the tortuous structure of splenic artery (**Figures 6** and **7**).

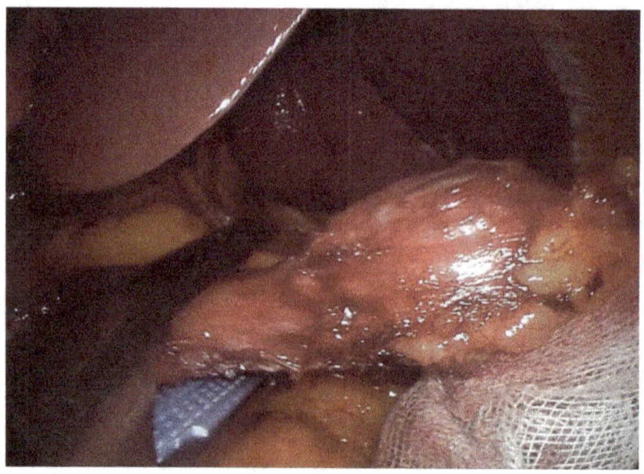

Figure 6. Transection of duodenum.

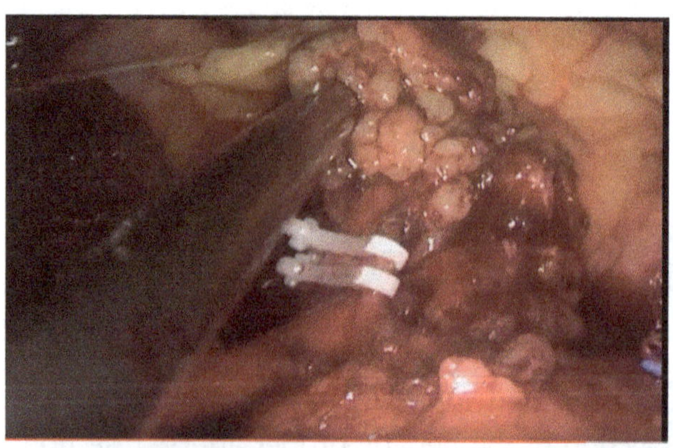

Figure 7. Dissection of number 7, 8, and 9 lymphatic area.

3.2.2.3. Cardiac region

The lymph nodes in the cardiac region are located on both sides of the cardia and along the lesser curvature [1–3]. Hepatogastric ligament is opened by vessel sealing devices in the avascular area at the posterior wall of the gastric lesser curvature. Thus, the gastric lesser curvature is fully bared and dissection of the No. 3 lymph nodes is done. The left and right diaphragm crus are identified and the phrenoesophageal membrane is dissected. Lymph nodes No:1 and No:2 are excised. The abdominal part of the esophagus is bared 5 cm in the abdomen. Left and right vagal nerves divided (**Figure 8**).

3.2.2.4. Gastric resection and reconstruction

The reconstruction should be in different forms according to the extent of the resection. Proximal resection was performed with Endo GIA blue cartridge which is placed from 15 mm trocar. Trans oral OrVil™ (Covidien Mansfield, USA) is propagated from the esophagus and anvil is placed in the esophageal stump. Transvers mesocolon lifted and the small window open from the avascular area. Jejunal ans is divided at 20 cm from the Treitz ligament by Endo GIA blue cartridge. Esophagojejunostomy is done with 25 mm circular stapler if totally gastrectomy planned or gastrojejunostomy is performed with EndoGIA if subtotal gastrectomy intended. Jejunal stump is closed with Endo GIA blue cartridge. Laparoscopic reinforcement

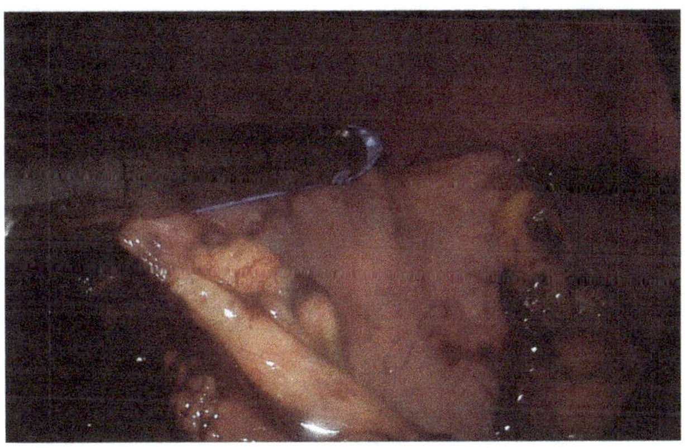

Figure 8. Dissection of cardiac lymphatic area.

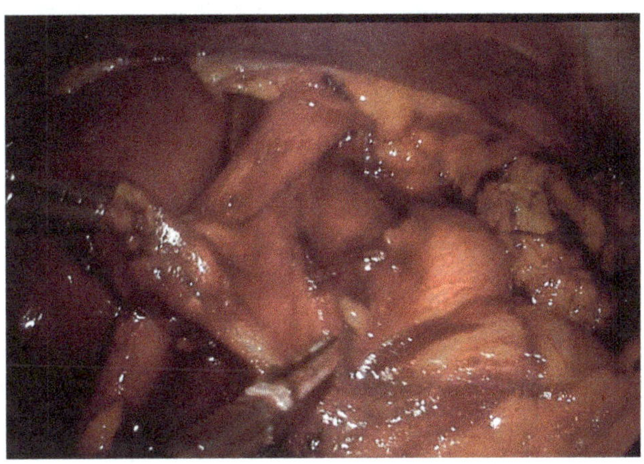

Figure 9. Proximal resection of stomach with EndoGIA.

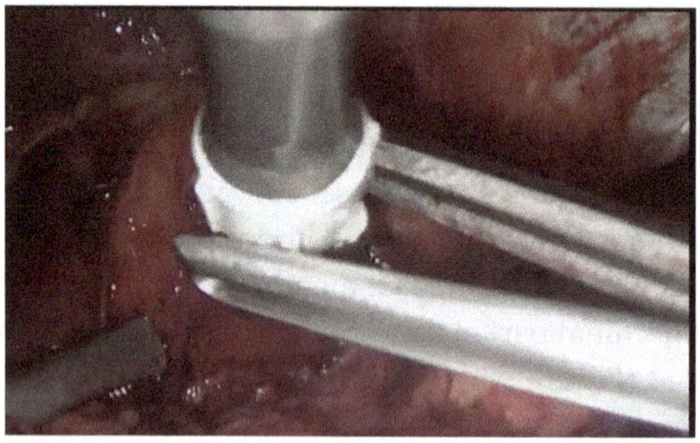

Figure 10. OrVil™ placement in the esophageal stump.

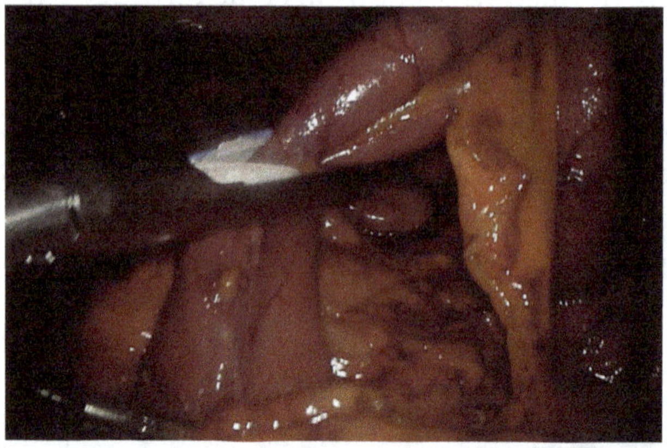

Figure 11. Division of jejunal ans 20 cm distal to the Treitz ligament.

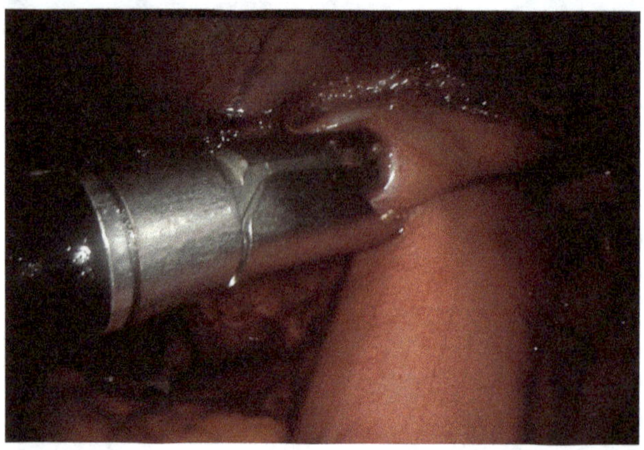

Figure 12. Gastrojejunostomy with EndoGIA.

sutures can be added if needed. Jejunum is fixed to the diaphragm crus. The jejunojejunostomy is also performed by means of a side to side Endo GIA blue cartridge stapler. Placement of the gastric tube is controlled laparoscopically. This tube is lowered until the distal part of the alimentary limb. A wound protector is placed into the defect, hence allowing for the extraction of the entire specimen, including the whole stomach and the omentum (**Figures 9–13, Table 4**).

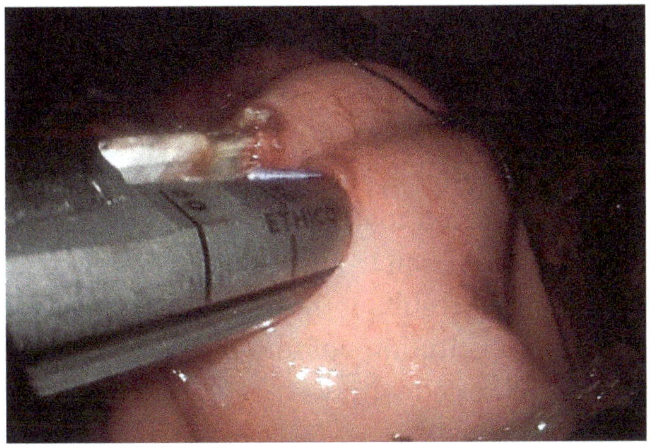

Figure 13. Jejunojejunostomy with EndoGIA.

Subtotal gastrectomy	Total gastrectomy

• Totally laparoscopic gastroduodenostomy (Billroth 1)
• Billroth 1 through mini laparotomy
• Billroth 1 with hand port
• Roux-en-Y Gastrojejunostomy
	• Roux-en-Y esophagojejunostomy
	• Hand-sewn anastomosis
	  • Laparoscopic
	  • Mini-laparotomy
	• Mechanical anastomosis
	  • Circular stapler
	  • Manually loaded anvil
	  • Transoral (OrVil™)

Table 4. Different reconstruction forms according to the resection types.

4. Post-operative outcomes

4.1. Early post-operative outcomes

Initial studies with laparoscopic gastrectomy consisted of mostly early GC and with growing experience it has been started to apply to later stages of the disease. Laparoscopic gastrectomy whether performed for early or advanced GC has advantages such as less blood loss, early ambulation, rapid recovery of bowel movement, and shorter hospitalization compared to open surgery [28–31]. Complication rates of laparoscopic gastrectomy for early GC ranged from 4.2 to 23.3% and these results did not differ from open surgery [29, 32–34]. In the latest ongoing clinical trials, short-term results have been shared. While, laparoscopic surgery for advanced GC has a complication rate of 16.4%, it is 24.3% for open surgery [35–37]. These studies will be finalized in 2018. In an ongoing study in Japan, short-term results have revealed incidence of anastomotic leakage rate as 4.7% for laparoscopic surgery in advanced stage [37]. In the retrospective studies, anastomotic leakage rate during LS for advanced GC was reported to range from 1.1 to 2.7% [30, 38–40]. But this risk should be evaluated appropriately.

4.2. Late post-operative outcomes

According to single-center studies, after laparoscopic gastrectomy for early GC, the morbidity rates ranged from 10 to 14.8% and mortality rates from 0 to 1.1% [6, 41, 42]. Regarding laparoscopic gastrectomy for AGC, the morbidity rates ranged from 8.0 to 24.2% but there was no significant difference compared to open surgery [30, 39, 40]. There are ongoing randomized phase-II and III studies in Asian Countries. They are expected to give scientifically more reliable results [30, 35]. Initial results indicate that LS for advanced GC is feasible and safe but surgeon experience and institution volume play important role on patient outcome. Long-term outcomes should be clarified with well-established studies.

Author details

Talha Sarigoz[1*], Inanc Samil Sarici[2], Ozgul Duzgun[3] and Mustafa Uygar Kalayci[4]

*Address all correspondence to: sarigozt.md@gmail.com

1 Department of General Surgery, Sason State Hospital, Batman, Turkey

2 Department of General Surgery, Kanuni Sultan Suleyman Training and Research Hospital, Istanbul, Turkey

3 Division of Surgical Oncology, Department of General Surgery, Umraniye Training and Research Hospital, Istanbul, Turkey

4 Department of General Surgery, Kanuni Sultan Suleyman Training and Research Hospital, Istanbul, Turkey

References

[1] Global Burden of Disease Cancer C, Fitzmaurice C, Allen C, Barber RM, Barregard L, Bhutta ZA, et al. Global, regional, and national cancer incidence, mortality, years of life lost, years lived with disability, and disability-adjusted life-years for 32 cancer groups, 1990 to 2015: A systematic analysis for the global burden of disease study. JAMA Oncology. 2017;**3**(4):524-548

[2] Lutz MP, Zalcberg JR, Ducreux M, Ajani JA, Allum W, Aust D, et al. Highlights of the EORTC St. Gallen International Expert Consensus on the primary therapy of gastric, gastroesophageal and oesophageal cancer—Differential treatment strategies for subtypes of early gastroesophageal cancer. European Journal of Cancer. 2012;**48**(16):2941-2953

[3] Kitano S, Iso Y, Moriyama M, Sugimachi K. Laparoscopy-assisted Billroth I Gastrectomy. Surgical Laparoscopy & Endoscopy. 1994;**4**(2):146-148

[4] Billroth T. Offenes schreiben an Herr, Dr. L. Wittelshöfer. Wiener Medizinische Wochenschrift. 1881;**26**:731

[5] Brar S, Law C, McLeod R, Helyer L, Swallow C, Paszat L, et al. Defining surgical quality in gastric cancer: A RAND/UCLA appropriateness study. Journal of the American College of Surgeons. 2013;**217**(2):347-357. e1

[6] Kitano S, Shiraishi N, Fujii K, Yasuda K, Inomata M, Adachi YA. Randomized controlled trial comparing open vs laparoscopy-assisted distal gastrectomy for the treatment of early gastric cancer: An interim report. Surgery. 2002;**131**(1 Suppl):S306-S311

[7] Son T, Hyung WJ, Lee JH, Kim YM, Noh SH. Minimally invasive surgery for serosa-positive gastric cancer (pT4a) in patients with preoperative diagnosis of cancer without serosal invasion. Surgical Endoscopy. 2014;**28**(3):866-874

[8] Lee J, Kim W. Long-term outcomes after laparoscopy-assisted gastrectomy for advanced gastric cancer: Analysis of consecutive 106 experiences. Journal of Surgical Oncology. 2009;**100**(8):693-698

[9] Huscher CG, Mingoli A, Sgarzini G, Brachini G, Binda B, Di Paola M, et al. Totally laparoscopic total and subtotal gastrectomy with extended lymph node dissection for early and advanced gastric cancer: Early and long-term results of a 100-patient series. American Journal of Surgery. 2007;**194**(6):839-844. discussion 44

[10] Xuan Y, Hur H, Byun CS, Han SU, Cho YK. Efficacy of intraoperative gastroscopy for tumor localization in totally laparoscopic distal gastrectomy for cancer in the middle third of the stomach. Surgical Endoscopy. 2013;**27**(11):4364-4370

[11] Park DJ, Lee HJ, Kim SG, Jung HC, Song IS, Lee KU, et al. Intraoperative gastroscopy for gastric surgery. Surgical Endoscopy. 2005;**19**(10):1358-1361

[12] Nakagawa M, Ehara K, Ueno M, Tanaka T, Kaida S, Udagawa H. Accurate, safe, and rapid method of intraoperative tumor identification for totally laparoscopic distal gastrectomy: Injection of mixed fluid of sodium hyaluronate and patent blue. Surgical Endoscopy. 2014;**28**(4):1371-1375

[13] Kim HI, Hyung WJ, Lee CR, Lim JS, An JY, Cheong JH, et al. Intraoperative portable abdominal radiograph for tumor localization: A simple and accurate method for laparoscopic gastrectomy. Surgical Endoscopy. 2011;**25**(3):958-963

[14] Kawakatsu S, Ohashi M, Hiki N, Nunobe S, Nagino M, Sano T. Use of endoscopy to determine the resection margin during laparoscopic gastrectomy for cancer. The British Journal of Surgery. 2017

[15] Mariette C, De Botton ML, Piessen G. Surgery in esophageal and gastric cancer patients: What is the role for nutrition support in your daily practice? Annals of Surgical Oncology. 2012;**19**(7):2128-2134

[16] Zheng HL, Lu J, Zheng CH, Li P, Xie JW, Wang JB, et al. Short- and long-term outcomes in malnourished patients after laparoscopic or open radical gastrectomy. World Journal of Surgery. 2017

[17] Chen QY, Huang CM, Zheng CH, Li P, Xie JW, Wang JB, et al. Do preoperative enlarged lymph nodes affect the oncologic outcome of laparoscopic radical gastrectomy for gastric cancer? Oncotarget. 2017;**8**(5):8825-8834

[18] Tjeertes EK, Hoeks SE, Beks SB, Valentijn TM, Hoofwijk AG, Stolker RJ. Obesity—A risk factor for postoperative complications in general surgery? BMC Anesthesiology. 2015;**15**:112

[19] Loffer FD, Pent D. Laparoscopy in the obese patient. American Journal of Obstetrics and Gynecology. 1976;**125**(1):104-107

[20] Yasuda K, Inomata M, Shiraishi N, Izumi K, Ishikawa K, Kitano S. Laparoscopy-assisted distal gastrectomy for early gastric cancer in obese and nonobese patients. Surgical Endoscopy. 2004;**18**(8):1253-1256

[21] Kim MG, Yook JH, Kim KC, Kim TH, Kim HS, Kim BS, et al. Influence of obesity on early surgical outcomes of laparoscopic-assisted gastrectomy in gastric cancer. Surgical Laparoscopy, Endoscopy & Percutaneous Techniques. 2011;**21**(3):151-154

[22] Lee HJ, Kim HH, Kim MC, Ryu SY, Kim W, Song KY, et al. The impact of a high body mass index on laparoscopy assisted gastrectomy for gastric cancer. Surgical Endoscopy. 2009;**23**(11):2473-2479

[23] Son SY, Jung DH, Lee CM, Ahn SH, Ahn HS, Park DJ, et al. Laparoscopic gastrectomy versus open gastrectomy for gastric cancer in patients with body mass index of 30 kg/m^2 or more. Surgical Endoscopy. 2015;**29**(8):2126-2132

[24] Zong L, Wu A, Wang W, Deng J, Aikou S, Yamashita H, et al. Feasibility of laparoscopic gastrectomy for elderly gastric cancer patients: Meta-analysis of non-randomized controlled studies. Oncotarget. 2017;**8**(31):51878-51887

[25] Huang C-M, Zheng C-H. Summary of anatomy and physiology of perigastric lymphatic system. In: Huang C-M, Zheng C-H, editors. Laparoscopic Gastrectomy for Gastric Cancer: Surgical Technique and Lymphadenectomy. Dordrecht: Springer Netherlands; 2015. pp. 1-6

[26] Japanese Gastric Cancer A. Japanese gastric cancer treatment guidelines 2010 (ver. 3). Gastric Cancer. 2011;**14**(2):113-123

[27] RH T, Li P, Xie JW, Wang JB, Lin JX, Lu J, et al. Development of lymph node dissection in laparoscopic gastrectomy: Safety and technical tips. Transl. Gastroenterología y Hepatología. 2017;**2**:23

[28] Kim YW, Baik YH, Yun YH, Nam BH, Kim DH, Choi IJ, et al. Improved quality of life outcomes after laparoscopy-assisted distal gastrectomy for early gastric cancer: Results of a prospective randomized clinical trial. Annals of Surgery. 2008;**248**(5):721-727

[29] Kim HH, Hyung WJ, Cho GS, Kim MC, Han SU, Kim W, et al. Morbidity and mortality of laparoscopic gastrectomy versus open gastrectomy for gastric cancer: An interim report—A phase III multicenter, prospective, randomized trial (KLASS trial). Annals of Surgery. 2010;**251**(3):417-420

[30] Hu Y, Huang C, Sun Y, Su X, Cao H, Hu J, et al. Morbidity and mortality of laparoscopic versus open D2 distal Gastrectomy for advanced gastric cancer: A randomized controlled trial. Journal of Clinical Oncology. 2016;**34**(12):1350-1357

[31] Hayashi H, Ochiai T, Shimada H, Gunji Y. Prospective randomized study of open versus laparoscopy-assisted distal gastrectomy with extraperigastric lymph node dissection for early gastric cancer. Surgical Endoscopy. 2005;**19**(9):1172-1176

[32] Lee JH, Han HS, Lee JHA. Prospective randomized study comparing open vs laparoscopy-assisted distal gastrectomy in early gastric cancer: Early results. Surgical Endoscopy. 2005;**19**(2):168-173

[33] Hosono S, Arimoto Y, Ohtani H, Kanamiya Y. Meta-analysis of short-term outcomes after laparoscopy-assisted distal gastrectomy. World Journal of Gastroenterology. 2006; **12**(47):7676-7683

[34] Adachi Y, Shiraishi N, Shiromizu A, Bandoh T, Aramaki M, Kitano S. Laparoscopy-assisted Billroth I gastrectomy compared with conventional open gastrectomy. Archives of Surgery. 2000;**135**(7):806-810

[35] Lee H-J, Hyung WJ, Yang H-K, Han SU, Park Y-K, An JY, et al. Morbidity of laparoscopic distal gastrectomy with D2 lymphadenectomy compared with open distal gastrectomy for locally advanced gastric cancer: Short term outcomes from multicenter randomized controlled trial (KLASS-02). Journal of Clinical Oncology. 2016;**34**(15_suppl):4062

[36] Kinoshita T, Kaito A. Current status and future perspectives of laparoscopic radical surgery for advanced gastric cancer. Transl. Gastroenterología y Hepatología. 2017;**2**:43

[37] Inaki N, Etoh T, Ohyama T, Uchiyama K, Katada N, Koeda K, et al. A multi-institutional, prospective, phase II feasibility study of laparoscopy-assisted distal gastrectomy with D2 lymph node dissection for locally advanced gastric cancer (JLSSG0901). World Journal of Surgery. 2015;**39**(11):2734-2741

[38] Kim W, Song KY, Lee HJ, Han SU, Hyung WJ, Cho GS. The impact of comorbidity on surgical outcomes in laparoscopy-assisted distal gastrectomy: A retrospective analysis of multicenter results. Annals of Surgery. 2008;**248**(5):793-799

[39] Shinohara T, Satoh S, Kanaya S, Ishida Y, Taniguchi K, Isogaki J, et al. Laparoscopic versus open D2 gastrectomy for advanced gastric cancer: A retrospective cohort study. Surgical Endoscopy. 2013;**27**(1):286-294

[40] Park DJ, Han SU, Hyung WJ, Kim MC, Kim W, Ryu SY, et al. Long-term outcomes after laparoscopy-assisted gastrectomy for advanced gastric cancer: A large-scale multicenter retrospective study. Surgical Endoscopy. 2012;**26**(6):1548-1553

[41] Kitano S, Shiraishi N, Uyama I, Sugihara K, Tanigawa N, Japanese Laparoscopic Surgery Study Group. A multicenter study on oncologic outcome of laparoscopic gastrectomy for early cancer in Japan. Annals of Surgery. 2007;**245**(1):68-72

[42] Kim MC, Kim W, Kim HH, Ryu SW, Ryu SY, Song KY, et al. Risk factors associated with complication following laparoscopy-assisted Gastrectomy for gastric cancer: A large-scale Korean multicenter study. Annals of Surgical Oncology. 2008;**15**(10):2692-2700

4

Laparoscopic Endoscopic Cooperative Surgery: Current Status and Perspective

Shunsuke Sakuraba

Abstract

Laparoscopic endoscopic cooperative surgery (LECS) is now performed worldwide as a result of the invention of new operative techniques. It is seromuscular resection by laparoscopy for gastric submucosal tumors such as gastrointestinal stromal tumors (GISTs). Endoscopic dissection of the mucosal to the submucosal layer determines the appropriate incision line, resects the tumor, and closes the visceral wall defect. Various minimally invasive LECS techniques are now well established. LECS-associated techniques, adaptation of them, and challenges for the future are reviewed in this chapter.

Keywords: LECS, SMT, GIST

1. Introduction

In the last decade, LECS has been performed all over the world in association with the invention of new operative techniques. Approaches are grouped into three major categories: laparoscopy-assisted endoscopic resection (LAER) in which resection is performed primarily by the endoscopic team under laparoscopic control; endoscope-assisted laparoscopic resection (EALR), where the laparoscopic teams perform the resection under endoscopic monitoring; and combined laparoscopic endoscopic resection (CLER), which is performed by the laparoscopic and the endoscopic teams. Description of these approaches and the details about CLER, especially LECS, nonexposed endoscopic wall-inversion surgery (NEWS), and a combination of laparoscopic endoscopic approaches to neoplasia with a nonexposure technique (CLEAN-NET) are described in the following chapters. Various LECS techniques for GIST are recently established, and the application of this approach to early stage gastric cancer, which is difficult to resect with the ESD technique because of severe scars or ulcers, is described. LECS for other organs such as the duodenum or colorectum is also being attempted, but only with expert technique and specialist knowledge. LECS plus biopsy of sentinel lymph node for early gastric cancer is planned as a clinical trial.

1.1. Laparoscopy-assisted endoscopic resection

Endoscopic resection is performed under laparoscopic control [1–3]. The endoscopist performs an endoscopic mucosal resection (EMR) or endoscopic submucosal dissection (ESD) with laparoscopic assistance (**Figure 1**). Laparoscopic support has many advantages. First, when accidental complications such as perforation or massive bleeding occur during the endoscopic resection, laparoscopic surgeons can treat them immediately. Second, if the endoscopist has difficulty in resecting the tumor as a result of tumor location, the laparoscopic team can reposition the stomach with manipulation of the serosal side. Although laparoscopy-assisted endoscopic resection (LAER) requires a laparoscopic team and general anesthesia in addition to endoscopy, the advantage is greater safety; therefore, perforation risk is high in ESD because of massive tumor or duodenal location, LAER is preferred. Irino et al. reported LECS for duodenal tumors in three patients using LAER, demonstrating feasibility of this approach [4]. A unique point of their method is that the laparoscopist places seromuscular sutures to reinforce the thinned duodenal wall in order to prevent postoperative perforation or bleeding. Seromuscular reinforcement is performed for all cases. As such, these techniques can be grouped into the CLER. The perforation rate for duodenal-ESD is still much higher than for gastric-ESD, esophageal-ESD and colorectal-ESD [5–10], so LAER or CLER are good alternatives.

1.1.1. Endoscope-assisted laparoscopic resection

In this category, laparoscopic surgeons mainly resect the tumor with endoscopic support as follows:

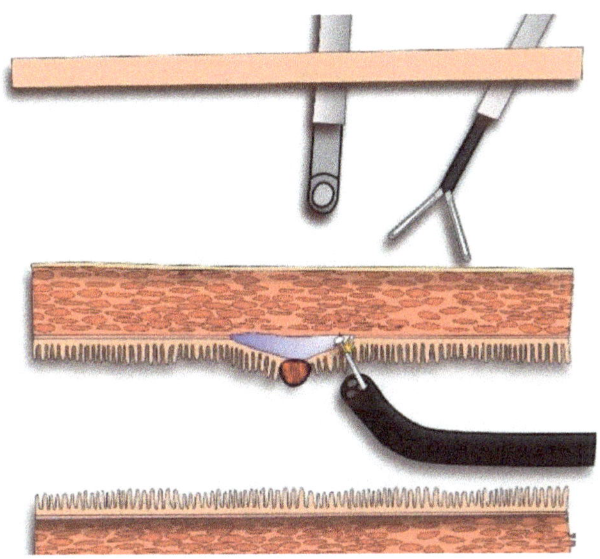

Figure 1. The endoscopist performs an endoscopic mucosal resection (EMR) or endoscopic submucosal dissection (ESD) with laparoscopic assistance.

1. Endoscope-assisted wedge resection:

   Under endoscopic monitoring, tumor location is confirmed, and blood vessels in the excision area around the tumor are prepared and if necessary the omentum is dissected, and the greater curvature of the stomach is mobilized by the laparoscopist. Several seromuscular sutures are placed around the lesion (**Figure 2**) and by pulling the stitches upward with laparoscopic forceps (**Figure 3**), the tumor is removed with laparoscopic linear stapling devices (**Figures 4** and **5**). According to laparoscopic surgeons, the staple line can be reinforced with a hand sewing suturing. The abovementioned technique is the most commonly combined surgery in the world, with more than 500 cases published [11–17]. Although the complication rate is 0–3% [11], the main problem can be excessive gastric resection by the laparoscopic linear stapling devices resulting in transformation or stenosis.

2. Endoscope-assisted laparoscopic transluminal (transgastric) surgery:

   When the tumor is located along the posterior gastric wall, it is difficult for the laparoscopist to obtain a visual field, so a transgastric technique is often used. Under endoscopic monitoring, the laparoscopic surgeons make an incision in the anterior abdominal wall (**Figures 6** and **7**). The laparoscopic team directly confirms the lesion and removes it with

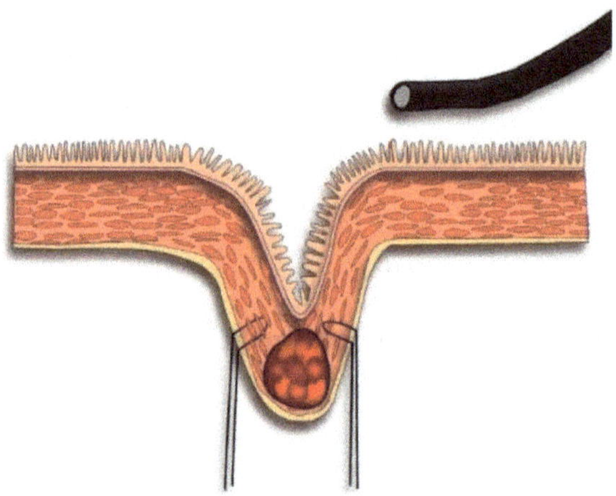

Figure 2. Several seromuscular sutures are placed around the lesion.

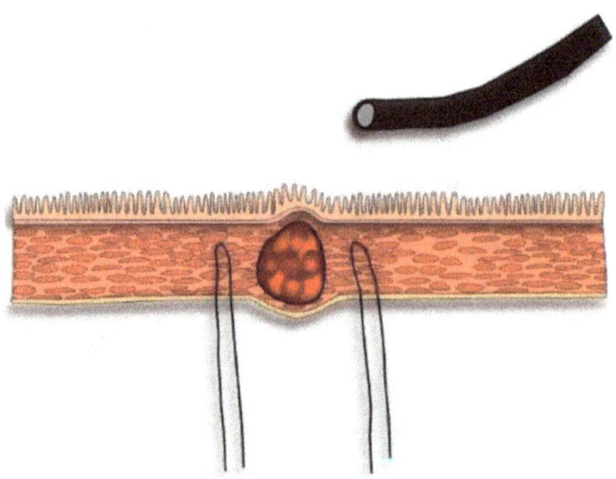

Figure 3. Surgeons pull the stitches upward with laparoscopic forceps.

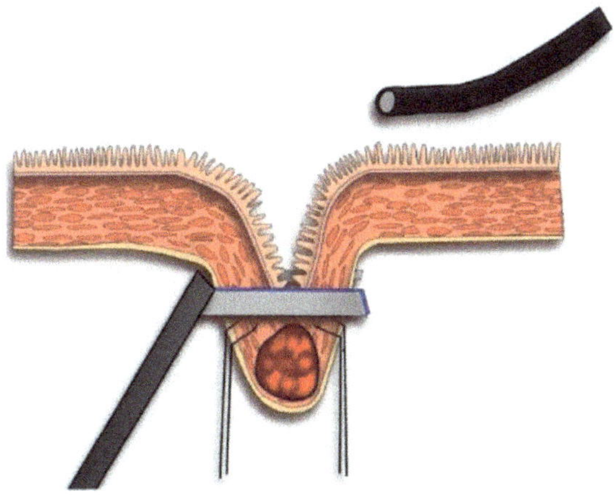

Figure 4. The appropriate incision line is determined under endoscopic monitoring.

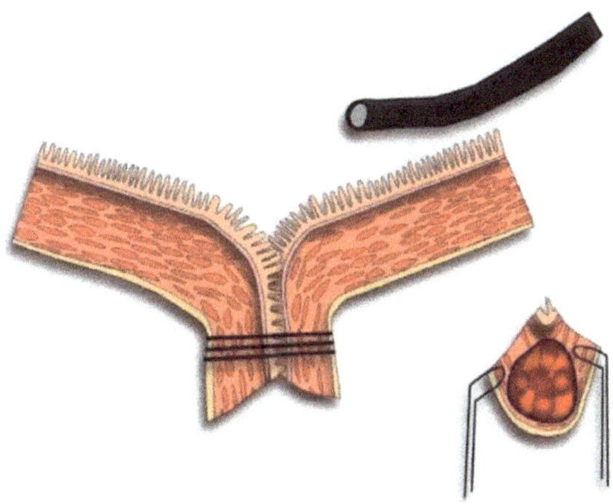

Figure 5. The tumor is removed with laparoscopic linear stapling devices.

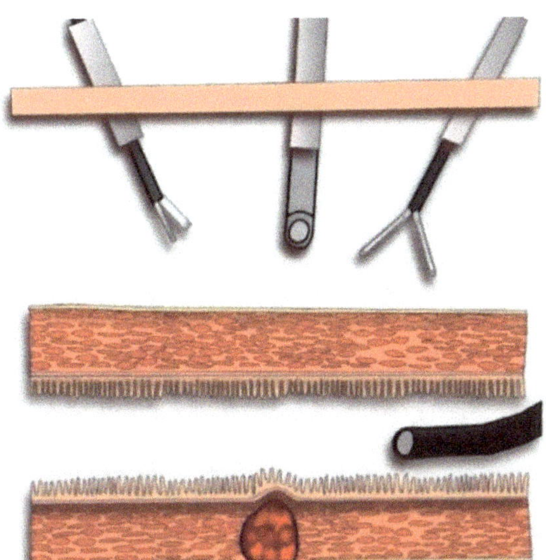

Figure 6. The tumor is located along the posterior gastric wall.

an inverted wedge resection using laparoscopic stapling devices. The opened gastric wall is closed with laparoscopic staplers or hand sewing sutures.

3. Endoscope-assisted laparoscopic intraluminal (intragastric) surgery:

   Indication for this technique is the same as for transgastric surgery approaching the posterior gastric wall. This technique was first reported by Ohashi et al. in [18], and a modified procedure was described by Dong et al. in [19]. All laparoscopic trocars are placed in the gastric cavity, penetrating both the abdominal and stomach walls. All trocars are fixed with balloon inflation of the stomach and the abdominal wall (**Figures 8** and **9**). The laparoscopist secures a visual field in the gastric lumen, and the tumor is removed by full-thickness resection or laparoscopic stapling devices. The trocar holes are closed with sutures or clips. **Figures 1–9** are excerpted from Dimitrios's report.

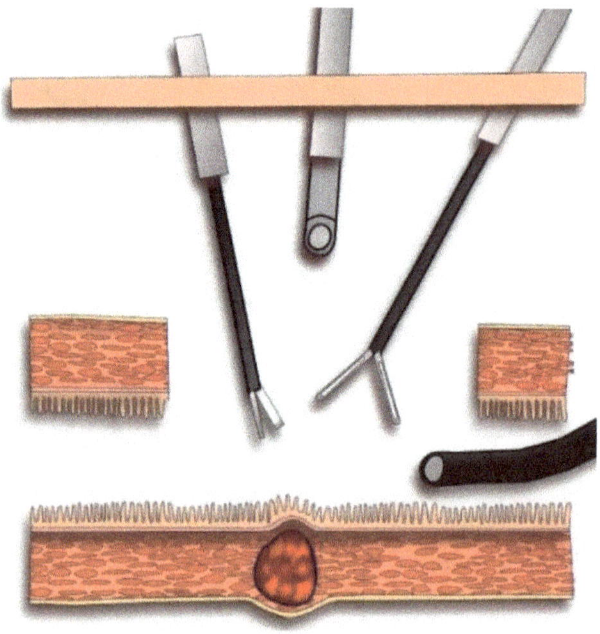

Figure 7. The laparoscopic surgeons make an incision in the anterior abdominal wall.

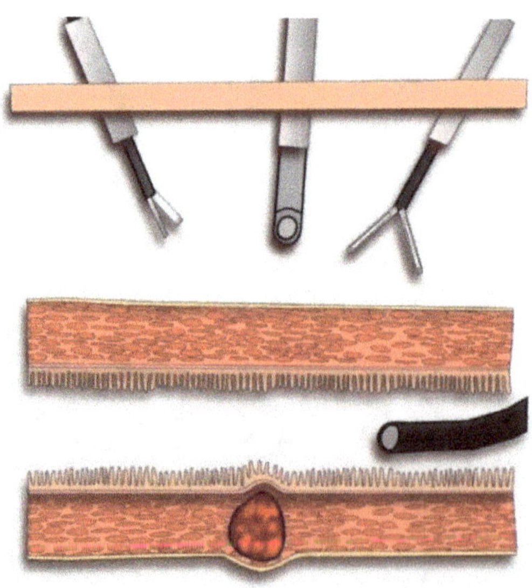

Figure 8. It is difficult for laparoscopist to approach the tumor.

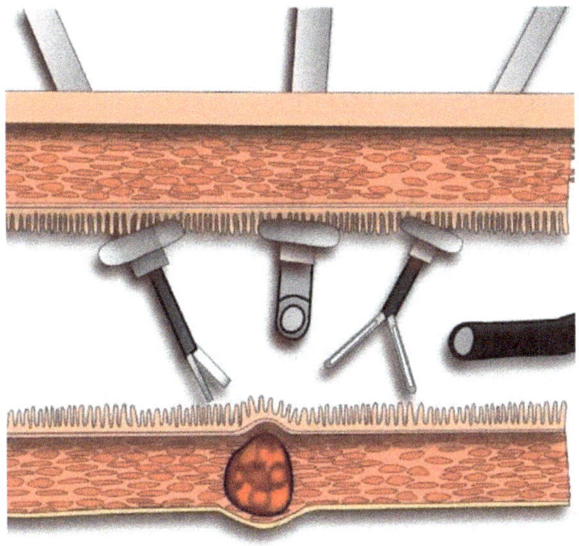

Figure 9. All laparoscopic trocars are placed in the gastric cavity, penetrating both the abdominal and stomach walls. All trocars are fixed with balloon inflation of the stomach and the abdominal wall. The **Figures 1-9** are excerpted from Dimitrios's report.

2. History of the LECS technique

Although surgical local resection with laparotomy or laparoscopic surgery is performed for gastric submucosal tumor (SMT), it is difficult when tumors are small or have an intramural growth pattern. It is difficult to determine the appropriate incision line from the abdominal cavity side, so excessive gastric resection might result in transformation or stenosis. LECS is a newly developed technique, first reported by Hiki et al. in [20] for local resection of GIST. This procedure is further categorized into CLER, which is an approach that combines ESD and laparoscopic gastric resection to determine the incision line, to resect the tumor and to close the stomach wall. As LECS can minimize the resected region and preserve the function of the stomach after surgery, the procedure was added to the national insurance list in Japan in 2014, and subsequently rapidly diffused throughout the surgical community [21–24]. Further applications of LECS then developed, so the first version is named classical LECS to distinguish it from subsequent modified LECS techniques. Classical LECS involves whole layer resection using laparoscopy and endoscopy. However, this technique may lead to contamination of and seeding of tumor cells into the peritoneal cavity, especially when the tumor is associated with an ulcer or epithelial lesion. To prevent peritoneal spread, modified LECS procedures now include inverted LECS with crown method [25], nonexposed endoscopic wall-inversion surgery (NEWS) [26] and a combination of laparoscopic endoscopic approaches to neoplasia with a nonexposure technique (CLEAN-NET) [27].

3. Classical LECS

Hiki et al. first reported classical LECS in 2006 [20] for local resection of GISTS in order to prevent excessive gastric resection followed by transformation, stenosis or stasis of food after surgery. In classical LECS, the incision line is determined by the endoscopist, and an endoscopic mucosal incision is made. Artificial perforation is performed by endoscopic forceps, and the seromuscular layer is dissected using laparoscopic and endoscopic forceps. The gastric wall defect is closed with laparoscopic stapling devices. Hiki described his LECS procedure in detail, and the following are excerpted from his writing.

1. "Tumor location was confirmed by intraluminal endoscopy." (**Figure 10**)
2. "Blood vessels in the excision area around the tumor were prepared by laparoscopy." (**Figure 11**)
3. "Endoscopic submucosal resection around the tumor and artificial perforation was performed." (**Figure 12**)
4. "Operation device was inserted into the perforation hole, and seromuscular dissection began by laparoscopy." (**Figure 13**)

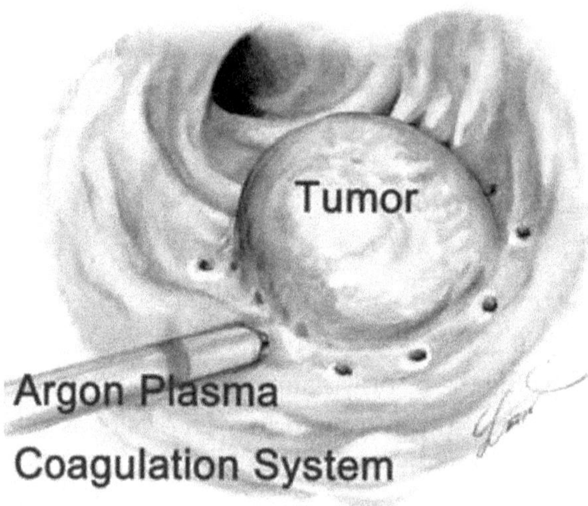

Figure 10. Tumor location was confirmed by intraluminal endoscopy.

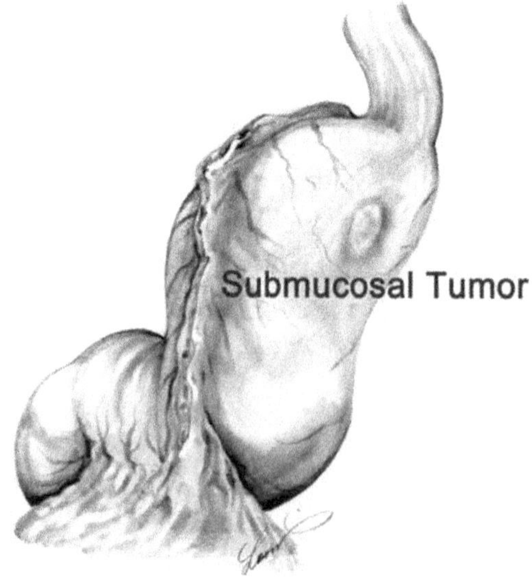

Figure 11. Blood vessels in the excision area around the tumor were prepared by laparoscopy.

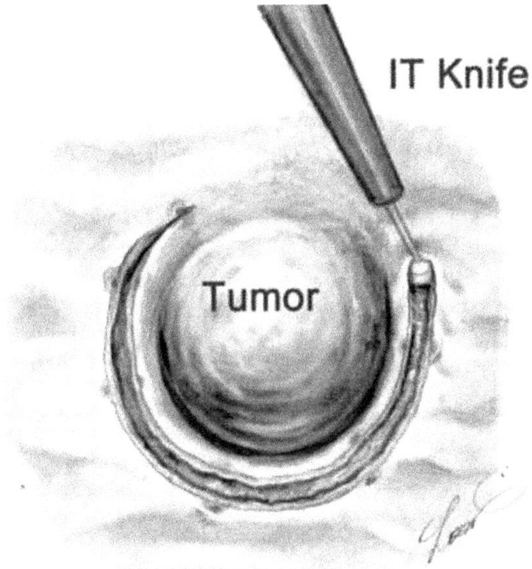

Figure 12. Endoscopic submucosal resection around the tumor and artificial perforation was performed.

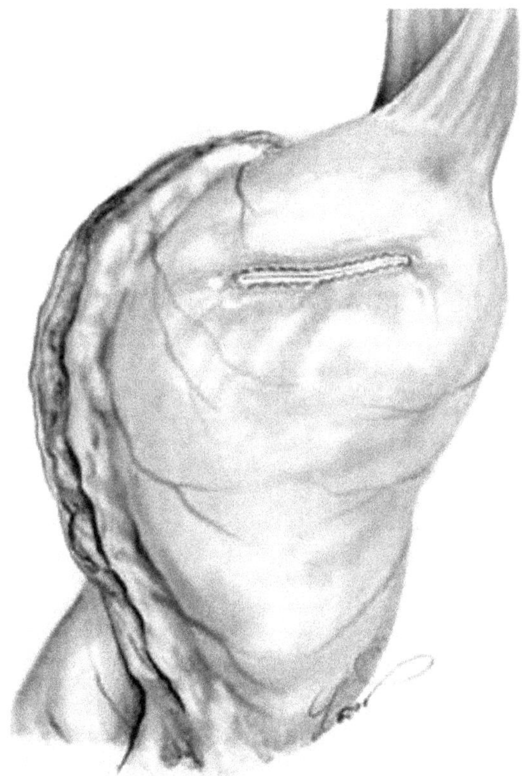

Figure 13. Operation device was inserted into the perforation hole, and seromuscular dissection began by laparoscopy.

5. "After resecting the tumor, the incision line was closed using laparoscopic stapling devices." (**Figures 14** and **15**). **Figures 10–15** are excerpted from Hiki's report.

Although modified LECS techniques are used, the Hiki procedure is a basic concept that is employed throughout low invasive surgery for GISTs. By minimizing the resected region,

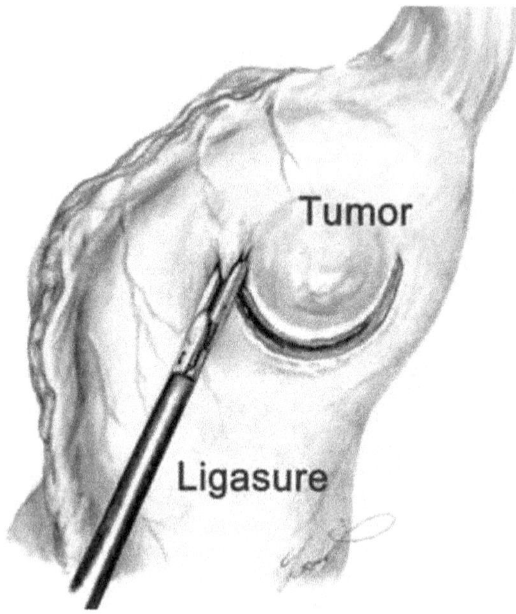

Figure 14. After resecting the tumor, the incision line was closed using laparoscopic stapling devices.

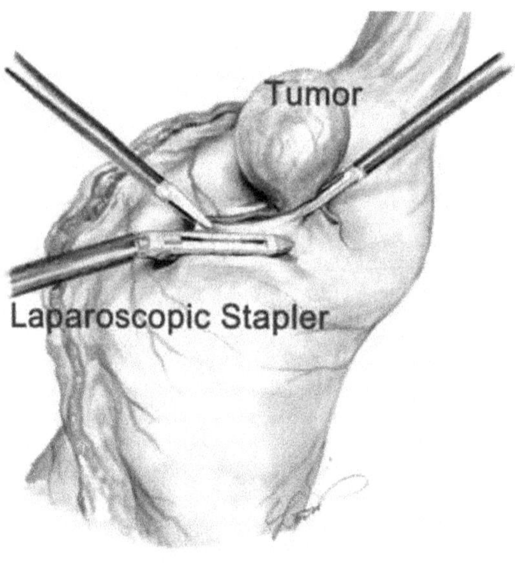

Figure 15. LECS technique can minimize the resected region. The **Figures 10-15** are excerpted from Hiki's report.

LECS makes it possible to preserve the postoperative function of the stomach. Hiki maintains that removal of the tumor must be performed carefully with a specimen retrieval bag in order to prevent peritoneal and port-site dissemination of tumor.

4. LECS with crown method

In order to reduce the transmural communication during the operation, Nunobe et al. reported the crown method and inverted LECS [25]. By pulling up the incision line of the stomach with several stitches, abdominal cavity contamination is prevented. This technique was named crown method because pulled-up stomach wall looks like a crown (**Figure 16**). Using the traction of the stitch, the resected specimen is inverted to the intragastric cavity. This technique

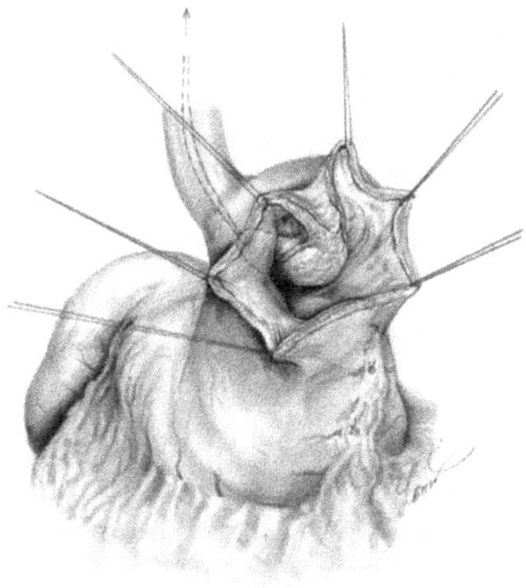

Figure 16. Surgeons pull up the incision line of the stomach with several stitches and pulled up stomach wall looks like a crown.

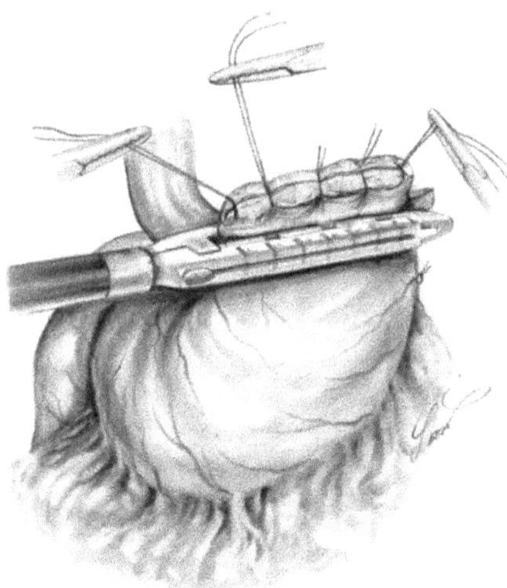

Figure 17. The stitches are also used as a supporting tool when the incision line is closed with a laparoscopic stapling device. The **Figures 16** and **17** are excerpted from Nunobe's report.

was named inverted LECS. Inverted LECS with crown method is not only useful for preventing tumor seeding into peritoneal cavity, but also for securing the visual field during the operation. The stitches are also used as a supporting tool when the incision line is closed with a laparoscopic stapling device (**Figure 17**). Although nonexposed endoscopic wall-inversion surgery (NEWS) [26] and a combination of laparoscopic endoscopic approaches to neoplasia with a nonexposure technique (CLEAN-NET) [27] are described later as nonexposure procedures, inverted LECS with crown method has few limitations such as tumor size or tumor location in comparison with NEWS or CLEAN-NET. As such, it can make it possible to remove the tumor without the contamination of abdominal cavity. **Figures 16** and **17** are excerpted from Nunobe's report.

5. NEWS

Classical LECS with crown method is an improved technique that reduces the risk of cancer cell dissemination. However, it can be difficult to completely prevent the contamination because of transmural communication during the procedure. Nonexposed endoscopic wall-inversion surgery (NEWS) was first reported by Goto et al. in 2011 with the goal of minimizing transmural communication during the operation [26]. They performed NEWS in an *ex vivo* porcine model and described the usefulness of this procedure. By inverting the tumor into the inside of the stomach without opening the gastric lumen, complete resection with nonexposure was achieved. The procedure is as follows:

1. "Markings around a model lesion are made with electrocautery knife."

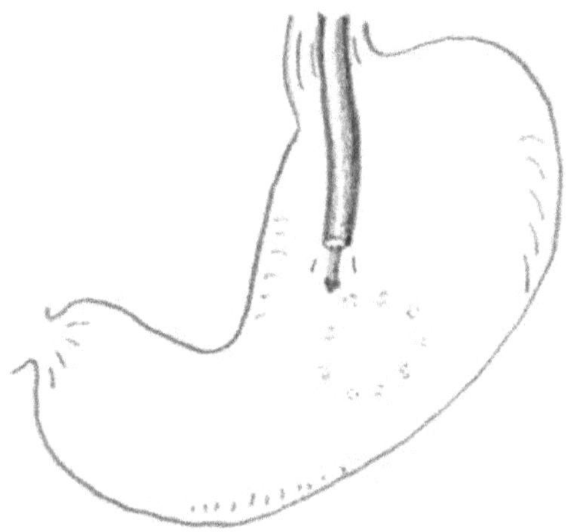

2. "A circumferential seromuscular incision is made from the outside."

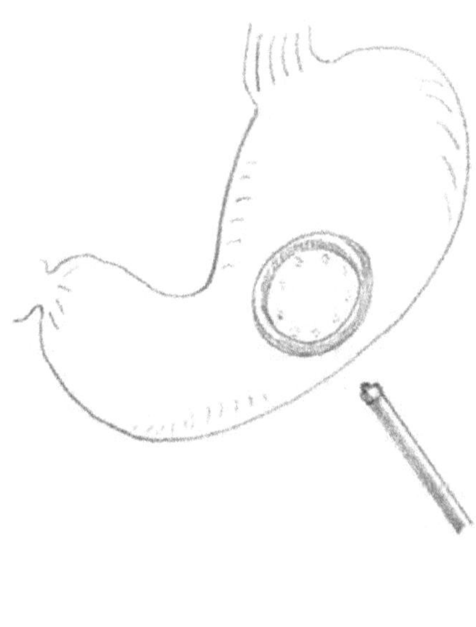

3. "The muscle layer is linearly sutured at approximately 5 mm intervals with the lesion inverted into the inside."

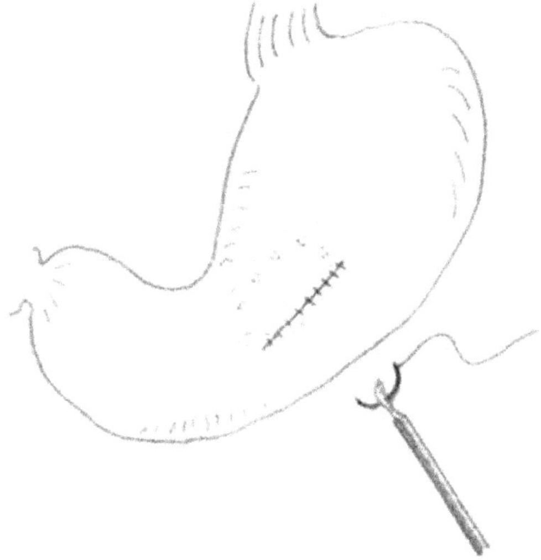

4. "A circumferential mucosubmucosal incision is performed from inside with electrocautery knife guided by the endoscope." These figures are excerpted from Goto's report.

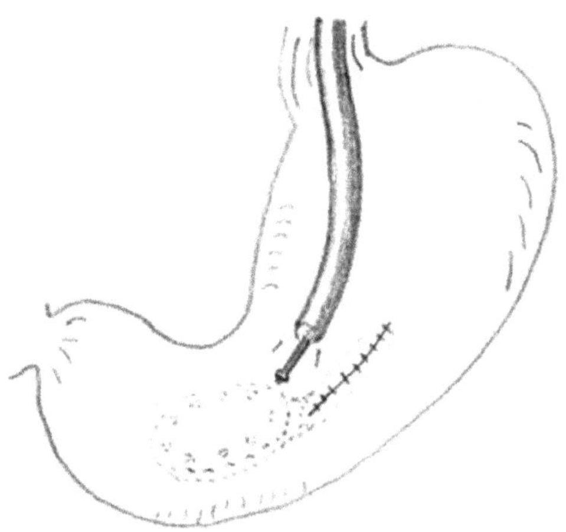

He reported NEWS for three lesions (one anterior wall, one lesser curve and one posterior wall of the gastric body) using porcine stomach, and complete resection was achieved for all lesions safely and without perforation or air leakage. Nonexposure techniques such as NEWS and CLEAN-NET are adequate for SMT without ulceration as well as SMT with ulceration or even early gastric cancer. In his report, the maximal specimen size was 50 mm; however, there is a limit of removable tumor size. Because the resected tumor is removed through the pharynx by the endoscope, solid tumor such as GIST over 30 mm is thought to be difficult to retrieve.

6. CLEAN-NET

A combination of laparoscopic endoscopic approaches to neoplasia with a nonexposure technique (CLEAN-NET) was first reported by Inoue et al. in [27]. This procedure also involves a nonexposure technique like NEWS, but with a difference. By preserving the continuity of the mucosa, the mucosa works as a barrier (a clean net), to prevent abdominal cavity contamination and seeding of tumor cells into the peritoneal cavity. The specimen is lifted from the peritoneal cavity, so it is retrieved laparoscopically. Inoue actively performs endoscopic and laparoscopic full-thickness resection for not only GISTs but also for early gastric cancer. The procedures are described below.

1. "Endoscopic markings are placed on the surrounding mucosa of the lesion with electrocautery knife."

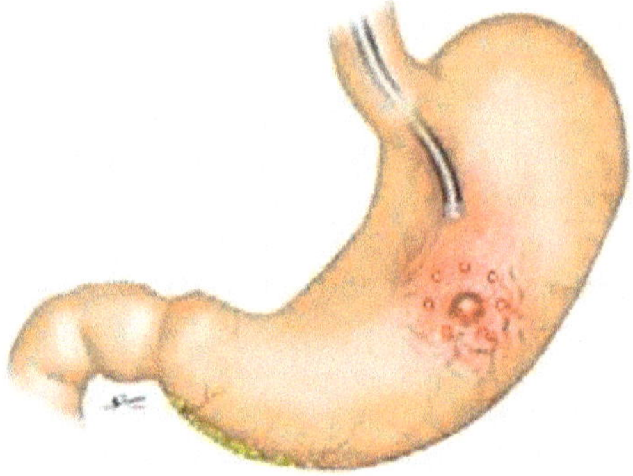

2. "The mucosal layer is fixed onto the seromuscular layer using four stay sutures."

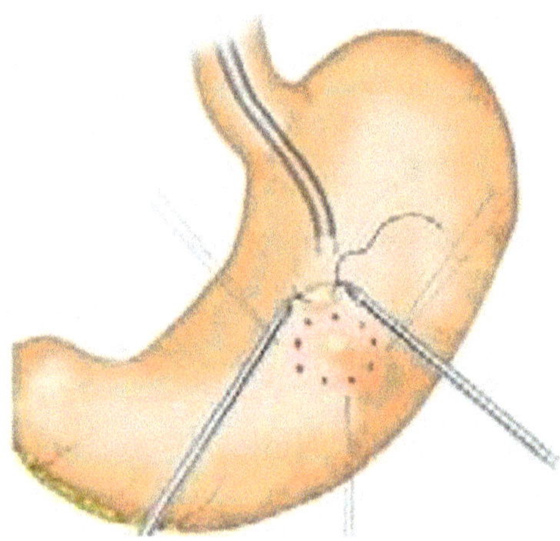

3. "By pulling four stitches upward with laparoscopic forceps, selective seromuscular dissection outside the four stiches is performed using a laparoscopic electrocautery knife."

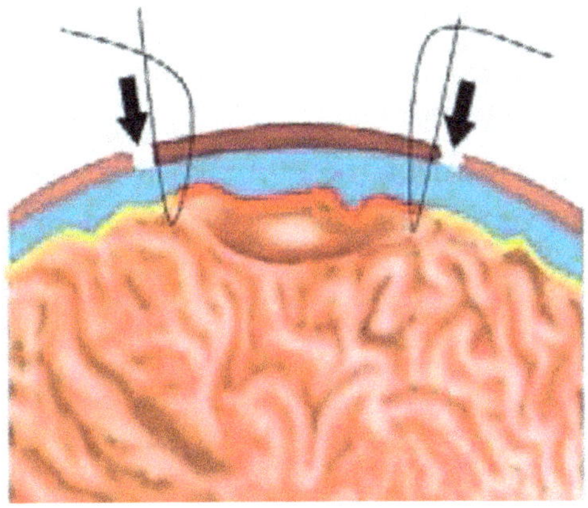

4. "A full-layer specimen is lifted by four stay sutures. This process allows a wider cancer-free margin around a full-thickness lesion."

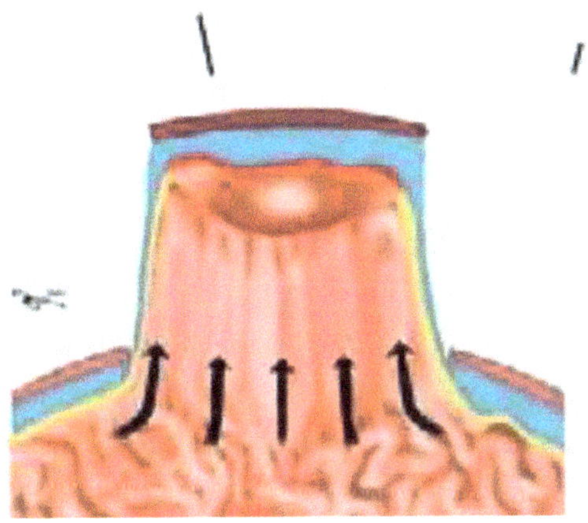

5. "A full-layer resection using a mechanical stapler is performed and the resected tumor is removed from abdominal cavity side." These figures are excerpted from Inoue's report.

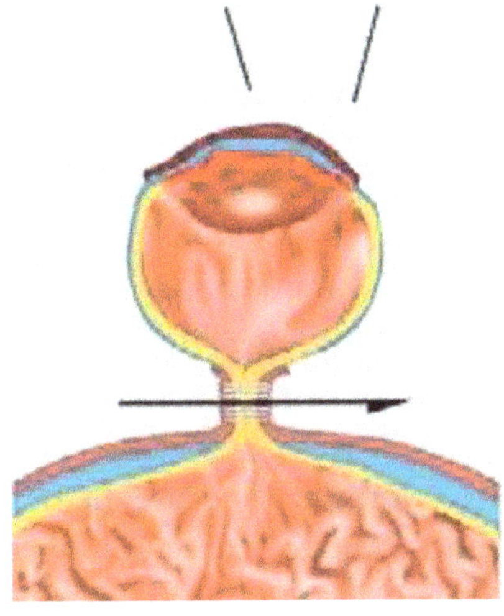

The abovementioned procedure with nonexposure technique is advantageous for epithelial tumor and GIST with ulceration. CLEAN-NET also makes it possible to secure a sufficient margin around the tumor and to resect lymph nodes together with the tumor if it is located at either the lesser or greater curvature of the stomach. Because the CLEAN-NET procedure needs the process that the mucosal layer stretches without breaking apart, a large tumor is thought to be difficult to resect.

7. Laparoscopy-assisted endoscopic full-thickness resection

This technique was reported by Abe et al. in [28]. The same procedure as LECS technique is applied; however, the endoscopist plays an important role in resecting the tumor. The endoscopic team starts full-thickness resection around the tumor, and after two-thirds of the resection is performed, the laparoscopic team finishes the full-thickness resection with laparoscopic devices.

7.1. LECS for duodenal tumors

There are some limitations with LECS for removal of duodenal tumors. First, anatomical elements such as the pyloric ring, Vater's papilla and the third to fourth portion make it difficult to perform. Second, there are a few reports of lymph node metastasis from submucosal invading duodenal cancers or carcinoids, so partial resection is controversial. Small submucosal tumors, duodenal adenomas, or intramucosal carcinomas at duodenal bulb or the opposite side of the papilla are indications for LECS. The basic concept of gastric LECS also applies to duodenum LECS [4, 29]. The difficulty in mobilizing organs and closing the defected walls needs to be advanced.

7.2. LECS for colorectal tumors

LECS for colorectal tumors is not often used. We rarely experience GISTs in the colorectum, and in many cases the laparoscopist must achieve adequate mobilization which may be difficult in colorectal-LECS. Some researchers have reported the laparoscopy-assisted endoscopic resection (LAER) for colorectal tumors [30–32], and as the combined laparoscopic endoscopic resection (CLER). Fukunaga et al. reported LECS for laterally spreading colorectal tumors, which are difficult to resect by the ESD technique because of submucosal fibrosis or multiple surrounding diverticula [33] (**Figures 18** and **19**). He suggested several concerns about his technique: limitation for tumors located on the mesenteric side, strictures after surgery, and contamination of the abdominal cavity by bowel contents. He proposed several adjustments in his report. Indications for colorectal LECS are the same as for colorectal ESD. Tumors that would be difficult to resect endoscopically are good indications for both. **Figures 18** and **19** are excerpted from Fukunaga's report.

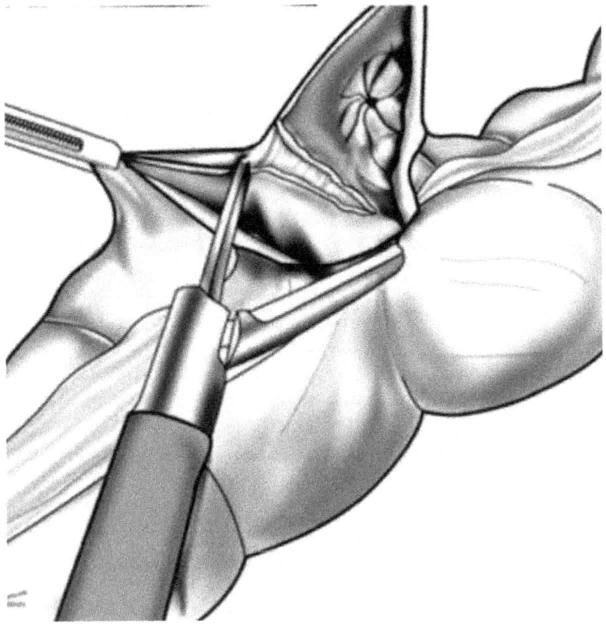

Figure 18. A laparoscopic coagulating system is used to dissect the full thickness of the colon wall along the submucosal line created by endoscopic dissection.

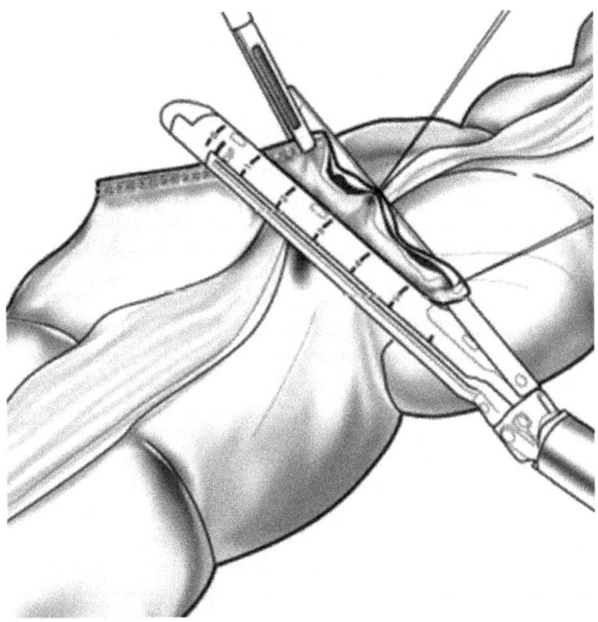

Figure 19. The incision line was closed using laparoscopic stapline devices. The **Figures 18** and **19** are excerpted from Fukunaga's report.

7.3. LECS plus biopsy to sentinel lymph node for early gastric cancer

The application LECS has progressed from resection of gastric submucosal tumors to early stage gastric cancer. The current therapeutic adaptation is for removal of low-risk lymph node metastases. Further, there still remains the possibility of lymph node metastasis in treating

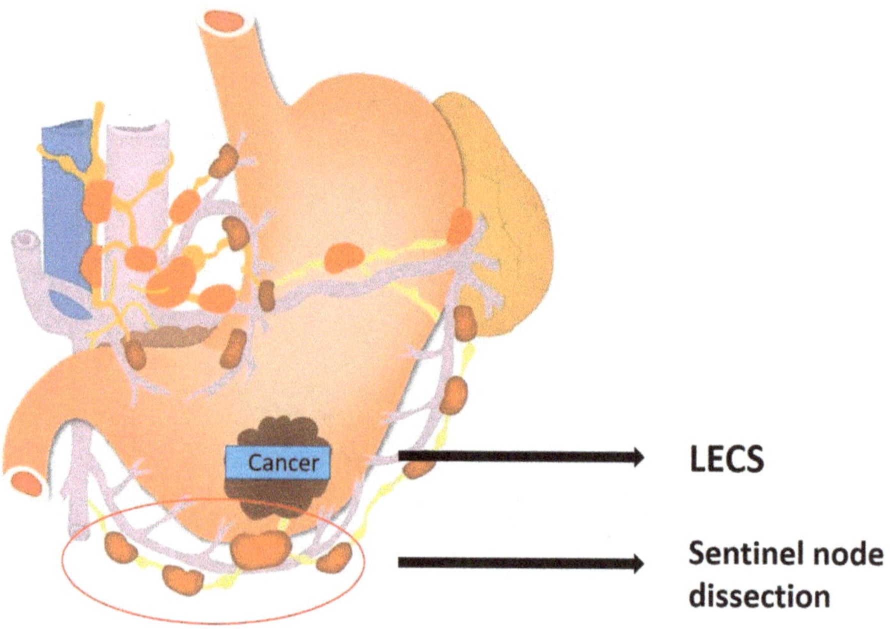

Figure 20. By combining LECS technique and sentinel node biopsy, LECS with lymph node dissection might become possible in the future.

gastric cancer. On the other hand, some researchers reported the utility of sentinel node biopsy in patients with gastric cancer [34–36]. Although gastric lymphatic drainage is often complicated, by using the dual tracer method with radiolabeled tin colloid and blue dye, Kitagawa reported that the sentinel node detection rate was 97.5% (387 of 397) and the accuracy of nodal evaluation for metastasis was 99% (383 of 387) in cT1 and tumors <4 cm [36]. These facts implicate that by combining LECS technique and sentinel node biopsy, LECS with lymph node dissection might become possible in the future (**Figure 20**). More research and clinical trials about LECS and biopsy to sentinel lymph node for early gastric cancer are expected.

Author details

Shunsuke Sakuraba

Address all correspondence to: lunlun8shunsuke@gmail.com

Department of Surgery, Juntendo Shizuoka Hospital, Shizuoka, Japan

References

[1] Qiu WQ et al. Minimally invasive treatment of laparoscopic and endoscopic cooperative surgery for patients with gastric gastrointestinal stromal tumors. Journal of Digestive Diseases. 2013;**14**:469-473

[2] Acker S et al. Laparoscopic-assisted endoscopic resection of a gastric leiomyoma. European Journal of Pediatric Surgery Reports. 2014;**2**:003-006

[3] Kato M et al. Local resection by combined laparoendoscopic surgery for duodenal gastrointestinal stromal tumor. Diagnostic and Therapeutic Endoscopy. 2011;**2011**:645609

[4] Irino T et al. Laparoscopic-endoscopic cooperative surgery for duodenal tumors: A unique procedure that helps ensure the safety of endoscopic submucosal dissection. Endoscopy. 2015;**47**(4):349-351

[5] Ohara Y et al. Enormous postoperative perforation after endoscopic submucosal dissection for duodenal cancer successfully treated with filling and shielding by polyglycolic acid sheets with fibrin glue and computed tomography-guided abscess puncture. Clinical Journal of Gastroenterology. 2017;**10**:524-529

[6] Fujihara S et al. Management of a large mucosal defect after duodenal endoscopic resection. World Journal of Gastroenterology. 2016;**22**(29):6595-6609

[7] Tsujii Y et al. Clinical outcomes of endoscopic submucosal dissection for superficial esophageal neoplasms: A multicenter retrospective cohort study. Endoscopy. 2015;**47**: 775-783

[8] Shin KY et al. Clinical outcomes of the endoscopic submucosal dissection of early gastric cancer are comparable between absolute and new expanded criteria. Gut and Liver. 2015; **9**:181-187

[9] Repici A et al. Efficiency and safety of endoscopic submucosal dissection for colorectal neoplasia: A systematic review. Endoscopy. 2012;**44**:137-150

[10] Toyonaga T et al. Endoscopic submucosal dissection cases in the esophagus, stomach, and colorectum: Complication rates and long-term outcomes. Surgical Endoscopy. 2013;**27**: 1000-1008

[11] Ntourakis D et al. Cooperative laparoscopic endoscopic and hybrid laparoscopic surgery for upper gastrointestinal tumors: Current status. World Journal of Gastroenterology. 2015;**21**(43):12482-12497

[12] Kang WM et al. Laparoscopic-endoscopic cooperative surgery for gastric submucosal tumors. World Journal of Gastroenterology. 2013;**19**:5720-5726

[13] Privette A et al. Laparoscopic approaches to resection of suspected gastric gastrointestinal stromal tumors based on tumor location. Surgical Endoscopy. 2008;**22**:487-494

[14] Wilhelm D et al. Simultaneous use of laparoscopy and endoscopy for minimally invasive resection of gastric subepithelial masses—Analysis of 93 interventions. World Journal of Surgery. 2008;**32**:1021-1028

[15] Huguet KL et al. Laparoscopic gastric gastrointestinal stromal tumor resection: The mayo clinic experience. Archives of Surgery. 2008;**143**:587-590; discussion 591

[16] Marano L et al. Combined laparoscopic-endoscopic "Rendez-vous" procedure for minimally invasive resection of gastrointestinal stromal tumors of the stomach. The American Surgeon. 2011;**77**:1100-1102

[17] Sasaki A et al. Tailored laparoscopic resection for suspected gastric gastrointestinal stromal tumors. Surgery. 2010;**147**:516-520

[18] Ohashi S et al. Laparoscopic intraluminal (intragastric) surgery for early gastric cancer. A new concept in laparoscopic surgery. Surgical Endoscopy. 1995;**9**:169-171

[19] Dong HY et al. Modified laparoscopic intragastric surgery and endoscopic full-thickness resection for gastric stromal tumor originating from the muscularis propria. Surgical Endoscopy. 2014;**28**:1447-1453

[20] Hiki N et al. Laparoscopic and endoscopic cooperative surgery for gastrointestinal stromal tumors dissection. Surgical Endoscopy. 2008;**22**(7):1729-1735

[21] Hiki N et al. Laparoscopic endoscopic cooperative surgery. Digestive Endoscopy. 2015;**27**: 197-204

[22] Matsuda T et al. Laparoscopic endoscopic cooperative surgery (LECS) for the upper gastrointestinal tract. Translational Gastroenterology and Hepatology. 2017;**2**(40)

[23] Hiki N et al. Function-preserving gastrectomy for early gastric cancer. Annals of Surgical Oncology. 2013;**20**:2683-2692

[24] Matsuda T et al. Feasibility of laparoscopic and endoscopic cooperative surgery for gastric submucosal tumors (with video). Gastrointestinal Endoscopy. 2016;**84**:47-52

[25] Nunobe S et al. Successful application of laparoscopic and endoscopic cooperative surgery (LECS) for a lateral-spreading mucosal gastric cancer. Gastric Cancer. 2012;**15**(3):338-342

[26] Goto O et al. New method of endoscopic full-thickness resection: A pilot study of non-exposed endoscopic wall-inversion surgery in an ex vivo porcine model. Gastric Cancer. 2011;**14**(2):183-187

[27] Inoue H et al. Endoscopic mucosal resection, endoscopic submucosal dissection, and beyond: Full-layer resection for gastric cancer with non-exposure technique (CLEAN-NET). Surgical Oncology Clinics of North America. 2012;**21**(1):129-140

[28] Abe N et al. Successful-treatment of early stage gastric cancer by laparoscopy-assisted endoscopic full-thickness resection with lymphadenectomy. Gastrointestinal Endoscopy. 2008;**68**:1220-1224

[29] Otowa Y et al. Safe management of laparoscopic endoscopic cooperative surgery for superficial non-ampullary duodenal epithelial tumors. Endoscopy International Open. 2017;**5**(11):E1153-E1158

[30] Wilhelm D et al. Combined laparoscopic-endoscopic resections of colorectal polyps: 10-year experience and follow-up. Surgical Endoscopy. 2009;**23**:688-693

[31] Wood JJ et al. Laparo-endoscopic resection for extensive and inaccessible colorectal polyps: A feasible and safe procedure. Annals of the Royal College of Surgeons of England. 2011;**93**:241-245

[32] Yan J et al. Treatment for right colon polyps not removable using standard colonoscopy: Combined laparoscopic-colonoscopic approach. Diseases of the Colon and Rectum. 2011; **54**:753-758

[33] Fukunaga Y et al. New technique of en bloc resection of colorectal tumor using laparoscopy and endoscopy cooperative (laparoscopy and endoscopy cooperative surgery – colorectal). Disease of the Colon and Rectum. 2014;**57**:2

[34] An JY et al. Which factors are important for successful sentinel node navigation surgery in gastric cancer patients? Analysis from the SENORITA prospective multicenter feasibility quality control trial. Gastroenterology Research and Practice. 2017;**2017**:1732571, 7 pages

[35] Huang L et al. Feasibility and diagnostic performance of dual-tracer-guided sentinel lymph node biopsy in cT1-2N0M0 gastric cancer: A systematic review and meta-analysis of diagnostic studies. World Journal of Surgical Oncology. 2017;**15**:103

[36] Kitagawa Y et al. Sentinel node mapping for gastric cancer: A prospective multicenter trial in Japan. Journal of Clinical Oncology. 2013;**31**(29):3704-3710

5

The Role of Esophagus in Voice Rehabilitation of Laryngectomees

Ljiljana Širić, Marinela Rosso and Aleksandar Včev

Abstract

The total laryngectomy is a standard procedure of laryngeal carcinoma treatment which leaves multiple persistent consequences on a laryngectomized person. After laryngectomy, all of patients cannot speak loudly, and 10–58% patients have a dysphagia. In such changed anatomical condition, the esophagus has a key function in two of three primary approaches to voice—speech rehabilitation of laryngectomized patients: esophageal and tracheoesophageal speech therapy method because one of these is the only acceptable solution of substitute alaryngeal speech. In esophageal speech, the esophagus has the role of speech air reservoirs since the respiratory and digestive pathways are permanently separated after the procedure. In the production of tracheoesophageal speech, the tracheoesophageal fistula and the esophagus allow the recommunication of these pathways and the use of air from the lungs for speech. There are several prerequisites for successful esophageal and tracheoesophageal speech. After tracheoesophageal puncture and insertion, the tracheoesophageal prosthesis may occur different complications in the early or late postoperative period in 10–60% of patients. The quality of alaryngeal voice is very different from the quality of laryngeal voice, but allows communication to laryngectomees.

Keywords: esophageal speech, laryngectomy, tracheoesophageal speech, voice prosthesis, voice rehabilitation

1. Introduction

The esophagus is a long, flexible muscular tube that starts as the continuation of the pharynx with the upper esophageal sphincter and ends with the lower esophageal sphincter as the junction with the stomach. Topographically, it is divided into three regions: cervical, thoracic and abdominal [1].

The function of the upper esophageal sphincter is to prevent breathed air from entering into the esophagus and to stop reflux of esophageal content into the pharynx to prevent airway aspiration, and the function of lower esophageal sphincter is to prevent gastroesophageal reflux.

The function of the esophagus is very simple: to actively transport solids and liquids from the pharynx to the stomach. It has no digestive, absorptive, metabolic, or endocrine functions, but in some people, esophagus takes another very important function [2]. These people are laryngectomized persons. Namely, after total laryngectomy, the lower respiratory tract is permanently separated from the upper respiratory tract. The breathing function begins and ends in the permanent tracheostoma, and the upper respiratory tract loses its function [3]. In such anatomical condition, the esophagus has a key function in two of three primary approaches to speech rehabilitation of laryngectomized patients: esophageal and tracheoesophageal speech therapy method. The upper part of the esophagus gets the function as some kind of air activator, and the pharyngoesophageal segment gets the function of the voice generator, thus allowing the function of the voice resonators.

2. Total laryngectomy

The standard options of laryngeal carcinoma treatment are surgery, radiotherapy, chemotherapy, or a combination of these modalities. When a conservation surgery is not indicated due to the tumor stage and localization, or due to patient's general medical condition, then total laryngectomy is considered. This surgical procedure implies a surgical removal of the entire larynx, from the hyoid bone to the second tracheal ring, and the lymph nodes on the ipsilateral or bilateral side. After removal of the larynx, the circular defect in the anterior wall of the pharynx is reconstructed and sutured to the base of the tongue. Inferiorly, resected distal part of trachea is brought forward and sutured to the skin edges forming permanent tracheostoma. Postoperative care after total laryngectomy includes nasogastric tube feedings and maintenance of tracheostoma. If the tracheostoma is satisfactory in size and shape, it is preferable not to use laryngectomy tube in the tracheostoma. Alaryngeal speech training may begin as early as 3 weeks after operation. Postlaryngectomy aphonia is one of the most devastating outcomes of total laryngectomy, and effective voice is critical to the successful prevention of psychological, social and economic consequences of totally laryngectomized individuals [4].

After total laryngectomy, there is a defect of hypopharynx that needs to be reconstructed. The base of tongue then makes anastomosis with neopharynx. Sometimes there is a retraction of the base of tongue, changed tonus of the pharyngoesophageal segment, an extension of a part of pharynx and esophageal stenosis, which can cause dysphagia in 10–58% of cases [5]. Reconstruction of the upper esophageal segment and the hypopharynx is essential for the swallowing function and alaryngeal phonation. In addition, radiotherapy and postoperative infection increases the risk of occurrence of scarring and stenosis of the oropharyngeal segment, causing dysphagia and odynophagia. Postoperative radiotherapy causes other problems such as reduced sense of taste, xerostomia, muscle fibrosis and tooth loss, which increases dysphagic disorders. Therefore, laryngectomees often need to modify their way of nutrition [6].

2.1. Voice rehabilitation after laryngectomy

Total laryngectomy leaves a number of significant and permanent anatomic and physiological-functional changes. One of them is the impossibility of loud laryngeal speech. Laryngectomy is the removal of vocal cords which are the vibrating source of sound, and it causes changes in the anatomic structures of the resonator, whereas tracheotomy prevents the use of the lungs as a physiological source of energy for the phonation. Patient is temporarily socially deprived which diminishes the quality of life and brings with it the limitations in other life spheres. Postoperatively, achieved by rehabilitation, a future alaryngeal voice will be created in the area where esophagus transitions into hypopharynx, under the influence of the airflow that causes the mucosa vibration [5]. This area is called neoglottis or pseudoglottis, and it is a pharyngoesophageal segment, anatomical structure in the area of the upper aerodigestive tract [7].

Rehabilitation of voice after removal of larynx has been known for more than 150 years [8]. The first well-known description of the possible way of producing alaryngeal voice was given by Czermak in 1859. He established an alaryngeal voice by redirecting the airflow from the endotracheal tube through a tube into the mouth of the laryngectomized patient [9]. After Billroth performed his first laryngectomy in 1873, his assistant, Gussenbauer, equipped the patient with a pneumatic device which had the function of a speech machine [8, 10, 11]. In the mid-nineteenth century, rehabilitation was discovered by establishing an esophageal voice. At the same time, various mechanical devices were used to transmit vibrations and thus allowed loud speech [12, 13]. In the mid-twentieth century, the first tracheoesophageal fistula was made, which allowed the air stream to reach the upper part of the esophagus and the pharynx [14]. A few years later, a voice prothesis was developed according to the principle of a one-way permeable valve that allows the airflow from the trachea into the esophagus and prevents the passage of food and fluid from the esophagus into the trachea.

Back a few decades, the world trend is the earliest possible rehabilitation of voice and speech after laryngectomy. The beginning and type of rehabilitation depend on the health, psychosocial and socioeconomic status of the patient [15].

Patients have three methods of substitute voice and speech:

1. Production of tracheoesophageal voice by insertion of a tracheoesophageal prosthesis.
2. Production of an esophageal voice.
3. Use of mechanical generators of acoustic vibrations [16].

3. Esophagus and esophageal speech

3.1. History of the esophageal speech

The use of esophagus as a speech tank for the purpose of rehabilitation of laryngectomized persons first occurs during the nineteenth century. In 1909, Gutzmann called this rehabilitation method an esophageal speech [17]. The method is the most natural way for the laryngectomized persons to have the alaryngeal phonation, which has made it the most commonly used method for many years. Although satisfying a number of factors is a prerequisite, Seeman considers the appropriate level of motivation to be the key factor for mastering the esophageal speech, and that most motivated patients successfully adopt this mode of substitution [17].

3.2. Prerequisites for successful esophageal speech

This method creates a new air reservoir used for speech within the esophagus of a lower capacity than the physiological one, which is the source of the sound wave. The capacity of the upper part of the esophagus after surgery is 60–80 ml of air [18], and the sound wave is generated by vibrations of the pharyngoesophageal segment in neoglottis, which allows the production of the esophageal voice. The exact localization of the pharyngoesophageal segment vibrations differs from author to author, and vibrations are possible from the base of the tongue to the upper esophageal sphincter, but most authors suggest that the most common vibrations of the pharyngoesophageal cavity vibration are at the level of the fifth, sixth and seventh cervical vertebrae, while Seeman feels that vibrations are at the level of the cricopharyngeal muscle at the height of the fifth cervical vertebra or where the pharyngoesophageal obstruction is the greatest [17].

In order for alaryngeal phonation to be possible (production of speech without the larynx), an appropriate tonus of pharyngoesophageal segment, more precisely the cricopharyngeal muscle, is needed. In determining the degree of tonus available, today there are two evaluation tools:

- Taub's insufflation test.
- Modified Taub's test.

When using Taub's Insufflation Test, the examiner places the nasal catheter into the esophagus, using the Polyzer balloon to insufflate the air to the catheter. If the tonus is appropriate, the patient will be able to phonate, and the test will then record a positive result. The reference limit of the phonation pressure is 22 mmHg, which allows the 10 s alaryngeal phonation, or speech production in the range of 10–15 syllables in one inspiration. The phonation pressure is measured with a manometer. In cases where there is hypertonicity, the patient is not able to produce an alaryngeal voice, and the test registers a negative result [19].

The self-blowing test (modified Taube test) has been used for 33 years and was invented by Blom and Singer. The difference is that the other end of the nasal catheter is introduced into the tracheostoma and in this way allows an independent insufflation of the air from the tracheostoma to the esophagus. The result is recorded as positive when the patient can alaryngeally phonate for at least 8 s [20].

The negative result in these tests indicates undesirable hypertonicity of the muscle which prevents the phonation, and requires surgical intervention in the form of cricopharyngeal myotomy [20]. Muscle hypotonicity is also undesirable because it may interfere with alaryngeal phonation, but it often results in a very weak intensity of the alaryngeal voice. As the voice of low intensity does not meet the daily communication requirements, the hypotonicity can be compensated by external compression or surgical intervention.

In addition to the appropriate muscular tonus of the pharyngoesophageal segment, the person who will be rehabilitated with the esophageal speech must have a satisfactory level of certain cognitive abilities. Considered among the most important cognitive abilities are the appropriate intellectual status and the motivation of a person, but the conative factors are also significant. When choosing modality, psychosocial and socioeconomic factors are also important. The person who will learn the esophageal speech should be highly motivated for the process of rehabilitation, be patient enough, cognitively superior, and live in an empathetic and supportive family and social environment. Socioeconomic status should be as high as necessary for regular attendance at a speech-language therapy in continuity. Regarding the health status, people who will learn the esophageal speech should be of a good general health and somatic status, and the primary disease should be under good local control, which means removing any suspicion of local recurrence. Certainly, a significant influence on the possibility of this modality has the auditory status of the patient, and the level of hearing should be appropriate to the chronological age of the person, at the hearing level of 20–55 dB [5]. Any hearing impairment above 55 dB affects the communication function significantly and disables the adequate reception of the information from the speech-language therapist, thereby making it difficult and slowing down the process of rehabilitation.

Doyle classified contraindications for the learning of the esophageal speech in four categories [17, 21, 22]:

1. Certain physical factors
   - local recurrence of illness.
   - extensive reconstruction operation.
2. Certain psychological status
   - the presence of psychological problems and psychopathology.
3. Socioeconomic factors
   - inability to attend a therapy at least three times a week.
4. The necessity of speaking
   - immediately after laryngectomy, the necessity to speak loudly for a certain reason.

3.3. Functional features of the esophageal speech

The acoustic parameters of the esophageal voice in the literature vary depending on the researchers, the selected research method, the measuring instrument, the measuring criteria, the sample of subjects, and the environmental and computer program conditions in which the measurement was performed. The fundamental frequency, or the height of the esophageal voice, is reduced, the frequency range is reduced, and the acoustic parameters determining the timbre of the voice also differ significantly from the regular laryngeal voice [5, 23, 24]. Such values of acoustic parameters form a rough and breathy voice, subjectively experienced. In addition, the time for turning on the voice is prolonged and the maximum time of the phoning is significantly reduced. According to prosodic features, the melody of the esophageal voice is more uniform and variable, lexical stress is not realized or is partially realized, frequent undesirable respiratory pauses are often present and the tempo of speaking is slower [5].

Sociofunctional features of the esophageal voice, which also make the advantage of this rehabilitation modality are: both hands free during speech and being less noticeable to the environment during speech, spontaneous and natural way of alaryngeal speech without additional surgery and insertion of foreign bodies, independence of prosthetic aids, the ability to speak without high consumption of material resources. On the other hand, the features that make up its shortcomings are: long periods of rehabilitation, lack of regular and continuous attendance at rehabilitation, discontinuous speech and additional undesirable noise during speech, especially tracheal noise during inspiration, which interfere with the intelligibility of the pronounced words [25].

3.4. Rehabilitation: educational process of learning the esophageal speech

The rehabilitation and education process starts with an individual preoperative counseling and patient preparation for a postoperative rehabilitation. A duration of the preoperative patient preparation varies depending on the individual's needs. During this period, the patient is given education on all the consequences of tracheotomy and total laryngectomy, pulmonary and speech aids for laryngectomized persons and modalities of speech-language rehabilitation. In addition, an oncological team of experts together with the patient decides on a single rehabilitation method.

The onset of postoperative speech-language therapy depends on a number of factors, such as further oncological treatment (primarily the need for radiotherapy), general health condition, psychological condition, and neuromotor capabilities of the patient. The optimal time to start postoperative rehabilitation is considered 40 days (approximately 6 weeks after surgery) unless postoperative radiotherapy is indicated [26]. However, Remacle and Demard state that rehabilitation can be started earlier, immediately after cicatrization, usually 3 weeks after the operation [17]. If postoperative radiotherapy is indicated, rehabilitation is delayed as long as acute consequences of radiation that hamper the process of rehabilitation are present. Of course, rehabilitation should begin within 6 months of surgery [26]. The total duration of rehabilitation is different and individual.

Early postoperative rehabilitation phase lasts 1 month from the onset of therapy, and primary focus of the therapy is on relaxation techniques and respiratory - rehabilitation operators in physiological breathing onto a tracheostoma to avoid, initially always present, tracheal noise at later phonation.

At this stage, the patient is also educated on how to achieve a ructus. Achieving a ructus is taught by two basic principles in one of three available methods. The first principle is based on the correct technique of injecting speech air into the esophagus, and the other is based on the proper technique of eructation of speech air. **Figure 1** shows the scheme of esophageal voice production.

There are several different methods of introducing speech air into the esophagus used in clinical speech therapy, namely: deglutition, inhalation, injection, blocking, Portman's, Tartapan's, and their combinations [5, 17, 22].

In 1900, Gottstein created and described the deglutition/swallowing method, and Gutzmann supplemented and propagated it. The method requires inserting the required air for the alaryngeal phonation according to the principle of swallowing or air ingestion as a bolus which causes eructation. This is considered the initial method because it allows a volitional ructus, but it affects the rhythm of speech and substantially slows it down, which is its disadvantage. As air swallowing, that is, "dry swallowing" is limited, it is recommended to consume the fluid during therapy [17].

In 1922, Seeman described the inhalation method, also referred to as aspirational or suctioning method. It requires a few swift inhalations that cause a sudden drop in intraoral pressure, which allows aspiration of air from the oral cavity into pharynx, and into the esophagus and relaxation of the pharyngoesophageal segment. When the pressures get equal, the air suction is stopped, the aspirated air is eructated and sounded through the pharyngoesophageal segment. Initially, the vocals are articulated, followed by the syllables made of a combination of gutural/h/ and vocals. Sometimes, the use of the method is followed by hyperventilation. There are several modifications of this method in the world.

The injectable or occlusive method was formed by collecting the experiences of patients who noticed that the easiest way for them to loudly articulate occlusives and syllables combined from occlusives and vocals is alaryngeally. The method requires sufficient pressure of the tongue which causes air compression in the oral cavity and pharynx and is injected into the

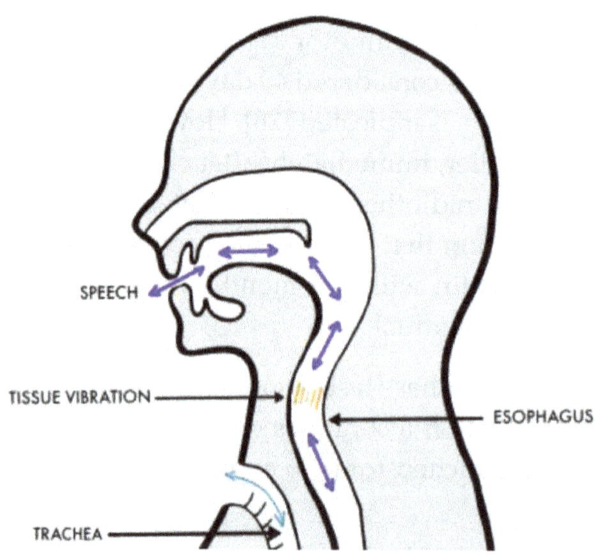

Figure 1. Esophageal voice production.

esophagus, and in the articulation of the labial, alveolar and guttural occlusive the air is liberated and affects the achievement of a satisfactory tonus of the pharyngoesophageal segment. In 1966, Diedrich and Youngstrom created a variation of this method by introducing certain modifications [17].

The blocking method was accomplished by performing several procedures of injectable method followed by specific articulator's movements and by changing the head position. The method involves injecting air from the oral cavity to the esophagus by lip occlusion causing anterior blockage with simultaneous posterior repositioning of the base of the tongue and inferior mandibular repositioning.

By combining several specific procedures from the deglutition and inhalation method, a new method was created by Portman, and was named after him as Portman's method. It requires a few fast-paced air inspirations that are followed by "edacious" deglutition of the air bolus to make speech air flow into the esophagus [22].

In addition, there is Tartapan's method, which is seldom used in clinical speech therapy practice, as well as other possible combinations of existing standard methods that are not specifically described.

4. Esophagus and tracheoesophageal speech

4.1. Tracheoesophageal puncture and tracheoesophageal prosthesis placement

Tracheoesophageal puncture is a surgical method of voice restoration after total laryngectomy that implies creation of a fistulous tract in tracheoesophageal wall—the wall that separates the trachea and esophagus, in the level of tracheostomy. This surgically created fistula which may be formed at the time of the total laryngectomy (primary tracheoesophageal puncture) or after the laryngectomized person has healed from surgery (secondary tracheoesophageal puncture). For satisfactory performance of the tracheoesophageal puncture, an adequate tracheostoma is preferable. The location of puncture is positioned in the midline, 5–10 mm below the mucocutaneous junction. A tracheoesophageal prosthesis is inserted into a fistula, as shown in **Figure 2** [4].

The prosthesis is an artificial device, mostly made of silicone. The purpose of the prosthesis, which is practically "one-way" valve is to allow air to be delivered from the lungs into the esophagus (**Figure 3**). At the same time, the leak of saliva and food in trachea is undesirable and prevented [27]. For this passage of air, good occlusion of the tracheostoma during phonation is necessary. During phonation, high intrathoracic pressure forces the valve to open and directs the air into the upper part of esophagus. Passing of this air into the pharynx and mouth produces vibrations in the mucosal wall of the pharyngoesophageal segment which generates sound. Resonation of the sound occurs in the pharynx, mouth and nose, with simultaneous articulation using the tongue, lips, and teeth.

The most important anatomical part responsible for alaryngeal voice formation is pharyngoesophageal segment. The vibrating pharyngoesophageal segment is the source of sound production and performs vocal cord function. The state of pharyngoesophageal segment made

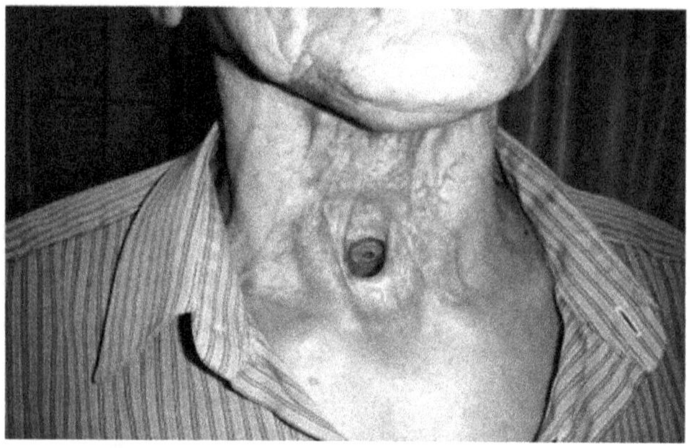

Figure 2. Tracheoesophageal fistula with inserted prosthesis.

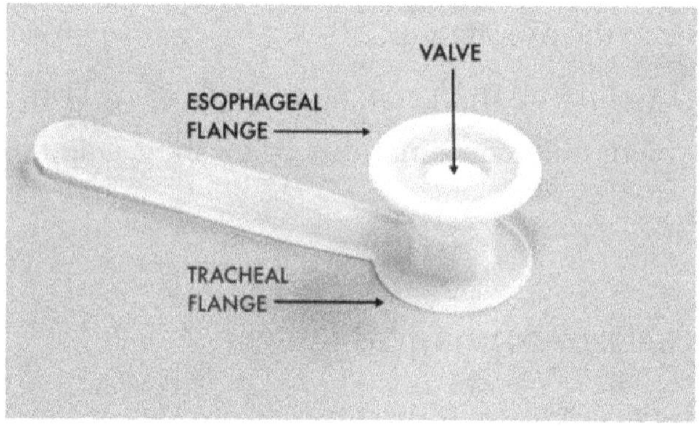

Figure 3. Tracheoesophageal prosthesis.

by the mucosa and surrounding fibers of the repaired cricopharyngeal, thyropharyngeal and the upper esophageal sphincter muscles is very important in voice production, and because of that it is important to preserve as much pharyngeal mucosa as possible at the time of laryngeal surgery [28]. Sometimes PE segment may be hypertonic, spastic or hypotonic. In case that hypertonicity or spasticity is a problem, cricopharyngeal myotomy, pharyngeal neurectomy, PES dilatation or botulinum toxin injection may be beneficial [29].

4.2. History of tracheoesophageal speech

The first experimental prostheses appeared in the second half of the last century, but due to initial structural defects, they could not be cleansed in detail from the secretion, resulting in an infection of the trachea and esophagus [30]. The first silicone tracheoesophageal prosthesis for commercial use was constructed in 1979 and its creators were Blom and Singer [31]. Due to its specific appearance, the prototype of the prosthesis was named duckbill. At the rounded esophageal end, an opening was located with the aim of one-way airflow from the trachea to the esophagus, and at the tracheal end, there was a rim with the extension and the possibility of sticking to the skin to prevent prosthesis from falling out. The second prototype of the prosthesis was created by introducing a one-way valve with a hinged door shape and reduced air resistance. The prostheses were built in secondarily, anterogradely through tracheostoma under general anesthesia. After this, other types of prostheses are created and developed, such as Hermann's prosthesis, Henley-Cohn's prosthesis, Staffieri's prosthesis, Traissac's prosthesis,

Nijdam's prosthesis, Ultra Voice prosthesis, Algaba prosthesis, and Provox prostheses [22]. The primary goal of the prosthesis development was to improve its structural and construction properties with the aim of achieving proper, safe and reliable use, adequate fixation of prosthesis within tracheoesophageal fistula, better prosthesis functionality in terms of low air resistance and greater resistance to fungal and bacterial infections. To date, different manufacturers' tracheoesophageal prostheses of perfected construction and design are available.

4.3. Prerequisites for successful tracheoesophageal voice and speech

The basic requirement for tracheoesophageal prosthesis is the absence of distant metastases or local recurrence [22]. The ability to produce tracheoesophageal voice implies the formation of tracheoesophageal fistula and the insertion of the prosthesis within the tracheoesophageal fistula, which is the surgical method of voice rehabilitation [5].

Andrews, according to Kazi, provides the following indicative criteria of patient's status for inserting the tracheoesophageal prosthesis: motivation, mental stability, sufficient level of comprehension and understanding of the changes in anatomy and functional mechanism of prosthesis and its use, appropriate manual and motor skills, the adequate vision status necessary for the maintenance of the prosthesis, the adequate tonus of hypopharynx, i.e., the absence of stenosis of the hypopharynx, the positive insufflation Taub's test, the tracheostoma of a neat appearance, i.e., the appropriate shape (minimum diameter of 15 mm) and depth, and sufficient lung capacity [32].

4.4. Functional characteristics of tracheoesophageal speech

The tracheoesophageal fistula allows communication between the trachea and esophagus, which is important for the speech because the patient uses the lungs as the air reservoir required for the phonation, which makes the speech more fluent [33], of more appropriate melody and pace with better achieved stresses and fewer respiratory pauses. Although, by acoustic measurements, the fundamental frequency is lowered, and the values of the parameters that determine the timbre are elevated, unlike the esophageal voice, the intensity or volume is greater, and the maximum time of the phonation is longer [5, 24]. If a tracheostoma is occluded manually, patient's hand will be occupied, but this is not necessary because an automatic speech valve can be used for occlusion. The advantage of this method is the duration of rehabilitation, which is considerably shorter than the esophageal speech learning process. The greatest disadvantages of the method are the need to replace prosthesis over a certain period of time and the possibility of developing various speech prosthesis complications or tracheoesophageal fistulas. The average life of the prosthesis is 3–6 months [34].

4.5. Rehabilitation: educational process of learning the tracheoesophageal speech

The rehabilitation process varies depending on the type of prosthesis insertion, whether it is primary, primary postponed or secondary, but the overall process lasts shorter than the esophageal speech learning process. During the tracheoesophageal voice production, it is necessary to occlude the tracheostoma. At the beginning of the rehabilitation, the tracheostoma is occluded with a non-dominant hand, usually by a thumb, to achieve the best occlusion. The complete occlusion of tracheostoma allows the air from the lungs to be directed through the

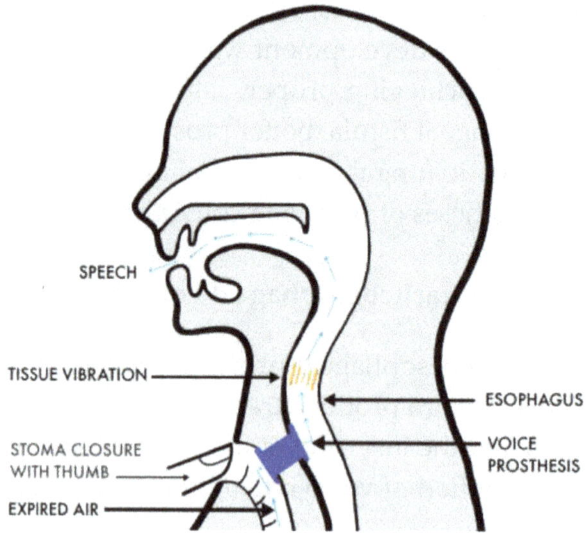

Figure 4. Tracheoesophageal voice production.

trachea and the esophagus into the oral cavity, thereby creating vibration of the pharyngoesophageal segment and the production of tracheoesophageal speech, while simultaneously preventing undesirable tracheal noise. Rehabilitation begins with rehabilitation-methodical operators of relaxation of the whole body, especially the neck and head, and operators of proper, relaxed, alaryngeal phonation. Once a satisfactory tracheoesophageal phonation is established, the production of this voice articulates the syllables in a combination of silent guttural occlusive and a vocal and then all other sounds. When the patient successfully uses tracheoesophageal voice and speech on a daily basis as the only mean of communication, attention is paid to the details. In order to fix the lack of a free hand, an automatic speech valve is used. The automatic speech valve consists of a plastic casing inside which is located the membrane for controlling the flow of the economical amount of air and the filter for maintaining the temperature and humidity of the air [34].

Rehabilitation ends when a patient can produce spontaneous speech without significant difficulties, that is, when tracheostoma is well-occluded, a voice of satisfactory quality, speech is intelligible, and when the patient uses tracheoesophageal speech as the main mean of communication. **Figure 4** shows the scheme of tracheoesophageal voice production.

The assessment of the performance of voice-speech rehabilitation is performed using the Harrison and Robillard-Schultz scales for assessing tracheoesophageal voice and speech, including a sub-scale for assessing the maintenance of tracheoesophageal prosthesis [35].

4.6. Tracheoesophageal puncture and tracheoesophageal prosthesis complications

Complications may occur in the early or late postoperative period in 10–60% of patients [34, 36, 37] and may be divided into:

1. Complications of tracheoesophageal puncture.
2. Complications of tracheoesophageal fistula.
3. Complications of tracheoesophageal prosthesis.

Complications of tracheoesophageal puncture are complications resulting from the surgical procedure itself, and among them are tracheostoma of inadequate form, size and depth, inadequate tonus of the pharyngoesophageal segment (hypotonicity or hypertonicity) [38] and the formation of pseudoepiglottis or pseudo-vallecula [39].

Complications of tracheoesophageal fistula occur in later postoperative period, most commonly the same patient having several different complications. Among these complications are the atrophy of the tracheoesophageal wall, tracheal mucosa granulation, esophageal mucosa hypertrophy, increase in diameter of tracheoesophageal fistulae, dislocation of the voice prosthesis and leakage of the esophagus from the voice prosthesis into the trachea [40]. Inadequate size of voice prosthesis causes pressure on the esophageal and tracheal mucosa and may result in fibromatous reactions [39]. Several cases of decubitus of the back esophageal wall have been reported due to the incompatibility of the length of the tracheoesophageal fistula with the length of the voice prosthesis.

The complications of the tracheoesophageal prosthesis are the release of one-way prosthesis valves, resulting in leakage of the esophagus through the voice prosthesis into the trachea [41, 42], and the creation of biofilm in the voice prosthesis due to its use during several months [43, 44].

5. Conclusion

The physiological function of the esophagus in healthy people is very simple: to actively transport solids and liquids from the pharynx to the stomach. It has no digestive, absorptive, metabolic, or endocrine functions, but in laryngectomized persons, esophagus takes one more function. In such changed anatomical condition, the esophagus has a key role in voice—speech rehabilitation of laryngectomized patients because the esophageal and tracheoesophageal speech are the only acceptable solution of substitute alaryngeal speech. The esophagus gets very important function at alaryngeal phonation as air reservoir, the upper esophageal sphincter gets the function as air activator and the pharyngoesophageal segment gets the function of the voice generator, thus allowing the function of the voice resonators.

Acknowledgements

We would like to thank Ms. Mirna Brunčić for translating this text.

Notes

The figures are from the author's own source.

Author details

Ljiljana Širić[1]*, Marinela Rosso[2] and Aleksandar Včev[3]

*Address all correspondence to: ljsiric@gmail.com

1 Department of Otorhinolaryngology and Head and Neck Surgery, University Hospital Centre Osijek, Osijek, Croatia

2 Polyclinic Rosso, Osijek, Croatia

3 Faculty of Medicine, J. J. Strossmayer University of Osijek, Osijek, Croatia

References

[1] Sabiston DC, Sellke FW, Del NPJ, Swanson SJ. Sabiston & Spencer Surgery of the Chest. Philadelphia: Saunders/Elsevier; 2010

[2] Rice TW. Esophagus. In: Norton JA et al, editors. Surgery. Berlin, Heidelberg: Springer; 2001

[3] Hilgers FJM, Ackerstaff AH. Comprehensive rehabilitation after total laryngectomy is more than voice alone. Folia Phoniatrica et Logopaedica. 2000;**52**:65-73

[4] Shah JP, Patel SG. Head and Neck Surgery and Oncology. Edinburgh: Mosby; 2003

[5] Širić Lj. Utjecaj vrste alaringealne fonacije na akustičke parametre glasa i prozodijske elemente govora. [Doktorska disertacija]. Osijek: Sveučilište J. J. Strossmayera Osijek, Medicinski fakultet; 2017

[6] Rosso M. Utjecaj kazeta za održavanje vlažnosti i temperature zraka na morfološki i funkcionalni status donjih dišnih putova laringektomiranih osoba. [Doktorska disertacija]. Osijek: Sveučilište J. J. Strossmayera Osijek, Medicinski fakultet; 2015

[7] Van der Torn M. A sound-producing voice prosthesis [Doctoral dissertation]. Amsterdam: Vrije University Medical Center; 2005

[8] Hirokazu S, Takahashi H. Voice generation system using an intra-mouth vibrator for the laryngectomee [Master's thesis]. Japan: University of Tokyo; 2000

[9] Czermak J. Uber die Sprache bei luftdichter Verschliessung des Kehlkopfs. Wien: Sitzungsberichte der kaiserlichen Academie der Wissenschafter mathematischnaturwissenschaftliche Classe; 1859

[10] Gussenbauer C. Ueber die erste durch Th. Billroth am Menschen ausgefuerte Kehlkopf – Extirpation und die Anwendung eines Kuenstlichen Kehlkopfes. Archiv Fur Klinische Chirurgie. 1874;**17**:343-356

[11] Weir N. Otolaryngology: An Illustrated History London: Butterworths; 1990

[12] Struebbing PDL. Pseudostimme nach Ausschaltung des Kehlkopfs, speziell nach Extirpation desselben. Deutsche Medizinische Wochenschrift. 1988;**14**:1061

[13] Struebbing PDL. Erzeugung einer (natuerlichen) Pseudo – Stimme bei einem Manne mit totaler Extirpation des Kehlkopfes. Archiv Fur Klinische Chirurgie. 1889;**38**:142

[14] Lowry LD. Artificial larynges: a review and development of a prototype selfcontained intra-oral artificial larynx. Laryngoscope. 1981;**91**(8):1332-1355

[15] Fagan JJ, Lentin R, Oyarzabal MF, Isaacs S, Sellars SL. Tracheoesophageal speech in a developing worldcommunity. Archives of Otolaryngology – Head & Neck Surgery. 2002;**128**(1):50-53

[16] Brown DH, Hilgers FJM, Irish JC, Balm AJ. Postlaryngectomy voice rehabilitation: State of the art at the millennium. World Journal of Surgery. 2003;**27**(7):824-831

[17] Stanković DP. Fonijatrijska rehabilitacija laringtomisanih pacijenata uspostavljanjem ezofagusnog glasa i govora modificiranom Semanovom metodom [Doktorska disertacija]. Beograd: Univerzitet u Beogradu, Medicinski fakultet; 1997

[18] Mahieu HF. Voice and speech Rehabilitation following laryngectomy [Doctoral thesis]. Groningen: Rijk University Groningen; 1988

[19] Taub S, Bergner LH. Air bypass voice prosthesis for vocal rehabilitation of laryngectomees. American Journal of Surgery. 1973;**125**:748-756

[20] Blom ED, Singer MI, Hamaker RC. A prospective study of tracheo-oesophageal speech. Archives of Otolaryngology-Head and Neck Surgery. 1986;**112**:440-447

[21] Doyle PC. Foundations of voice and speech Rehabilitation following laryngeal Cancer San Diego: Singular Publishing Group Inc; 1994

[22] Dragičević D. Govorna rehabilitacija totalno laringektomisanih pacijenata ugradnjom vokalnih proteza [Doktorska disertacija]. Medicinski fakultet Novi Sad: Novi Sad; 2013

[23] Milutinović Z. Studija glasa posle lečenja karcinoma larinksa. Nova knjiga: Beograd; 1985

[24] Širić LJ, Šoš D, Rosso M, Stevanović S. Objective assessment of tracheoesophageal and esophageal voice using acoustic analysis of voice. Collegium Antropologicum 2012;**36**: 111-114

[25] Štajner-Katušić S. Glas i govor nakon totalne laringektomije. Grafostil: Zagreb; 1998

[26] Mumović GM. Konzervativni tretman disfonija. Medicinski fakultet Novi Sad: Novi Sad; 2004

[27] Blom ED, Hamaker RC. Tracheoesophageal voice restoration following total laryngectomy. In: Myers EN, Suen J, editors. Cancer of the Head and Neck. 3rd ed. Philadelphia: W.B. Saunders Company; 1996. pp. 839-852

[28] Kotby MN, Hegazi MA, Kamal I, Gamal El Dien N, Nassar J. Aerodynamics of the pseudo-glottis. Folia Phoniatrica et Logopaedica. 2009;**61**:24-28

[29] Arenaz B, Rydell R, Westin U, Olsson R. The pharyngoesophageal segment in laryngectomees with non-functional voice: Is it all about spasm? Journal of Otology & Rhinology. 2016;**5**:4. DOI: 10.4172/2324-8785.1000287

[30] Hilgers FJM, Ackerstaff AH, Balm AJ, et al. Development and clinical evaluation of a second-generation voice prosthesis (Provox 2), designed for anterograde and retrograde insertion. Acta Oto-Laryngologica. 1997;**117**(6):889-896

[31] Singer MI, Blom ED. An endoscopic technique for restoration of voice after laryngectomy. Annals of Otology. 1980;**89**:529-533

[32] Andrews JC, Mickel RA, Hanson DG, Monahan GP. Major complications following tracheoesophageal puncture for voice rehabilitation. The Laryngoscope. 1987;**97**:562-567

[33] Lorenz KJ, Groll K, Ackerstaff AH, Hilgers FJM, Maier H. Hands-free speech after surgical voice rehabilitation with a Provox voice prosthesis: Experience with the Provox free hands HME tracheostoma valve system. European Archives of Oto-Rhino-Laryngology. 2006;**264**(2):151-157

[34] Capaccio P, Schnidler A, Tassone G, Ottaviani F. Comparative study of esophageal and tracheo-esophageal voice by digital spectrographic analysis. Acta Phoniatrica Latina. 2001;**23**:322-326

[35] Op de Coul B, Hilgers F, Balm A, Tan I, van den Hoogen F, Van Tinteren H. A decade of postlaryngectomy vocal rehabilitation in 318 patients: A single institutions experience with consistent application of provox indwelling voice prostheses. Archives of Otolaryngology – Head & Neck Surgery 2000;**126**:1320-1328

[36] Lukinović J, Bilić M, Raguž I, Živković T, Kovač-Bilić L, Prgomet D. Overview of 100 patients with voice prosthesis after total laryngectomy-Experience of single institution. Collegium Antropologicum. 2012;**36**:99-102

[37] Malik T, Bruce I, Cherry J. Surgical complications of tracheo-oesophageal puncture and speech valves. Current Opinion in Otolaryngology & Head and Neck Surgery. 2007;**15**:117-122

[38] Brok H, Stroeve R, Copper M, Schouwenburg P. The treatment of hypertonicity of the pharyngo-oesophageal segment after laryngectomy. Clinical Otolaryngology. 1998;**23**: 302-307

[39] Đanić Hadžibegović A. Utjecaj ekstraezofagealnog refluksa na učestalost komplikacija i kvalitetu glasa bolesnika s govornom protezom [Doktorska disertacija]. Zagreb: Sveučilište u Zagrebu, Medicinski fakultet; 2013

[40] Balm AJM, Van den Brekel MWM, Tan IB, Hilgers FJM. The indwelling voice prosthesis for speech rehabilitation after total laryngectomy: A safe approach. Otolaryngologia Polska. 2011;**65**:402-409

[41] Soolsma J, Van den Brekel M, Ackerstaff A, Balm A, Tan I, Hilgers F. Long-term results of Provox ActiValve, solving the problem of frequent Candida and "Underpressure"-related voice prosthesis replacements. Laryngoscope. 2008;**118**:252-257

[42] Leder SB, Acton LM, Kmiecik J, Ganz C, Blom ED. Voice restoration with the advantage tracheoesophageal voice prosthesis. Otolaryngology and Head and Neck Surgery. 2005;**133**:681-684

[43] Smith A, Buchinsky FJ, Post JC. Eradicating chronic ear, nose and throat infections. Otolaryngology and Head and Neck Surgery. 2011;**144**:338-347

[44] Mahieu H, Van Saene J, Den Besten J, Van Saene H. Oropharynx decontamination preventing Candida vegetations on voice prostheses. Archives of Otolaryngology – Head & Neck Surgery. 1986;**112**:1090-1092

6

Adjuvant Chemotherapy of Gastric Cancer

Byoung Jo Suh

Abstract

Adjuvant chemotherapy is a standard treatment for operable gastric cancer. However, the preferred treatment varies by geographical region. Southwestern Oncology Group (SWOG) conducted a, randomized trial of adjuvant chemotherapy for patients with surgically resected gastric cancer. The 3-year survival rates were 50% in the chemoradiotherapygroup and 41% in the surgery group. The Medical Research Council Adjuvant Gastric Infusional Chemotherapy (MAGIC) trial that compared perioperative chemotherapy with the ECF regimen (epirubicin, cisplatin, and 5-fluorouracil) and patients with surgery alone had a 5-year survival rate of 36 and 23%. The Adjuvant Chemotherapy Trial of TS-1 for Gastric Cancer (ACTS-GC) showed that the 3-year overall survival rate was 80.1% in the S-1 group and 70.1% in the surgery-only group in stage II or III gastric cancer patients who underwent a D2 gastrectomy. An analysis of the Capecitabine and Oxaliplatin Adjuvant Study in Stomach Cancer (CLASSIC) study showed 3-year disease-free survival, 74% in the chemotherapy and surgery group and 59% in the surgery-only group in the patients with stage II–IIIB gastric cancer who had D2 gastrectomy. In conclusion, for all patients with stage II and III gastric cancer, standard D2 gastrectomy and adjuvant chemotherapy are strongly recommended for improved survival rates.

Keywords: gastric cancer, D2 lymph node dissection, chemotherapy

1. Introduction

Gastric cancer is the second most common cause of cancer-related death worldwide [1]. Radical operation is the main treatment for gastric cancer, but the recurrence rate following surgery is high due to the early dissemination of cancer cells via the lymphatic system (about 40–80% in advanced gastric cancer) [1, 2]. In East Asia, especially Japan and Korea, D2 lymph node dissection is the standard treatment for operable gastric cancer [3, 4].

However, in the Western world, D2 gastrectomy is not as widely performed as in Japan and Korea [5]. Western surgical studies have shown that most patients present with tumors that penetrated the submucosa; they have a 5-year survival rate of 20–30% [6]. Postoperative chemotherapy is a standard treatment component of resectable gastric cancer and has improved patient outcomes [3, 4]. Treatment results of adjuvant chemotherapy may depend on the interaction between residual cancers and anticancer drugs. The Japanese recommendation for adjuvant chemotherapy is based on the Adjuvant Chemotherapy Trial of TS-1 for Gastric Cancer (ACTS-GC) study, which showed a survival benefit with adjuvant chemotherapy after D2 gastrectomy compared with surgery alone [4]. This study showed a survival benefit for stage II and IIIA gastric cancer [4]. However, the FLAGS trial for advanced gastric cancer or gastroesophageal cancer that compared cisplatin and S-1 versus cisplatin and fluorouracil in non-Asian countries did not prolong overall survival [7]. In Korea, adjuvant immunochemotherapy in advanced gastric cancer patients, who had undergone radical subtotal gastrectomy for stage III gastric cancer has been performed. For immunotherapy, a *Streptococcus pyogenes* preparation (picibanil) was followed by MF (mitomycin C and 5-FU) in the late 1990s and early 2000s [3, 8]. The Capecitabine and Oxaliplatin Adjuvant Study in Stomach Cancer (CLASSIC) study was designed to compare the effect of adjuvant capecitabine plus oxaliplatin after D-2 gastrectomy with stage II or III gastric cancer [1]. Although adjuvant chemotherapy is a standard treatment option for operable gastric cancer, there have been some differences concerning methods of chemotherapy and survival data between the Western world (Europe and North America) and East Asia (Korea and Japan). Therefore, this article summarizes the adjuvant chemotherapy for resectable gastric cancer using a medical literature review.

2. Treatment results with adjuvant chemotherapy

Treatment results of adjuvant chemotherapy may depend on the interaction between residual tumor and anticancer drugs. The tumor burden should be reduced as much as possible to obtain the most optimal survival benefit of adjuvant chemotherapy [10]. As compared to Western countries, the high survival rate in East Asia might have resulted from a selection of early-stage patients and radical operations, including systematic lymph node dissection [10]. The Southwestern Oncology Group (SWOG) conducted a two-armed prospective, randomized trial of adjuvant chemotherapy for patients with gastric adenocarcinoma surgically resected to negative margins (**Table 1**). Most patients (54%) had undergone a D0 dissection, which is less than a complete dissection of the N1 nodes. The chemotherapy regimen included fluorouracil, 425 mg/m^2 of body-surface area per day, and leucovorin, 20 mg, followed by radiotherapy of 4500 cGy of radiation at 180 cGy/day. The median survival time in the surgery group was 27 months as compared with 36 months in the chemoradiotherapy group [5]. The 3-year survival rates were 50% in the chemoradiotherapy group and 41% in the surgery-only group [5, 11]. The 503-patient United Kingdom National Cancer Research Institute (NCRI) Medical Research Council Adjuvant Gastric Infusional Chemotherapy (MAGIC) trial was the first randomized trial to demonstrate the survival benefit from the use of perioperative chemotherapy for patients with resectable gastric cancer compared with surgery alone.

Study	Regimen (surgery + chemotherapy surgery alone)	No. of patients	3-YSR (%)	5-YSR (%)
Macdonald et al. [5]	5FU + leucovorin + radiotherapy	281	50	40
	Control	275	41	30
Cunningham et al. [6]	Epirubicin + cisplatin +5FU	250	45	36
	Control	253	30	23
Sakuramoto et al. [4, 9]	S-1	529	80	71
	Control	530	61	70
Bang et al. [1, 2]	Capecitabine + oxaliplatin	520	83	78
	Control	515	78	69

YSR, year survival rate.

Table 1. Adjuvant chemotherapy compared to the surgical control of curative resection of stomach cancer.

The patients who received perioperative chemotherapy with the ECF regimen (epirubicin, cisplatin, and 5-fluorouracil, 5FU) had a 5-year survival of 36%, compared with 23% in patients treated with surgery alone [12] (**Table 1**). Kim et al. evaluated 10,783 consecutive patients who underwent operation for gastric cancer [3]. The prognostic significance of treatment modality (surgery alone, surgery + chemotherapy, surgery + immunotherapy + chemotherapy <immunochemotherapeutic treatment>) was evaluated for stage III gastric cancer. The protocol for immunochemotherapy was as follows: Picibanil (a *Streptococcus pyogenes* preparation; Tokyo, Japan), mitomycin C 4 mg/50 kg, and 5-FU 500 mg/50 kg. They concluded that radical lymph node dissection, with more than 25 resected lymph nodes, improved survival in patients with stage II and IIIc disease; as postoperative adjuvant therapy, immunochemotherapy was most effective in patients with stage III disease. There were significant differences in survival in stage III patients; the 5-year survival rates were 44.8% for the immunochemotherapy group, 36.8% for the surgery + chemotherapy group, 36.8% for the surgery + chemotherapy group, and 27.1% for the surgery-alone group [3]. In the meta-analysis, which assessed entitled adjuvant chemotherapy after curative resection for gastric cancer in Non-Asian patients, Earle et al. concluded adjuvant chemotherapy may produce a small survival benefit of borderline statistical significance in patients with curatively resected gastric carcinoma [13]. Sakuramoto et al. reported that patients with stage II or III gastric cancer who underwent gastrectomy with extended (D2) lymph node dissection were randomly assigned to undergo surgery followed by adjuvant chemotherapy with S-1 or to undergo surgery only. The analysis of the follow-up data showed that the 3-year overall survival rate was 80.1% in the S-1 group and 70.1% in the surgery-only group [4]. Consecutive results of the ACT-GC trial showed the overall survival rate at 5 years was 71.1% in the S-1 group and 61.1% in the surgery-only group (**Table 1**) [9]. In the Capecitabine and Oxaliplatin Adjuvant Study in Stomach Cancer (CLASSIC) trial, the patients with stage II–IIIB gastric cancer who had curative D2 gastrectomy were randomly assigned to receive adjuvant chemotherapy of eight cycles of oral capecitabine (1000 mg/m^2 twice daily on days 1–14 of each cycle) plus intravenous oxaliplatin (130 mg/m^2 on day 1 of each cycle) for 6 months or surgery only. The 3-year disease-free survival was 74% in the chemotherapy and surgery group and 59% in the surgery-only group. They concluded that adjuvant capecitabine plus oxaliplatin treatment after curative D2 gastrectomy should be considered as a treatment option for patients with operable gastric cancer [1].

3. Discussion

Adjuvant chemotherapy is a standard treatment option for operable gastric cancer and improves patient outcomes, but the preferred treatment differs by geographical region [10]. The recommended adjuvant treatment is chemoradiotherapy in the United States and perioperative chemotherapy in the United Kingdom and some parts of Europe [1, 5, 12]. The Japanese ACT-GC trial was the first large-scale randomized trial of adjuvant chemotherapy after curative resection with D2 gastrectomy [4]. In the Republic of Korea, the CLASSIC trial was the second large-scale randomized trial after D2 gastrectomy [1]. The survival rate of two Asian large-scale randomized trials was substantially higher than in the US Intergroup-0116 and UK MAGIC trials (78% in the CLASSIC trial, 80% in ACT-GC vs. 30–40% in the Intergroup-0116 and MAGIC trials) [1, 4, 5, 12]. Most recurrences after surgery of gastric cancer occurred within 3 years of surgery [14]. The duration of adjuvant chemotherapy differed from previous studies. Kim et al. had adjuvant chemotherapy for 24 months [3]. The ACT-GC trial had adjuvant chemotherapy for 12 months [4]. CLASSIC trial had adjuvant chemotherapy 6 months [1]. The duration of adjuvant chemotherapy after surgery was different, although similar survival results were present in two clinical trials. Kim et al. reported that radical lymph node dissection, with more than 25 resected lymph nodes, improved survival in patients with stage II and IIIa disease [3]. Postoperative immunochemotherapy was most effective in patients with stage II and III disease [3]. The favorable outcomes of Asian studies were a result of the consistent adoption of D2 gastrectomy and the quality control of surgery using video techniques [1, 4]. But postoperative chemoradiotherapy in the United States and perioperative chemotherapy in Europe is not based on D2 gastrectomy. In the Intergroup-0116 study, quality assessment was done for radiotherapy before the initiation of this treatment [5]. However quality control of surgery was not done, because patients were usually identified postoperatively, and they could not require specific surgical procedures. Only 10% of the patients underwent a D2 dissection, while 36% had a D1 dissection, and 54% had a D0 lymphadenectomy (a resection in which not all of the N1 nodes were removed) [5]. The low long-term survival rate of stomach cancer patients in Western studies might result from excessive residual tumor left behind during surgery. The high survival rate in countries such as South Korea and Japan might be the reflection of the small amount of residual tumor due to radical gastrectomy and extensive lymph node dissection [10]. Songun et al. [15] reported that after a median follow-up of 15 years, D2 lymphadenectomy with strict quality control is associated with lower locoregional recurrence and gastric cancer-related death rates in patients with stage II and IIIa disease than D1 surgery; they recommended D2 resection as the standard surgical approach to resectable gastric cancer [15]. The CLASSIC and ACT-GC trials showed the effectiveness of postoperative adjuvant chemotherapy with S-1 and XELOX for stage II and III gastric cancer patients who underwent D2 gastrectomy [1, 4]. Biological aspects may cause the different gastric cancer results between

East Asia and the Western world. However, no significant differences in prognostic factors were reported between these two regions of the world. In conclusion, for all patients with stage II and III gastric cancer worldwide, standard D2 gastrectomy and adjuvant chemotherapy are strongly recommended for a better rate of survival.

Author details

Byoung Jo Suh

Address all correspondence to: oltx62@hanmail.net

Department of Surgery, Memorial Jin-Pok Kim Gastric Cancer Center, Haeundae Paik Hospital, Inje University College of Medicine, Busan, Korea

References

[1] Bang YJ, Kim YW, Yang HK, et al. Adjuvant capecitabine and oxaliplatin for gastric cancer after D2 gastrectomy (CLASSIC): A phase 3 open-label, randomised controlled trial. Lancet. 2012;**379**(9813):315-321

[2] Noh SH, Park SR, Yang HK, et al. Adjuvant capecitabine plus oxaliplatin for gastric cancer after D2 gastrectomy (CLASSIC): 5-year follow-up of an open-label, randomised phase 3 trial. The Lancet Oncology. 2014;**15**(12):1389-1396

[3] Kim JP, Lee JH, Kim SJ, Yu HJ, Yang HK. Clinicopathologic characteristics and prognostic factors in 10783 patients with gastric cancer. Gastric Cancer. 1998;**1**(2):125-133

[4] Sakuramoto S, Sasako M, Yamaguchi T, et al. Adjuvant chemotherapy for gastric cancer with S-1, an oral fluoropyrimidine. The New England Journal of Medicine. 2007; **357**(18):1810-1820

[5] Macdonald JS, Smalley SR, Benedetti J, et al. Chemoradiotherapy after surgery compared with surgery alone for adenocarcinoma of the stomach or gastroesophageal junction. The New England Journal of Medicine. 2001;**345**(10):725-730

[6] Cunningham D, Allum WH, Stenning SP, et al. Perioperative chemotherapy versus surgery alone for resectable gastroesophageal cancer. The New England Journal of Medicine. 2006;**355**(1):11-20

[7] Ajani JA, Rodriguez W, Bodoky G, et al. Multicenter phase III comparison of cisplatin/S-1 with cisplatin/infusional fluorouracil in advanced gastric or gastroesophageal adenocarcinoma study: The FLAGS trial. Journal of Clinical Oncology. 2010;**28**(9):1547-1553

[8] Oh SJ, Suh BJ, Park JK, Oh SD, Yu HJ. Prognostic discrepancy of the 6th and 7th UICC N classification for lymph node staging in gastric cancer patients after curative resection. Case Reports in Oncology. 2017;**10**(1):57-65

[9] Sasako M, Sakuramoto S, Katai H, et al. Five-year outcomes of a randomized phase III trial comparing adjuvant chemotherapy with S-1 versus surgery alone in stage II or III gastric cancer. Journal of Clinical Oncology. 2011;**29**(33):4387-4393

[10] Nakajima T. Review of adjuvant chemotherapy for gastric cancer. World Journal of Surgery. 1995;**19**(4):570-574

[11] Smalley SR, Benedetti JK, Haller DG, et al. Updated analysis of SWOG-directed intergroup study 0116: A phase III trial of adjuvant radiochemotherapy versus observation after curative gastric cancer resection. Journal of Clinical Oncology. 2012;**30**(19):2327-2333

[12] Chua YJ, Cunningham D. The UK NCRI MAGIC trial of perioperative chemotherapy in resectable gastric cancer: Implications for clinical practice. Annals of Surgical Oncology. 2007;**14**(10):2687-2690

[13] Earle CC, Maroun JA. Adjuvant chemotherapy after curative resection for gastric cancer in non-Asian patients: Revisiting a meta-analysis of randomised trials. European Journal of Cancer. 1999;**35**(7):1059-1064

[14] Deng J, Liang H, Wang D, Sun D, Pan Y, Liu Y. Investigation of the recurrence patterns of gastric cancer following a curative resection. Surgery Today. 2011;**41**(2):210-215

[15] Songun I, Putter H, Kranenbarg EM, Sasako M. van de Velde, Cornelis JH. Surgical treatment of gastric cancer: 15-year follow-up results of the randomised nationwide Dutch D1D2 trial. The Lancet Oncology. 2010;**11**(5):439-449

7

Reconstruction after Laparoscopic Distal Gastrectomy

Satoshi Kanda and Tetsu Fukunaga

Abstract

Laparoscopy-assisted distal gastrectomy (LADG) has advanced much in the past 10 years in the eastern countries, due to the high gastric cancer incidences. Reconstruction is the major hurdle for perfect laparoscopic distal gastrectomy (LDG). Initially, hand-associated or small incisional open laparotomy reconstruction, the so-called associated operation, was performed. A full laparoscopic operation is much better for the patient—small wound, less pain, and quick recovery. Several reconstruction methods have been developed by experts during more than 10 years. The question of what method is the best after distal gastrectomy is still controversial. This chapter focuses on the reconstruction methods in the total laparoscopy distal gastrectomy (LDG) operation, explains the merits and demerits of several methods, and introduces our original method, named augmented rectangle technique (ART).

Keywords: LDG, Billroth I and II, R-Y, delta, ART

1. Introduction

Gastric cancer operations have the most impact on food intake and body weight loss, resulting in more changes in patient's circumstances than any other surgery [1–3]. Its morbidity and mortality are, respectively, ranked fifth and third in the world—with the incidence in China, Japan, and Korea, the highest in the world. Even now, with chemotherapy and immunotherapy well progressed, surgery is still required for the curable treatment for that cancer [4, 5].

Laparoscopy-assisted distal gastrectomy (LADG) with gastroduodenostomy for early gastric cancer was first reported in 1994 by professor Kitano. Initially, hand-associated or small incisional open laparotomy reconstruction, the so-called associated operation, was performed. Full laparoscopic operation is much better for the patients, due to small wound, less pain, and quick recovery. According to the 12th Nationwide Survey of Endoscopic Surgery in Japan, in

2013, 52.7% of patients who underwent distal gastrectomy underwent laparoscopic surgery [1]. After distal gastrectomy, several reconstruction methods are available, and the choice of reconstruction is usually dependent on surgeons or institutions. There are three famous reconstruction methods, Billroth I and II and Roux-en-Y. Studies comparing gastroduodenostomy with gastrojejunostomy are still lacking and inconsistent; therefore, controversy remains regarding which method is the best after distal gastrectomy.

Billroth I gastroduodenostomy is one of most common reconstruction methods, and it offers advantages such as the following: (1) it is the only way to preserve the physiological root of the food passing through the duodenum, (2) it has technical simplicity during open surgery, and (3) it confers a lower incidence of internal hernia or adhesions. However, the risk of anastomotic failure is higher, and the laparoscopic gastrointestinal anastomosis involves a high degree of difficulty. Of course, if the size of gastric remnant is too small, Billroth I reconstruction cannot be done. These methods for total laparoscopic operation are the most difficult and have developed by experts during more than 10 years.

Billroth II gastrojejunostomy shares some pros and cons with the Billroth I and Roux-en-Y methods. It enables a wide stomach resection without anastomotic tension and is relatively easy during laparoscopic surgery. However, postoperative bile reflux into the remnant stomach is more frequent, and, although rare, afferent loop syndrome can develop.

Roux-en-Y gastrojejunostomy prevents bile reflux [1]. Other advantages over Billroth I are as follows. It is acceptable if the gastric remnant is too small to perform Billroth I, and there is less anastomotic tension. However, the high incidence of Roux stasis syndrome is one of its major drawbacks and, although rare, leakage of duodenal stump is a severe complication.

2. Billroth I

Billroth I is the most common and physiological reconstruction method after distal gastrectomy. For laparoscopy-assisted distal gastrectomy (LADG), Billroth I reconstruction can be performed by an extracorporeal or intracorporeal method. Initially, hand-associated or small incisional open laparotomy reconstruction, so-called associated operation, was performed. Due to an increasing number of laparoscopic gastrectomies, the laparoscopic technique has become possible for total laparoscopic distal gastrectomy (TLDG). This portion describes old extra-methods and new intra-methods.

2.1. Extracorporeal Billroth I anastomosis

Extracorporeal Billroth I anastomosis has several merits when compared to intracorporeal anastomosis. Tumor location is identified by palpitation. It is easily and rapidly performed like conventional open surgery, and it uses fewer staples than the intracorporeal anastomosis. For the problem of the cost, extracorporeal Billroth I is still the most common reconstruction method for LADG. Additionally, extracorporeal anastomosis is a procedure that should be considered as the first choice in view of safety in the inexperienced facility learning laparoscopic gastrectomy.

2.1.1. *Extracorporeal hemi-double stapling technique*

After lymph node dissection, a 4–6 cm minilaparotomy is made at the upper midline (**Figure 1**) [6]. The stomach is pulled out of the peritoneal cavity through the small incision, which is applied by a wound retractor (**Figure 2**). A purse-string instrument is applied to the duodenum distal to the resection line. A Lister forceps is applied just proximal to the purse-string clamp, and the duodenum is transected between the two clamps (**Figure 3**). The duodenal stump is unclamped and held by Alice forceps equally at three points. An anvil is inserted into the duodenal stump, and a purse-string suture is tied over the anvil (**Figure 4**). Then, the duodenal stump is returned to the abdominal cavity; at this time, the purse-string suture thread is clamped without cutting it, leaving the clamp outside of the abdominal cavity. The greater curvature side of the proximal resection margin is transited with an 80-mm linear stapler (**Figure 5**). Thereafter, an entry hole is made along the lesser curvature side of the previous staple line at the disbanded of 3 cm to the lesser curvature; the shaft of the circular stapler is introduced into the gastric remnant through the gastrostomy (**Figure 6**). The shaft is rotated toward the duodenum with the distal stomach, and then the trocar is advanced to penetrate the corner of the stapling line at the greater curvature (**Figure 7**). The trocar is connected to the anvil placed in the duodenum. The instrument is closed and fired, completing the end-to-end gastroduodenostomy. After checking for bleeding at the anastomotic line, the lesser curvature side of proximal resection margin is transected with another linear stapler (**Figure 8**).

2.1.2. *Extracorporeal end-to-side posterior wall method*

The distal gastrectomy procedure is the same as for the abovementioned method [6]. For resection of the proximal margin, the stomach is transected 5 cm from the greater curvature to the middle of the planned resection line using two clamps, and the remaining proximal resection is done using an 80-mm linear stapler. After distal gastrectomy, the head of the circular stapler is inserted into the remnant stomach through the opening of the greater curvature side of the proximal resection, which was temporarily clamped. The trocar is advanced

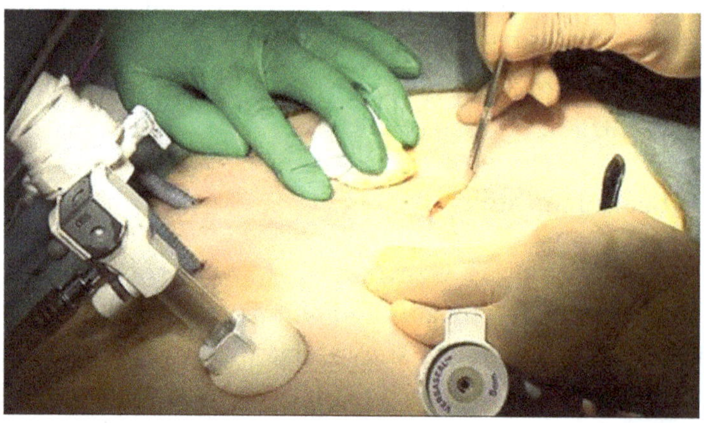

Figure 1. Extracorporeal hemi-double stapling technique – depiction of procedure as described in the text, step 1.

to pass through the posterior wall of the remnant stomach and then coupled on the anvil placed in the duodenum. The device is closed and fired, completing the end-to-side gastroduodenostomy. Finally, the opening in the remnant stomach is shuttered using an additional linear stapler.

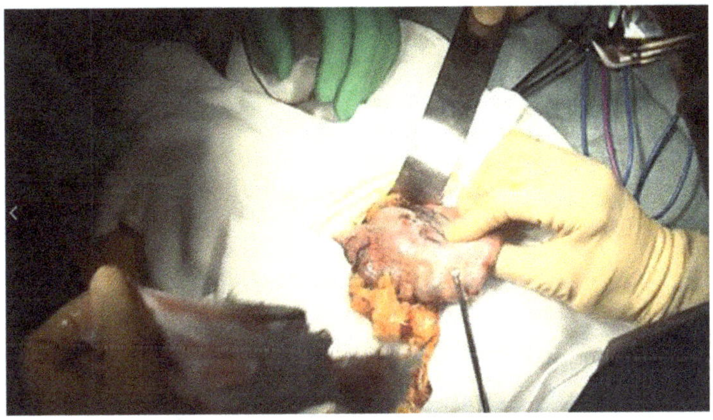

Figure 2. Extracorporeal hemi-double stapling technique – depiction of procedure as described in the text, step 2.

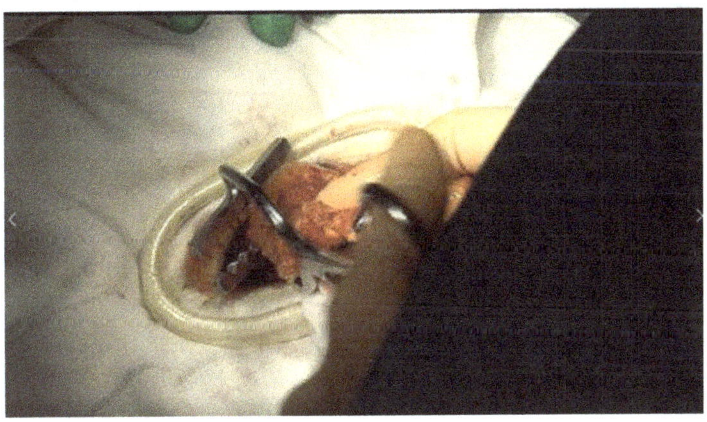

Figure 3. Extracorporeal hemi-double stapling technique – depiction of procedure as described in the text, step 3.

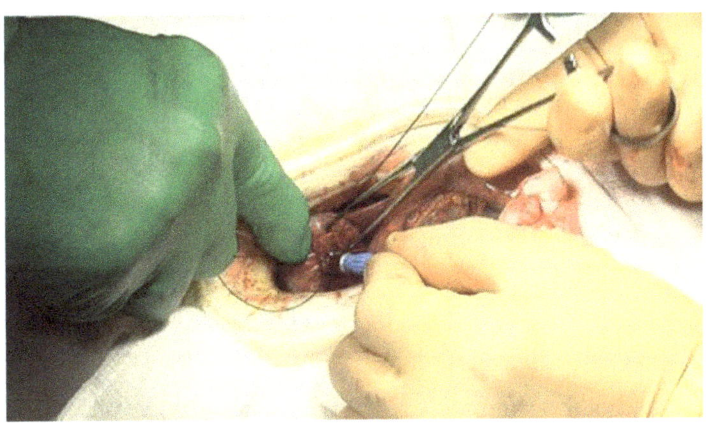

Figure 4. Extracorporeal hemi-double stapling technique – depiction of procedure as described in the text, step 4.

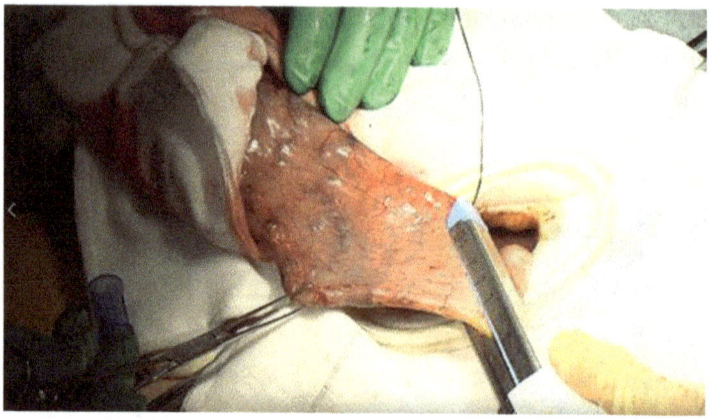

Figure 5. Extracorporeal hemi-double stapling technique – depiction of procedure as described in the text, step 5.

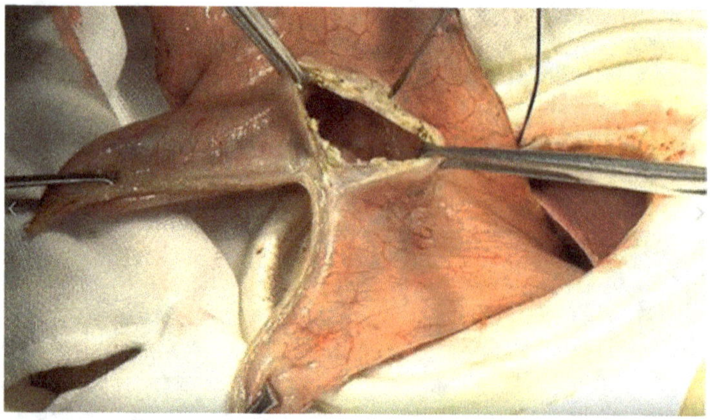

Figure 6. Extracorporeal hemi-double stapling technique – depiction of procedure as described in the text, step 6.

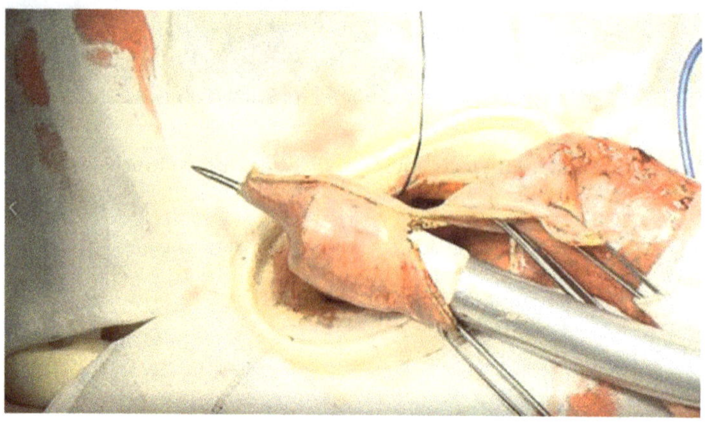

Figure 7. Extracorporeal hemi-double stapling technique – depiction of procedure as described in the text, step 7.

In this method, there is no overlap between the liner stapler and circular stapler, which is said to be likely to cause anastomotic leakage in general, but the possibility of an ischemic area remaining between the liner stapler and the circular stapler is considered a problem. In order to avoid this complication, it is said to set the place to puncture the back wall ten from liner stapler, but then the "dog's ear" deformation remains widely.

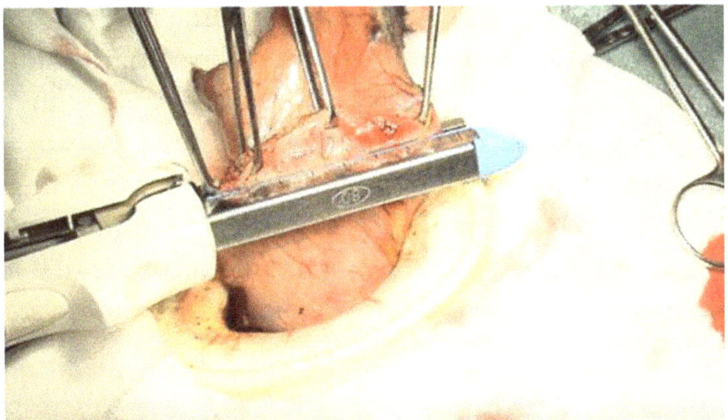

Figure 8. Extracorporeal hemi-double stapling technique – depiction of procedure as described in the text, step 8.

2.2. Intracorporeal Billroth I anastomosis

2.2.1. Delta-shaped anastomosis

The delta-shaped anastomosis originally created by Professor Kanaya is a functional end-to-end gastroduodenostomy technique using endoscopic linear staplers [7].

For the duodenal bulbus resection, the direction of the stapling is more vertical than the mesenteric-antimesenteric direction. End-to-end anastomosis is done vertically to maintain an enough blood supply to the anastomosis and to preserve a space for the jaw of 45-mm linear stapler to be inserted into the entry hole. Before stapler firing, the staple line on the remnant stomach is rotated to the left side, and the staple line on the duodenal stump is rotated to the right side to form a side-to-side gastroduodenostomy between the posterior wall of the remnant stomach and the posterior wall of the duodenum. After firing the stapler, a relatively large entry hole is made, and the operator checks for anastomotic bleeding through this hole. After transient approximation of the entry hole with clips, the hole is closed by two consecutive firings of a 45-mm liner stapler.

2.2.2. Intracorporeal triangular anastomotic technique (INTACT)

The other intracorporeal anastomosis method, novel intracorporeal triangular anastomotic technique, was reported by Omori et al. [8].

After all dissection of lymph nodes is finished, the stomach and duodenal bulb are staple-transected parallelly, and the resected stomach with dissected LNs is retrieved through the umbilical incision. Small entry holes are made on the greater curvature side, for each of the remnant stomach and the duodenal bulb, leaving a space almost 1 cm away from each stapling line. The cartridge side of the linear stapler (45-mm articulating medium/thick cartridge) is inserted to the transection line of the stomach. Then, the linear stapler fork side is carefully inserted into the bulb via the hole parallelly. This process makes The cartridge side is inserted parallel to the transection line of the stomach. The posterior walls, so-call V-shaped anastomosis, of both the gastric remnant and the bulbs, the dorsal side of the posterior suture line of the Billroth I. After arresting hemorrhage of the suture line, the entry hole is sutured by 2–3 points temporarily, avoiding slipping the liner staple. Finally, the entry hole is closed by a 45-mm linear stapler suture and created completing the anterior half of the anastomosis. The almost

60° anastomotic angle between the second anastomotic line and the first suture line is best designed for passing the food. This second anastomotic line length should be approximately 30 mm without the ventral staple lines. Thirdly, the linear staple with a 60-mm articulating medium/thick cartridge is placed in the direction toward the posterior wall and also placed almost perpendicular to the transection line of the stomach for resecting the blood less area. Those three staplers created the triangular anastomosis and simultaneously removed three staple lines of the duodenal transection line, the ventral line of the first anastomosis, the end of gastric transection line, and the ischemic tissues in between these staple lines. This technique yielded an end-to-end anastomosis of a triangular orifice [9].

2.2.3. *Augmented rectangle technique*

We have reported that laparoscopy-assisted distal gastrectomy (LADG) with extended lymph node dissection for gastric cancer was technically feasible and had favorable oncologic outcomes compared to the open gastrectomy [1, 10]. Unlike the extracorporeal anastomosis performed during the LADG, a standardized reconstruction method has not been established for the Billroth I (BI) gastroduodenostomy in the totally laparoscopic distal gastrectomy (LDG). A triangle anastomosis or a delta-shaped anastomosis is reported for the LDG without associated laparotomy. However, these two methods seem complicated for the LDG because of the need for stay sutures and further have the risks of ischemia or stenosis postoperatively. Therefore, we have developed an "augmented rectangle technique (ART)" as a new BI anastomosis performed during the LDG. The ART does not need stay sutures and therefore facilitates the LDG.

A 12-mm trocar for the laparoscope is inserted into the umbilicus. A 12-mm trocar is introduced into the left premaxillary line 1 cm below the costal margin. A second 12-mm trocar is inserted into the left midclavicular line 2 cm above the umbilicus. A 5-mm trocar is inserted into the right premaxillary line 1 cm below the costal margin. A third 12-mm trocar is placed by the camera assistant between the patient's legs (**Figure 9**).

Duodenal resection is performed with the surgeon's right hand using a 60-mm endoscopic linear stapler (ELS) from the greater curvature side of duodenum to lesser curvature side. The duodenum is transected just below the pyloric ring because it is necessary to preserve a long duodenum for anastomosis (**Figure 10**).

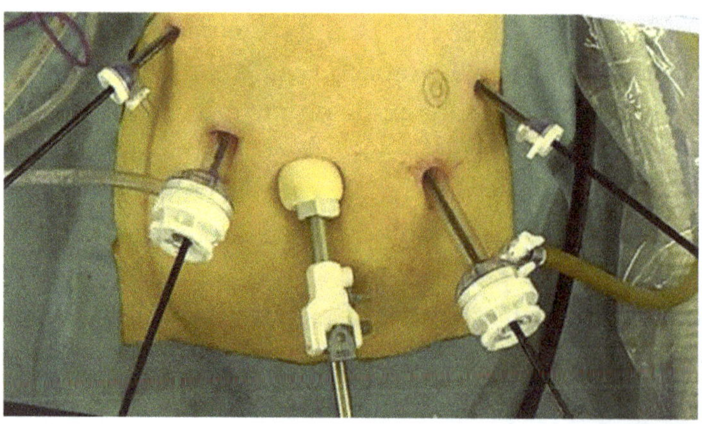

Figure 9. Augmented rectangle technique – depiction of procedure as described in the text, step 1.

Gastric resection is also done using two 60-mm ELS through the 12-mm trocar of the left lower quadrant from greater curvature to lesser curvature (**Figure 11**).

The superior duodenal vessels along the lesser curvature are transected to mobilize the duodenum (**Figure 12**).

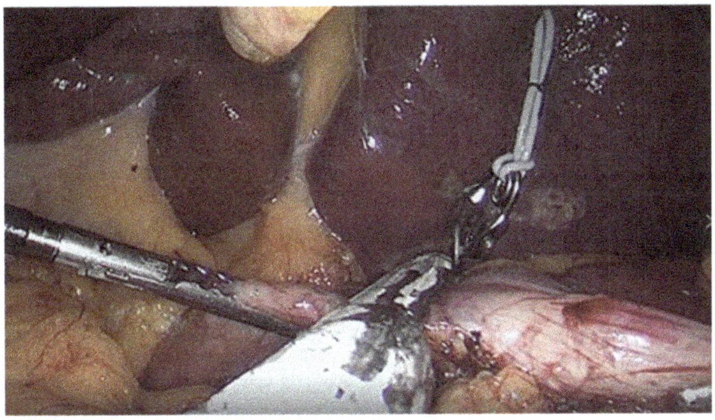

Figure 10. Augmented rectangle technique – depiction of procedure as described in the text, step 2.

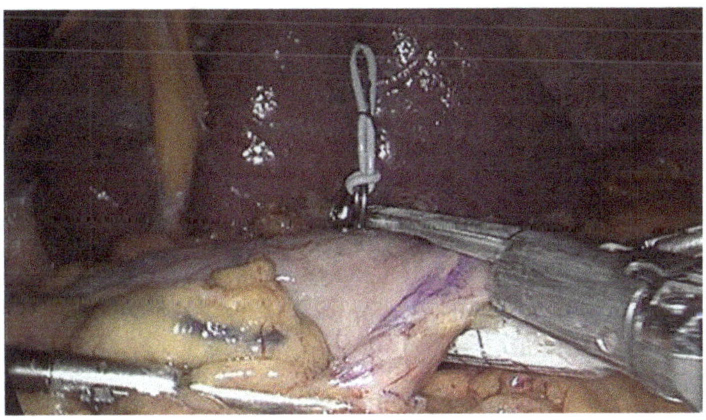

Figure 11. Augmented rectangle technique – depiction of procedure as described in the text, step 3.

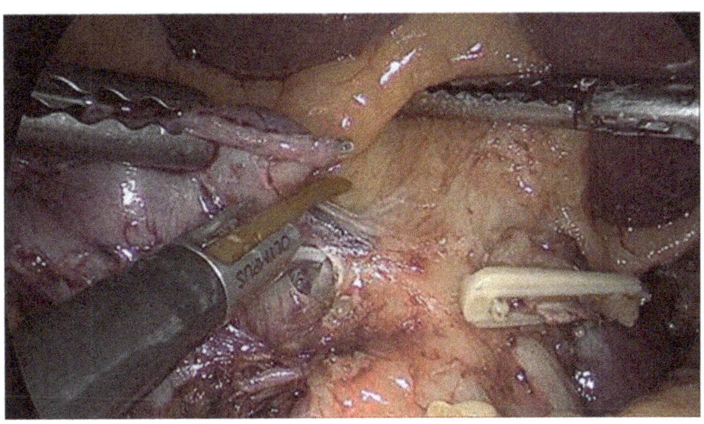

Figure 12. Augmented rectangle technique – depiction of procedure as described in the text, step 4.

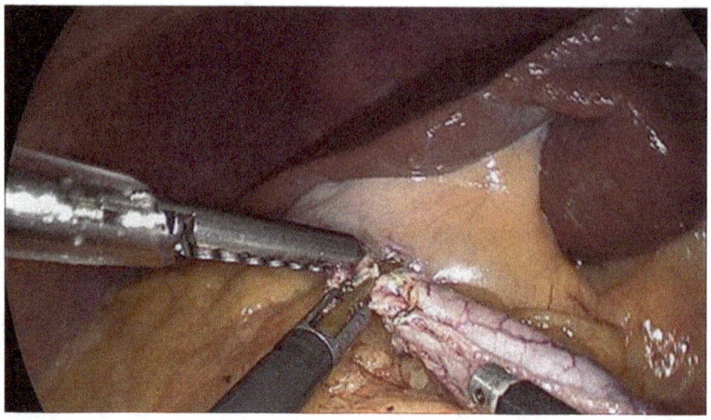

Figure 13. Augmented rectangle technique – depiction of procedure as described in the text, step 5.

An entry hole is made on the tip of the greater curvature side of the duodenal stump. The surgeon holds the tip of greater curvature side of the duodenal stump by his left hand located upside, and the assistant holds the tip of lesser curvature side of the duodenal stump by her right hand. Also, an assistant holds a suction by her left hand to prevent contamination by digestive tract contents in the abdominal cavity. A 5-mm incision is created in the previous stapled line at the greater curvature side of duodenal stump (**Figure 13**). Also, an entry hole is made on the tip of greater curvature side of remnant stomach (**Figure 14**).

The thicker cartridge fork of the 60-mm ELS is inserted into the stomach through the 12-mm trocar of the left lower quadrant. At this time, the tip of the ELS is pressed against the posterior gastric wall 2 cm away from the gastric resection margin, and the ELS is used to grasp the tissue close to the suture line near the ELS entry hole (**Figure 15**).

An ELS gently holding the posterior wall of the remnant stomach is rotated clockwise to the duodenal side, which is then ready for the gastroduodenostomy. The surgeon, who is standing on the patient's right, opens the ELS and moves its thinner jaw to cover the duodenum. The margin of resection at the lesser curvature end of the duodenum is rotated externally by 90° (**Figure 16**). The entire length of the ELS is inserted, and the device is then closed and

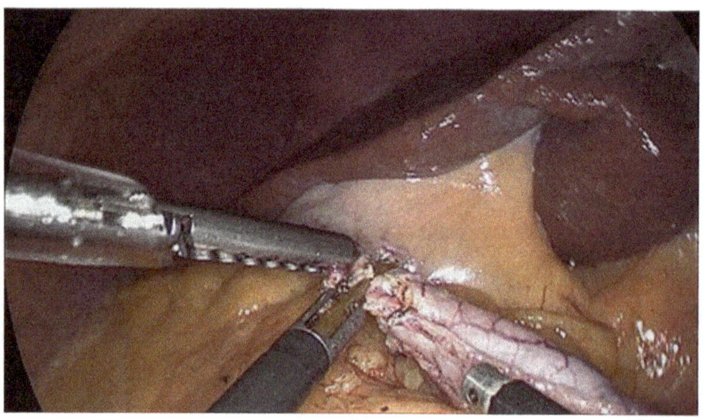

Figure 14. Augmented rectangle technique – depiction of procedure as described in the text, step 6.

fired. The ELS is withdrawn, the lumen is examined to confirm the absence of hemorrhage, and the residual duodenum and stomach are once again placed under adequate traction (**Figure 17**).

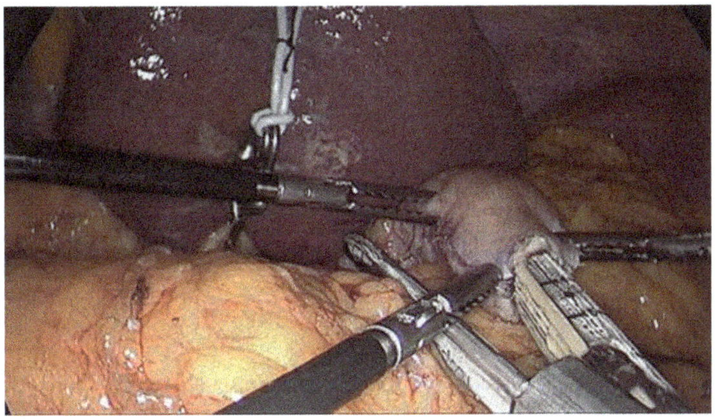

Figure 15. Augmented rectangle technique – depiction of procedure as described in the text, step 7.

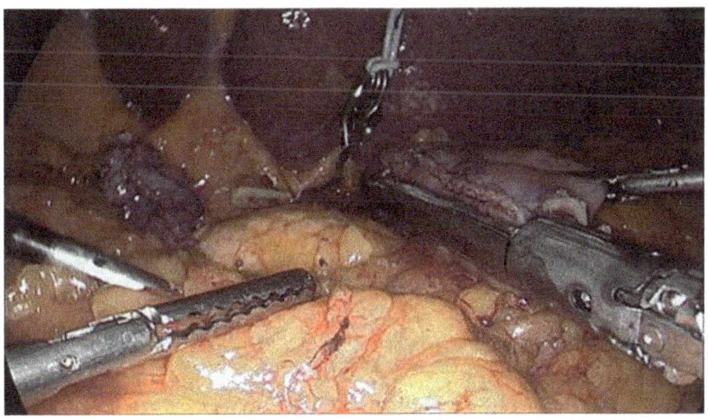

Figure 16. Augmented rectangle technique – depiction of procedure as described in the text, step 8.

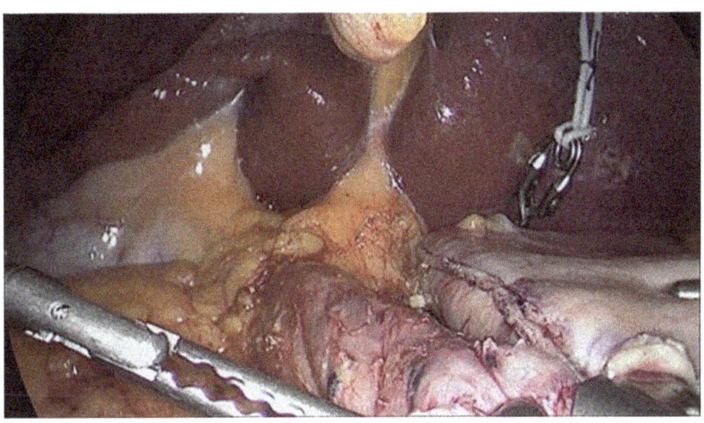

Figure 17. Augmented rectangle technique – depiction of procedure as described in the text, step 9.

Next, the insertion hole is closed, and a margin is created with the use of a 30-mm ELS. This margin is closed on this side to avoid the need for stapling the transected duodenal margin (**Figure 18**). The surgeon grasps the cranial ends of a V-shaped suture line created with the first ELS, and care is taken to ensure that the gastric and duodenal resection margins remain

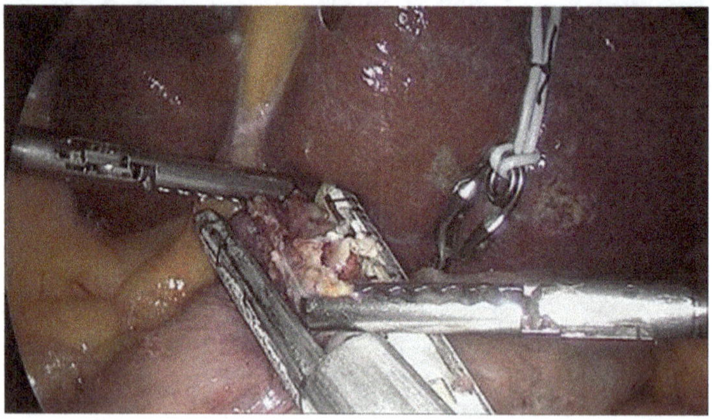

Figure 18. Augmented rectangle technique – depiction of procedure as described in the text, step 10.

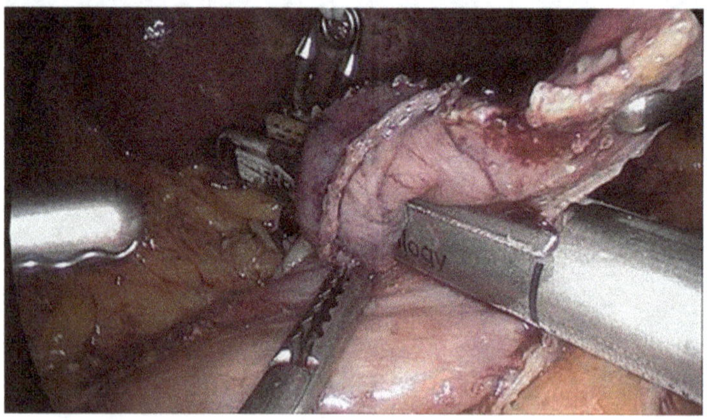

Figure 19. Augmented rectangle technique – depiction of procedure as described in the text, step 11.

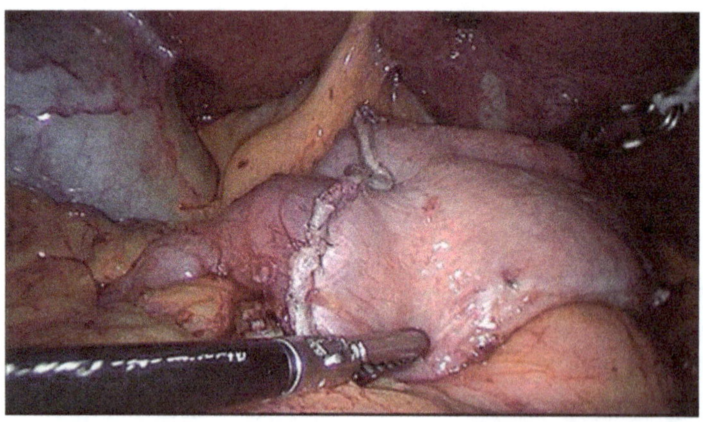

Figure 20. Augmented rectangle technique – depiction of procedure as described in the text, step 12.

close together. This creates the third side of a rectangle. Next, a 60-mm ELS is used to create the fourth side of the rectangle, while the entire stapled duodenal stump is being removed. The surgeon places caudolateral traction on the duodenal stump. Meanwhile, the assistant adjusts the position of the ELS to ensure overlap between the two suture lines, the first being along the second staple line and the second being along the gastric stump (**Figure 19**). With this suturing, the end-to-end anastomosis with an augmented rectangular gastroduodenal anastomotic stoma is complete (**Figure 20**).

3. Roux-en-Y reconstruction (RY)

Roux-en-Y reconstruction is one of the standard options after distal gastrectomy. In 1995, Kitano et al. used an extracorporeal gastrojejunostomy with manual suturing as a reconstruction procedure for distal gastrectomy. The improvements in stapling devices contributed to easy access to the site of operation. The advantage and disadvantage of RY reconstruction compared with Billroth I are as follows: prevention of bile reflex and reduction in incidence of anastomotic leakage.

3.1. Antecolic isoperistaltic RY reconstruction

A 12-mm trocar is inserted through the umbilical region by the open procedure, and then CO_2 pneumoperitoneum is established. A 12-mm trocar is introduced into the left pre-axillary line 1 cm below the costal margin. A 5-mm trocar is inserted into the left midclavicular line 2 cm above the umbilicus. The second 5-mm trocar is inserted into the right pre-axillary line 1 cm below the costal margin. Another 12-mm trocar is placed by the camera assistant between the patient's legs.

Laparoscopic mobilization of the stomach and lymph node dissection are carried out in a conventional procedure. The duodenum is divided distal to the pylorus with a 60-mm ELS; then, the stomach is divided with two ELSs. The specimen is removed through an extended 4-cm incision in the umbilical port. Following re-establishment of the pneumoperitoneum, the jejunum 20 cm distal to the ligament of Treitz is prepared for Roux limb, and the mesentery of this jejunum is divided for a distance of 8 cm. The prepared jejunum is then divided with an ELS to ensure a gastrojejunostomy without tension. A side-side jejunojejunostomy is fashioned 25 cm distal to the planed gastrojejunostomy using an ELS under direct vision through the umbilical incision. The jejunojejunostomy defect is closed with absorbable suture in an intermittent fashion. Following re-pneumoperitoneum, the jejunal limb is brought to the gastric remnant through an antecolic route. A right-oriented Roux limb is created such that the cut end of the Roux limb faces the greater curvature of remnant stomach. The jejunal limb is anastomosed to the greater curvature of remnant stomach side to side with an ELS; then, the site of entry hole is closed using an absorbable barbed suture. The duodenal stump is embedded with seromuscular suture and then fixed with the alimentary limb on the duodenal stump in a proper radian.

3.2. Antecolic antiperistaltic RY reconstruction

The duodenum and stomach are divided distal to the pylorus with three 60-mm ELSs. The specimen is removed through an extended 4-cm incision in the umbilical port. After re-pneumoperitoneum, the proximal jejunum is identified and divided 25 cm distal to the Treitz ligament, and the mesentery of the jejunum is divided. The jejunum is divided with a 60-mm ELS. Small holes are made at the tips of linear stapler of the greater curvature side of the remnant stomach and distal side of jejunal stump. The gastrojejunostomy is performed between the posterior wall of remnant stomach and antimesenteric border of the distal jejunum with a 60-mm ELS. The common entry hole is closed with a 60-mm ELS. The jejunojejunostomy is performed through an umbilical minilaparotomy with a 60-mm ELS and hand-sewn suture.

4. Billroth II anastomosis

A Billroth II gastrojejunostomy enables wide stomach resection without anastomotic tension and is relatively easy during laparoscopic surgery. However, postoperative bile reflex into the remnant stomach is bothersome, and although rare, afferent loop syndrome can develop. So, Billroth II is rarely performed in Japan, but according to a nationwide survey conducted in 2014 in Korea, Billroth II was the adopted reconstruction after distal gastrectomy in 35.8% of cases [2].

4.1. Surgical procedure of Billroth II gastrojejunostomy

Herein, a laparoscopy-assisted uncut Roux-en-Y operation after distal gastrectomy as reported by Uyama et al. is described [11].

A laparoscopic mobilization of the stomach and en bloc lymph node dissection is performed, with a 4-cm long minilaparotomy made on the upper abdomen, through which the en bloc mobilized stomach and lymph nodes were delivered and the stomach is transected.

Laparoscopy-assisted reconstruction is then started. First, the transverse colon is retracted cephalad to expose the ligament of Treitz, and the jejunum 25 cm distal to this ligament is delivered via the minilaparotomy. The position of the gastrojejunostomy, whose length is 4 cm, is determined. Next, a Braun anastomosis is created extracorporeally. A stapler without a blade is placed across the afferent jejunal limb just distal to the created Braun anastomosis. This stapler is closed and fired extracorporeally, which enables occlusion of the afferent jejunal lumen without division of the jejunum. Seromuscular sutures are placed on this staple line, and delivered jejunum is replaced into the abdominal cavity. The operation turns again to a laparoscopic procedure. The gastrojejunostomy is started while observing the created Braun anastomosis and stapling across the jejunum laparoscopically. The corner of the greater curvature of the stomach stump is cut, and a small hole is made on the site of the planned gastrojejunostomy, using laparoscopic coagulating shears.

One jaw of the endoscopic linear stapler is inserted into the jejunum and the other into the stomach. The device is closed and fired, creating a gastrojejunostomy. The firing of the stapler converts the two holes into one common entry hole, which is closed by a laparoscopic hand-sewn technique. Two seromuscular sutures are placed between the afferent loop and lesser curvature of the gastric remnant to lift up the afferent loop, with the aim of preventing food flowing into the afferent loop. Finally, the seromuscular suture between the stomach and efferent loop is placed on the top of created V-shaped anastomosis, because this is the weakest point, due to the remaining tension.

5. Discussion

Our policy of reconstruction after distal gastrectomy is as follows. The first choice is Billroth I reconstruction. If the remnant stomach is too small for Billroth I reconstruction, we perform isoperistaltic RY reconstruction.

To date, we have used ART in 160 patients who underwent laparoscopic distal gastrectomy for stomach cancer between December 2013 and August 2017. These included 50 women and 110 men, with a mean age of 69.5 years and a mean body mass index (BMI) of 21.8. D1+ lymphadenectomy was performed in 81 patients, and D2 lymphadenectomy in 79 patients. The mean operation time was 227 minutes, and the mean blood loss volume was 47.3 mL. There were no intraoperative complications associated with reconstruction of the gastrointestinal tract, and none of the patients required conversion to open surgery. There were also no postoperative complications, such as anastomotic leakage or stenosis, associated with the reconstruction, and the mean postoperative hospital stay was 12 days (**Table 1**). Postoperative endoscopic examinations typically confirmed a large, elliptical anastomotic stoma (**Figure 21**).

Sex
Age
Body mass index
Operation time
Intraoperative blood loss
Extent of lymph node dissection
D1+/D2
Clinical stage
I/II/III/IV
Conversion to open surgery
Postoperative complications
Anastomosis-related complications
Anastomotic leakage
Anastomotic hemorrhage
Delayed gastric emptying
Non-anastomosis-related complications
Pancreatic fistula
Intra-abdominal infection
Intraperitoneal hemorrhage
Surgical site infection
Time to oral intake
Postoperative hospital stay

Table 1. Characteristics of patients in whom ART-based anastomosis was performed ($n = 160$).

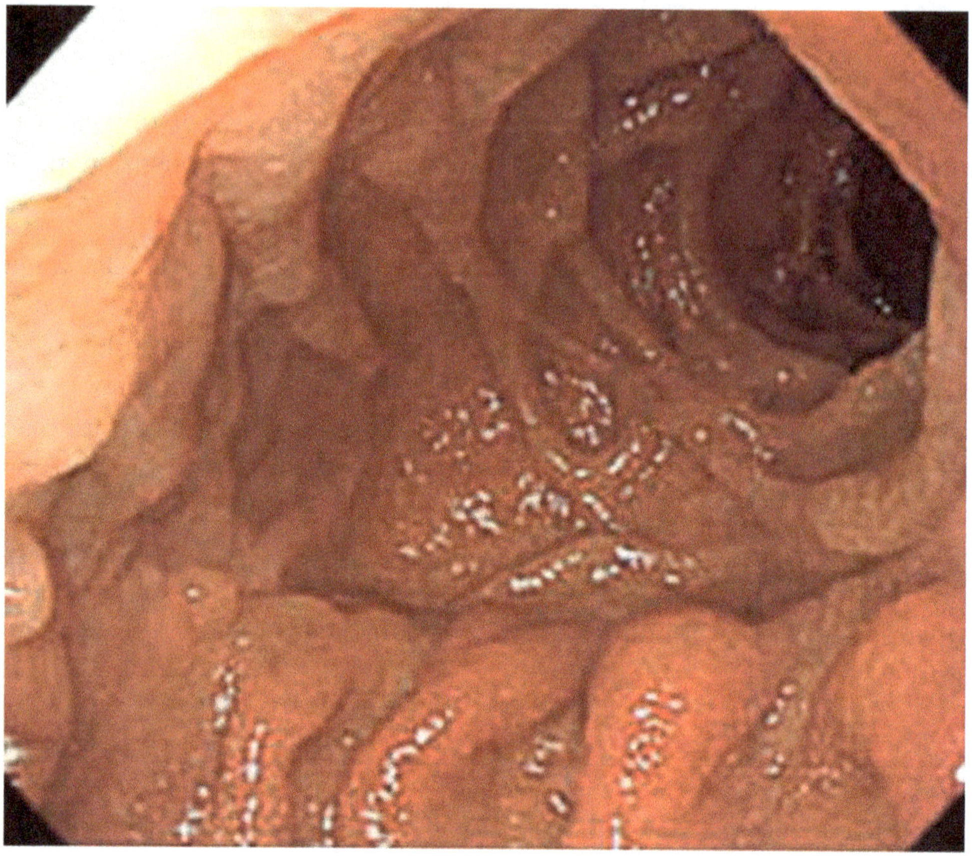

Figure 21. Elliptical anastomotic stoma in postoperative examination.

We performed antecolic isoperistaltic RY reconstruction in 52 consecutive patients who underwent laparoscopic gastrectomy for gastric cancer between April 2015 and December 2017. There were 32 women and 20 men, with a mean age of 70.4 years and mean body mass index of 22.3. D1+ lymphadenectomy was performed in 35 patients, and D2 lymphadenectomy in 17 patients. The mean operation time was 282 min, and the mean blood loss volume was 35.8 ml. All of the procedures were free of intraoperative complications. There were no postoperative complications, such as anastomotic leakage, intestinal obstruction, and duodenal stump leakage.

Author details

Satoshi Kanda* and Tetsu Fukunaga

*Address all correspondence to: st-kanda@juntendo.ac.jp

Gastroenterology and Minimally Invasive Surgery, Juntendo University, Tokyo, Japan

References

[1] Fukunaga T, Ishibashi Y, et al. Augmented rectangle technique for Billroth I anastomosis in totally laparoscopic distal gastrectomy for gastric cancer. Surgical Endoscopy. 2018. DOI: 10.1007/s00464-018-6266-1

[2] He Z, Zang L. Reconstruction after laparoscopic assisted gastrectomy: Technical tips and pitfalls. Translational Gastroenterology and Hepatology. 2017;**2**:66

[3] Japan Society for Endoscopic Surgery: 12th Nationwide Survey of Endoscopic Surgery in Japan. Journal of Japan Society for Endoscopic Surgery. 2014;**19**:495-640

[4] Bandoh T, Shiraishi N, et al. Endoscopic surgery in Japan: The 12th national survey (2012-2013) by the Japan Society for Endoscopic Surgery. Asian Journal of Endoscopic Surgery. 2017;**10**:345-353

[5] Clark CJ, Thirlby RC, Picozzi V, Schembre DB, Cummings FP, Lin E. Current problems in surgery: Gastric cancer. Current Problems in Surgery. 2006;**43**:566-670

[6] Kitano S, Yang H-K. Laparoscopic Gastrectomy for Cancer. Springer; 2012. pp. 89-93

[7] Kanaya S, Gomi T, et al. Delta-shaped anastomosis in totally laparoscopic billroth I gastrectomy: New technique of intraabdominal gastroduodenostomy. Journal of the American College of Surgeons. 2002;**195**:284-287

[8] Omori T, Matsuzawa T, et al. A simple and safe method for Billroth I reconstruction in single-incision laparoscopic gastrectomy using a novel intracorporeal triangular anastomotic technique. Journal of Gastrointestinal Surgery. 2014;**18**:613-616

[9] The Information Committee of Korean Gastric Cancer Association. Korean gastric cancer association nationwide survey on gastric cancer in 2014. Journal of Gastric Cancer. 2016;**16**(3):131-140

[10] Annals of Surgical Oncology. 2013;**20**:2676-2682

[11] Uyama I, Sakurai Y, et al. Laparoscopy-assisted uncut roux-en Y operation after distal gastrectomy for gastric cancer. Gastric Cancer. 2005;**8**:253-257

8

The Clinical Relevance of Gastroesophageal Reflux Disease and Laryngopharyngeal Reflux in Clinical Practice

Aragona Salvatore Emanuele,
Mereghetti Giada and Giorgio Ciprandi

Abstract

Gastric reflux may be considered a para-physiological event that may occur up to 50 times a day. It usually happens when gas (less commonly liquids) flow back from stomach into esophagus. However, when defense mechanisms leave, disease may progress. If the esophagus is the trigger, gastroesophageal reflux disease (GERD) emerges. The prevalence of GERD in the primary care setting seems to be even more evident when one considers that, in the United States, 4.6 million office encounters annually are primarily for GERD, whereas 9.1 million encounters include GERD in the top 3 diagnoses for the encounter. GERD constitutes also the most frequently first-listed gastrointestinal diagnosis in ambulatory care visits. In addition, the extraesophageal manifestations of reflux, including LPR, asthma, and chronic cough, have been estimated to cost $5438 per patient in direct medical expenses in the first year after presentation and $13,700 for 5 years. Presently, the newest alginate compounds renowned the interest in this attracting and stimulating area. In this regard, a new medical device (Marial®), unique still now possessing the indication for both GERD and LPR, has been recently launched in the Italian market, two large surveys were conducted in Italy: RELIEF, involving 86 otolaryngologists, and EMERGE, involving 56 gastroenterologists. The aims of these surveys were: (1) to define clinical characteristics, including previous treatment, of the patients referred to consultation; (2) to evaluate the reliability of RFS, GIS, and RSI questionnaires in real-world settings, such as specialist office; and (3) to investigate the patients' perception of efficacy of the prescribed therapy, based on the best practice and considering also the new medical device Comparing the patients' perception of treatment efficacy, reduction in RSI values for each single symptom before and after a 4 week-treatment with Marial® alone or with PPI in add-on in EMERGE and RELIEF patients are reported. Marial® alone treatment induced a statistically significant higher reduction in each single symptom in RELIEF patients than in EMERGE patients, with the exception of heartburn, chest pain, indigestion, or stomach acid coming up. Similar results were obtained evaluating the reduction in RSI values in patients treated with PPI in add-on that was able to determine a higher statistically significant decrease in RELIEF than in EMERGE patients in each single symptom, with the exception of heartburn, chest pain, indigestion, or stomach acid coming up.

Keywords: regenerative medicine, GERD, LPR

1. Background

Actually, gastric reflux may be considered a para-physiological event that may occur up to 50 times a day. It usually happens when gas (less commonly liquids) flow back from stomach into esophagus. However, when defense mechanisms leave, disease may progress. If the esophagus is the trigger, gastroesophageal reflux disease (GERD) emerges. On the other hand, laryngopharyngeal reflux (LPR) is considered an extraesophageal manifestation of the GERD. Both GERD and its extraesophageal manifestation are very common in clinical practice. Both disorders have a relevant burden for the society: many pharmaco-economic studies were conducted in the United States. In population-based studies, 19.8% of North Americans complain of GERD symptoms, including heartburn and regurgitation, at least weekly [1]. Likewise, in the late 1990s, GERD accounted for $9.3 to $12.1 billion in direct annual healthcare costs in the United States, higher than any other digestive disease. Consequently, acid-suppressive agents are still the leading pharmaceutical expenditure in the United States.

The prevalence of GERD in the primary care setting seems to be even more evident when one considers that, in the United States, 4.6 million office encounters annually are primarily for GERD, whereas 9.1 million encounters include GERD in the top 3 diagnoses for the encounter. GERD constitutes also the most frequently first-listed gastrointestinal diagnosis in ambulatory care visits [2, 3]. In addition, the extraesophageal manifestations of reflux, including LPR, asthma, and chronic cough, have been estimated to cost $5438 per patient in direct medical expenses in the first year after presentation and $13,700 for 5 years. Estimates of the economic burden of extraesophageal reflux have shown that expenditures for extraesophageal manifestations of reflux could surpass $50 billion, 86% of which could be attributable to pharmaceutical costs [2, 3]. In addition, the National Health Care Survey carried out by the Center for Disease Control and Prevention has reported that the main complaint for primary care patient visits was cough in 6.1%, throat symptoms in 4%, and asthma in 2.8% [4]. Within these visits for cough, asthma, and throat symptoms are contained the hidden prevalence of extraesophageal manifestations of GERD, which to date have not been adequately addressed from a medical or surgical perspective due to their perceived obscurity. Therefore, the gastric reflux, globally understood, represents a very important medical issue that deserves adequate attention in daily practice.

From a pathophysiological point of view, gastric reflux includes different mechanisms, such as the provocation and perception of reflux. The transient lower esophageal sphincter relaxations (TLESR), hiatus hernia, acid pocket, visceral hypersensitivity, and obesity represent important causes of gastric reflux. Impaired esophageal, and extraesophageal, mucosal integrity, poor esophageal clearance, and delayed gastric emptying could be associated with GERD development. In addition, another pathogenic factor is a neural reflex sustained by acid exposure: the so-called Reflex-Reflux [5].

Distinguishing whether cough, LPR, and asthma may be sustained by GERD remains difficult challenging for both the primary care physician and the specialist. The distinction between them is clinically relevant as treatment of GERD with the intent of improving or curing extraesophageal manifestation could be ineffective. To review the current literature on extraesophageal manifestations of reflux should assist in clinical decision making.

The Montreal Classification gave the most recent consensus definition of GERD. This document defines GERD as heartburn symptoms or complications resulting from the reflux of gastric contents into the esophagus, up to the oral cavity, and lungs [5]. GERD is again classified into two subgroups. The first subgroup is represented by GERD with heartburn symptoms but without endoscopic evidence of mucosal erosions (the so called Non-Erosive Reflux Disease or NERD). The second sub-group is GERD with heartburn symptoms accompanied by objective evidence of erosions, ulcers, and inflammation (the so called Erosive Reflux Disease or ERD) [6].

It has to be considered that functional heartburn might fall under endoscopic negative disease. However, it is important to note that it is a distinct entity from NERD. NERD is usually defined as typical reflux symptoms without evidence of reflux disease in endoscopy but abnormal acid exposure on the impedance-pH monitoring and is responsive to proton pump inhibitors - PPI [7, 8]. Functional heartburn on the other hand, as defined by Rome IV classification, is a retrosternal burning discomfort or pain refractory to anti-secretory therapy without presence of GERD, histopathologic abnormality, motility disorder or structural abnormality for at least 3 months with symptoms onset at least 6 months prior to the diagnosis [5].

As just defined, stomach content may also reflux outside of the esophagus into respiratory organs, such as extraesophageal reflux, including LPR. LPR is most commonly manifested as laryngeal symptoms such as coughing, hoarseness, dysphagia, globus, and sore throat, but there can be signs also of nose, sinus, ear, and eye involvement [9]. Epidemiological studies have shown that the prevalence of this LPR may be extremely high, that it has certain characteristics of an outbreak and that it is one of the most common causes of patient visits to their family medicine physicians, but also to otolaryngologists, gastroenterologists, pediatricians, pulmonologists, allergists, and psychiatrists [1, 10–13]. Today it has been proven that gastroesophageal reflux is not the only cause of LPR. LPR is a multifactorial syndrome with a vast clinical representation, during the disease and with complications, so it requires and deserves a multidisciplinary approach. Based on newly discovered findings about the specific pathogenesis of the disease, LPR may be considered a new clinical entity [11–13]. As once pointed out, GERD is caused by the lower esophageal sphincter dysfunction and the dysfunction of the stomach emptying mechanism. Esophageal mucosa has protective mechanisms against aggressive factors of the stomach content (mucosal barrier) and it remains intact when a physiological reflux occurs, which normally happens at night. However, laryngeal and pharyngeal mucosa do not possess the esophageal protective mechanisms, so acid and peptic activity of the stomach content quickly leads to mucosal lesions. Notably, laryngopharyngeal reflux occurs most commonly during the day as a result of the upper esophageal sphincter dysfunction. This aspect is intriguing as typical GERD symptoms usually occur in supine position and overnight. However, acidity of the stomach content is not the only cause of LPR. Pepsin with its proteolytic effects can be the determining factor. Other possible etiological factors are pancreatic proteolytic enzymes, bile salts, and bacteria [1, 13, 14]. Extraesophageal manifestations of stomach content reflux have only recently started being seen as important based on the assumption of their important role in causing respiratory tract diseases. In clinical practice, LPR is mostly not recognized because it may be a "silent reflux" and diagnostic and therapeutic protocols are still inadequate, so proper treatment is usually delayed. Laryngeal symptoms are the most common, so patients are managed by otolaryngologists. Indeed, otolaryngologists have developed the diagnostic Reflux Symptom Index (RSI) questionnaire based on the importance of certain disease symptoms and the Reflux Finding Score (RFS) based on frequency of pathological changes determined by laryngoscopy [15]. On the other hand, considering the high prevalence of the disease and uncharacteristic clinical image, most patients report to their family medicine physicians [14–17]. For family medicine physicians LPR represents an important medical problem and a challenge in fast diagnostics, proper treatment, and proper selection of patients who require additional multidisciplinary diagnostic procedures. Knowledge of pathogenic pathway of the disease and its clinical manifestations can help physicians in creating an adequate program for prevention, early diagnosis, and adequate therapy for LPR. In particular, it has to be considered that untreated LPR can be one of the etiological causes of laryngeal cancer. The development of the disease can be benign or malignant and life threatening, and all of its forms can considerably affect life quality in patients. Laryngeal pathological changes could be discovered with laryngoscopy, and some even with detailed esophagogastroscopy. These changes may include: edema, hyperemia, or erythema of the vocal chords and laryngeal edges, ventricular obliteration, granulation, presence of dense endolaryngeal secretion, and hypertrophy of the posterior commissure [10, 15]. As consequence, an appropriate diagnosis of LPR represents a challenge for general practitioner and specialists. A large number of clinical studies confirmed low specificity and sensitivity of diagnostic tests such as laryngoscopy, esophagogastroscopy, proximal pH monitoring (hypopharyngeal and oropharyngeal). Evaluation of symptoms using the Reflux Symptom Index is considered to be the basic diagnostic procedure. A newer method of measuring salivary pepsin (Pep-test) can confirm LPR diagnosis because its sensitivity and specificity is 87% [13]. In this regard, it has to be noted that pepsinogen is produced only in the stomach, so pepsin may be envisaged as a specific biomarker for gastric reflux. The Pep-test is a fast and non-invasive method and could have a wide variety of uses in primary health care.

LPR therapy is complex and requires also modification of the patient's lifestyle and habits. Body weight reduction and physical activity, quitting cigarettes and alcohol use are one of the first steps in lowering the intensity of symptoms in patients [17]. Nutritional interventions with correct food choices and bowel movement regulation lead to lowering dyspeptic complains, but also lower the number of reflux episodes. Emptying of the bowels causes lower intra-abdominal pressure, which leads to lower possibility of stomach content reflux into the esophagus, larynx and pharynx. Obesity, or more precisely high BMI, so including overweight, is an independent factor in stomach reflux occurrence because of its specific effect mechanism on the gastroesophageal juncture [17]. LPR treatment and management is supposed to reduce the acidity or stomach contents and neutralize acid-peptic activity in larynx, pharynx and esophagus. High dosages of PPI (proton pump inhibitors) have shown the best effects in reducing reflux in the course of 24 h. Alkaline water and alginates show a positive additional effect in lowering acid-peptic activity in the larynx and pharynx. Patients are supposed to have long-term treatment during the course of 6 months because of high sensitivity of the mucosal membrane in the stomach and pharynx. Difficult cases with a proven hiatal hernia can be considered for surgical treatment as well [6].

Therefore, acid suppression is the mainstay of therapy for gastric reflux, and PPIs are the most effective drug in this approach [18, 19]. Although PPIs are the treatment of choice for GERD, still approximately one-third of patients with GERD fail to respond symptomatically to a standard dose PPI, either partially or completely [20]. Actually, NERD accounts for 60–70% of GERD patients and is considered the most common presentation of GERD. However, only approximately 30–40% of NERD patients respond to a standard dose of PPIs, much lower than that in erosive esophagitis, and the low response rate to PPIs in NERD patients is the main contributor to the high portion of PPI failure phenomenon in GERD, and also LPR, management [21]. The mechanisms of failure of PPI therapy are complex and multifactorial [20, 22–24]. Consequently, other medications should be considered and used. In this context, alginates and histamine type-2 receptor antagonists (H2RAs) may provide additional benefit for symptom relief in patients with persistent symptoms despite PPI therapy and can be considered as add-on therapy for patients who fail with a PPI. However, because of the concern about tolerance, H2RA is suggested to be taken on demand or intermittently. PPI-refractory GERD (and LPR), defined as persistent reflux symptoms not responding to a double dose of a PPI therapy during a treatment period of at least 12 weeks, is an important issue in clinical practice and poses a great challenge for general practitioners, internists, gastroenterologists, and otolaryngologists [20]. Compliance with therapy should be verified first by the physician, and the presence of functional gastrointestinal disorders, psychological distress, functional heartburn or other esophagitis not related to reflux should also be carefully evaluated in these patients.

On the basis of these concepts, alginate may be considered a fruitful and relevant option in many patients with reflux disease. In particular, the knowledge about the utility of alginates derives from an interesting research area investigating the pathogenic role of the so-called "acid pocket." The acid pocket is a short zone of unbuffered highly acidic gastric juice that accumulates in the proximal stomach after meals. Serving as the source of acid reflux, the acid pocket increases the propensity for acid reflux by all conventional mechanisms, such as TLESR and hiatus hernia, and has been considered as an important cause of GERD [25, 26]. Alginate is an anionic polysaccharide occurring naturally in brown algae and has a unique property in the treatment of gastric reflux by eliminating the acid pocket. Alginate-antacid formulation can reduce postprandial symptoms by neutralizing the acidity of gastric contents. In addition to neutralizing the gastric acidity, more importantly, alginate and bicarbonate, usually contained in an alginate-based formulation, form a foamy gel that is like a raft floating on the surface of gastric contents after interacting with gastric acid, and this barrier-like gel displaces the acid pocket from the esophageal-gastric junction and protects both the esophageal and the upper respiratory mucosa from the acid and non-acid reflux by gel coating [27–30]. Like an antacid, an alginate-based formulation demonstrates an immediate onset of effect within 1 h of administration, which is faster than a PPI and H2RA [31]. Compared with antacids, an alginate-based formulation is more effective than an antacid in controlling postprandial esophageal acid exposure and quickly relieving reflux symptoms, including heartburn, regurgitation, vomiting and belching, with longer duration [32–34]. Alginate-based formulations are also non-inferior to omeprazole in achieving a heartburn-free period in moderate episodic heartburn [35]. Therefore, alginate has the special properties of protection of the esophageal and upper respiratory mucosa from acid and non-acid reflux and displacement of acid pocket away from the esophagus, all of which make alginate an attractive agent in the management of refractory reflux symptoms with a cause other than by acid, such as NERD [36]. Compared with placebo, an alginate-antacid formulation demonstrated superior relief of reflux symptoms including heartburn and regurgitation in both patients with NERD and erosive esophagitis in a double-blind randomized controlled trial [37]. In another double-blind randomized clinical trial comparing the efficacy of alginate to omeprazole in patients with NERD, alginate demonstrated non-inferiority to omeprazole and was as effective as omeprazole for symptomatic relief [38]. Furthermore, adding alginate to a PPI can significantly relieve heartburn compared to using a PPI alone in patients with NERD, suggesting an additional benefit of alginate as add-on therapy in the management of refractory symptoms [39].

Interestingly, in a meta-analysis study, six of nine randomized trials found no difference between the PPI and placebo groups for LPR, whereas three trials exhibited statistically significant results [1]. In a systemic review, three of four randomized controlled studies revealed that prokinetic agents significantly reduced LPR symptoms, but there were too many study limitations to draw firm conclusions [40]. In a small randomized controlled study, a liquid alginate suspension could achieve significant improvement in the symptom scores and clinical findings of LPR [41].

Therefore, on the basis of this discussed background, the management of suspected LPR is intriguing as it is very difficult, if even possible, to make a definitive diagnosis with the tools currently available [42]. If there is no doubt that many patients do have LPR symptoms, the probability of suspecting LPR, especially when typical reflux symptoms are lacking and PPIs do not improve symptoms, are low, mainly in non-specialist setting. LPR management is responsible of high economic burden mainly related to the prescription of PPIs, which may be, in most cases, not justified [3, 43, 44]. Therefore, in patients, initially visited by GP, who do not respond to a 2 to 3-month course of double dose PPI therapy, the role of the otolaryngologist is to document the presence of signs and symptoms suggestive of LPR with appropriate (i.e., validated and reproducible) investigations, namely fiber-endoscopy, and validated questionnaire (for example RSI and RFS). If LPR is documented, it is reasonable empirically testing these patients on PPIs to check for reflux control may be useful to select PPI-responder patients. If PPI are not adequate to control symptoms an add-on treatment should be prescribed. On the basis of the above-mentioned concepts, alginate could be a first-choice option. As a matter of the fact, as there is no specific and focused medication able to irreversibly inactivate pepsin and block acid production, other compounds have place in LPR management, including medical devices with barrier effect. In the current scenario, an effective supportive strategy may be constituted by compounds able to strengthen the epithelial barrier providing protection from acid and pepsin and promoting mucosal healing. In other words, an old concept could be revised for LPR therapy: the "cytoprotection" of mucosal tissues [45]. Mucosal cytoprotection was an ideal target of two main drug classes: prostaglandins and sucralfate. Many clinical trials supported this theory that met favorable impression some decades ago [46–49].

Presently, the newest alginate compounds renowned the interest in this attracting and stimulating area. In this regard, a new medical device (Marial®), unique still now possessing the indication for both GERD and LPR, has been recently launched in the Italian market. It is an innovative gel compound, containing magnesium alginate and E-Gastryal® (hyaluronic acid, hydrolyzed keratin, Tara gum, and Xantana gum). E-Gastryal® is a complex of phyto-polymers, Tara and Xantana gums, that are natural polysaccharides with high molecular weight and partially hydrosoluble, and able to provide viscosity to the solution and to generate a support frame where keratin peptide chains and hyaluronic acid anchor. Hyaluronic acid (HA) is a biopolymer with medium molecular weight characterized by optimal hygroscopic and hydrodynamic features. The chemical–physical properties of the polymeric complex confer mucoadhesiveness to E-Gastryal® so increasing the contact surface and the residence time on the mucous membranes of larynx, pharynx, and esophagus. In this context, hyaluronic acid is extremely bioavailable and able to carries out its activity aimed to induce repairing and regenerating the damaged epithelium. HA, by its hydrophilic essence, realizes a favorable milieu for cellular migration; in addition, HA, having a scavenger activity of free radicals, exerts a protective role towards oxide damage and proteolytic enzymes, such as pepsin.

Hydrolyzed keratin, an indigestible substance, increases the solidity and the resistance of E-Gastryal®, enhancing the barrier effect. Really, keratin abounds with cysteine, amino acid sulfide, that forms disulfide bridges extremely firm and able to link the amino acid chains, making an helical structure characterized by difficult dissolution and resistant to attack of acid and pepsin. The alginate has the peculiar property of a boating raft at the acid pocket and selectively inhibits pepsin by mannuronic acid, highly contained in the specific alginate [50]. In particular, this medical device contains magnesium alginate with high ratio mannuronic acid/glucuronic acid and with raised viscosity shaping a stable and compact raft.

For these reasons, two large surveys were conducted in Italy, involving both otolaryngologists and gastroenterologists. The aims were to define the patients' characteristics, including the clinical features, the assessment of treatments, and new therapeutic approaches in view of the new medical device Marial®.

2. Clinical experience

As pointed out, the gastroesophageal reflux is considered a normal physiological process that usually happens after eating in healthy infants, children, young people and adults. In contrast, gastroesophageal reflux disease occurs when the effect of GER leads to symptoms severe enough to merit medical treatment. In clinical practice, it is difficult to differentiate between GER and GERD, and the terms are used interchangeably by health professionals and families alike. There is no simple, reliable and accurate diagnostic test to confirm whether the condition is GER or GERD, and this in turn affects research and clinical decisions [50–52]. Furthermore, the term GERD covers a number of specific conditions that have different effects and present in different ways. This makes it difficult to identify the person who genuinely has GERD, and to estimate the real prevalence and burden of the problem. Nevertheless, regardless of the definition used, GERD affects many subjects, who commonly seek advice from primary, secondary or tertiary care. As a result, it constitutes a major health burden for the Health Service. Moreover, if gastric refluxate moves more proximally into the laryngopharynx, it is defined laryngopharyngeal reflux (LPR). LPR should be considered as part of extraesophageal reflux (EER), reflux involving structures other than, or in addition to, the esophagus, and airway reflux involving proximal gastric reflux into the airways. LPR contributes to several otorhinolaryngologic symptoms and inflammatory disorders, and probably also to neoplastic diseases of the laryngopharynx, and seems to be also as common in children and infants as adults.

From a diagnostic point of view, GERD and LPR diagnosis may be performed on a clinical ground as there is no gold-standard diagnostic tool. In this regard, some questionnaires may very fruitful in clinical practice: Reflux Finding Score (RFS) based on signs viewed by laryngoscopy, Reflux Score Index (RSI) based on reflux symptoms, and GERD Impact Scale (GIS) based on frequency of symptoms, as reported in the tables (**Tables 1–3**).

	None of the time	**A little of the time**	**Some of the time**	**All of the time**
	1	2	3	4
In the past week				
1. How often have you had the following symptoms				
a. Pain in chest/behind the breastbone?				
b. Burning sensation in your chest or behind the breastbone?				
c. Regurgitation or acid taste in your mouth?				
d. Pain or burning in upper stomach?				
e. Sore throat or hoarseness that is related to your heartburn or acid reflux?				
2. How often have you had difficulty in getting a good night's sleep because of your symptoms?				
3. How often have your symptoms prevented you from eating or drinking any of the foods you like?				
4. How often have your symptoms kept you from being fully productive in your job or daily activities?				
5. How often do you take additional medication other than what the physician told you to take (such as Gaviscon, Maalox)?				

Table 1. GERD Impact Scale (GIS).

Within the last month, how did the following problems affect you?	0 = no problem 5 = severe problem					
1. Hoarseness or a problem with your voice	0	1	2	3	4	5
2. Clearing your throat	0	1	2	3	4	5
3. Excess throat mucus or postnasal drip	0	1	2	3	4	5
4. Difficulty swallowing food, liquids, or pills	0	1	2	3	4	5
5. Coughing after you ate or after lying down	0	1	2	3	4	5
6. Breathing difficulties or choking episodes	0	1	2	3	4	5
7. Troublesome or annoying cough	0	1	2	3	4	5
8. Sensation of something sticking in your throat or a lump in your throat	0	1	2	3	4	5
9. Heartburn, chest pain, indigestion, or stomach acid coming up	0	1	2	3	4	5
RSI > 13 = Abnormal	Total					

Abbreviation: RSI, reflux symptom index.

Table 2. Reflux Symptom Index.

From a management point of view, the guidelines suggest to give advice about GER and reassure patients and caregivers. Patients with dyspepsia with mild–moderate symptoms and without severe complications, such as bleeding, painful complaints, vomiting, could be treated with empirical full-dose PPI therapy for 4 weeks. Patients with GERD could be treated with a full-dose PPI for 4 or 8 weeks. If symptoms recur after initial treatment, a PPI could be offered at the lowest dose possible to control symptoms. In addition, it is recommended to encourage people who need long-term management of dyspepsia symptoms to reduce their use of prescribed medication stepwise: by using the effective lowest dose, by trying 'as-needed' use when appropriate, and by returning to self-treatment with antacid and/or alginate therapy (unless there is an underlying condition or co-medication that needs continuing treatment). It is also necessary to advise people that it may be appropriate for them to return to self-treatment with antacid and/or alginate therapy (either prescribed or purchased over-the-counter and taken as needed). Finally, it is important to avoid long-term, frequent dose and continuous antacid therapy (it only relieves symptoms in the short term rather than preventing them).

On the basis of these considerations, proposed by guidelines, alginates may be considered as a valid and reasonable therapeutic option. A new medical device (Marial®), unique still now possessing the indication for both GERD and LPR, has been recently launched in the Italian market [53]. It is an innovative gel compound, containing magnesium alginate and E-Gastryal®. E-Gastryal® is a complex of phyto-polymers, keratin, Tara and Xantana gums, that are natural polysaccharides with high molecular weight and partially hydrosoluble, and able to provide viscosity to the solution and to generate a support frame where keratin peptide chains and hyaluronic acid anchor. Hyaluronic acid (HA) is a biopolymer with medium molecular weight characterized by optimal hygroscopic and hydrodynamic features. The chemical–physical properties of the polymeric complex confer mucoadhesiveness to E-Gastryal® so increasing the contact surface and the residence time on the mucous membranes of larynx, pharynx, and esophagus.

Subglottic edema	0 = absent
	2 = present
Ventricular edema	2 = partial
	4 = complete
Erythema/hyperemia	2 = arytenoids only
	4 = diffuse
Vocal-fold edema	1 = mild
	2 = moderate
	3 = severe
	4 = polypoid
Diffuse laryngeal edema	1 = mild
	2 = moderate
	3 = severe
	4 = obstructing
Posterior commissure hypertrophy	1 = mild
	2 = moderate
	3 = severe
	4 = obstructing
Granuloma/granulation tissue	0 = absent
	2 = present
Thicken laryngeal mucus	0 = absent
	2 = present

RFS, Reflux Finding Score. RFS > 7 suspect of laryngopharyngeal reflux (LPR).

Table 3. Reflux Finding Score.

Therefore, two large surveys were conducted in Italy: RELIEF, involving 86 otolaryngologists, and EMERGE, involving 56 gastroenterologists [54–56]. The aims of these surveys were: (1) to define clinical characteristics, including previous treatment, of the patients referred to consultation; (2) to evaluate the reliability of RFS, GIS, and RSI questionnaires in real-world settings, such as specialist office; and (3) to investigate the patients' perception of efficacy of the prescribed therapy, based on the best practice and considering also the new medical device.

The outcomes of these surveys are here presented and discussed. Now, we would draw the conclusive remarks from a pragmatic point of view. So, we compared the most relevant outcomes obtained by the two surveys.

First, we compared RSI questionnaires: at baseline, RSI questionnaire was filled by 1934 RELIEF patients and by 789 EMERGE patients. Globally, 594 (75.3%) EMERGE patients and 1250

(64.6%) RELIEF patients had positive RSI score. RSI values for each single symptom are analytically reported in **Figure 1**. The symptoms with the highest score were: heartburning, sensation of something sticking in the throat or a lump in the throat, and clearing throat, whereas breathing difficulties or choking episodes had the lowest score. The total score was 16 [14–20] in the EMERGE patients was significantly higher than in the RELIEFE patients: 16 [12–20] ($p < 0.001$; data not shown). Interestingly, RELIEF patients had significantly higher scores for some symptoms, including lump sensation, cough, dyspnea, hoarseness, and throat clearing, whereas EMERGE patients had higher scores for heartburn and difficult swallowing. So, the clinical features were really different in the two populations, such as GERD and LPR patients.

Considering the previous treatments, the frequency of past/current treatments in the EMERGE group (**Figure 2A**) was significantly higher than in RELIEF group (**Figure 2B**) patients ($p<0.0001$): this outcome underlines the more intense recourse to medical therapy in GERD patients than in LPR patients. Analyzing the treatment options, **Figure 3** shows the distribution of different types of treatments prescribed in the past (panel A, C) or currently used (panel B, D): monotherapy with PPI, PPI in add-on, and Miscellany in EMERGE (panel A, B) and RELIEF (panel C, D) patients. LPR patients were more frequently treated with PPI as monotherapy and with miscellany treatments, whereas GERD patients use more commonly PPI plus add-on, even though PPI alone are the first-choice therapy also in GERD. Considering the distribution of the new prescribed

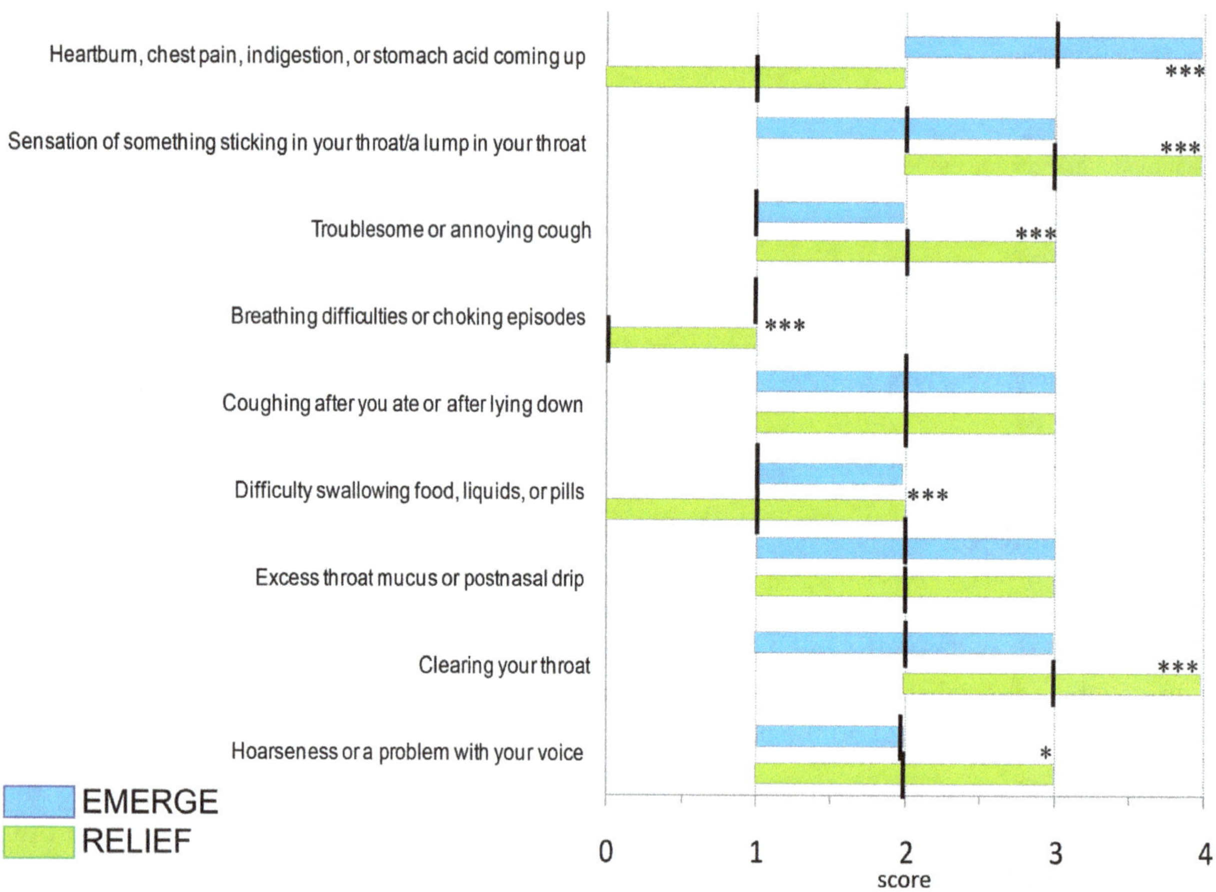

Figure 1. Reflux Symptom Index (RSI) as median values for each single symptom in the EMERGE (no. 789) and in the RELIEF population (no. 1934). Scores are reported as medians (bars) with lower and upper quartiles (boxes).

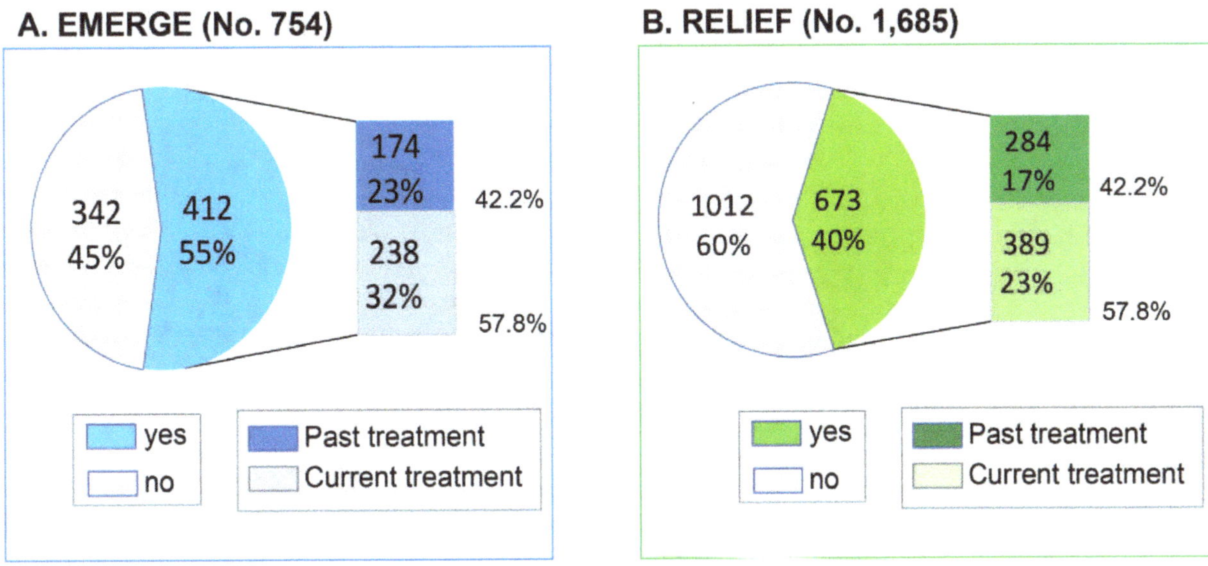

Figure 2. Distribution of the EMERGE (panel A) or RELIEF (panel B) patients according to the treatments: past, current, or never.

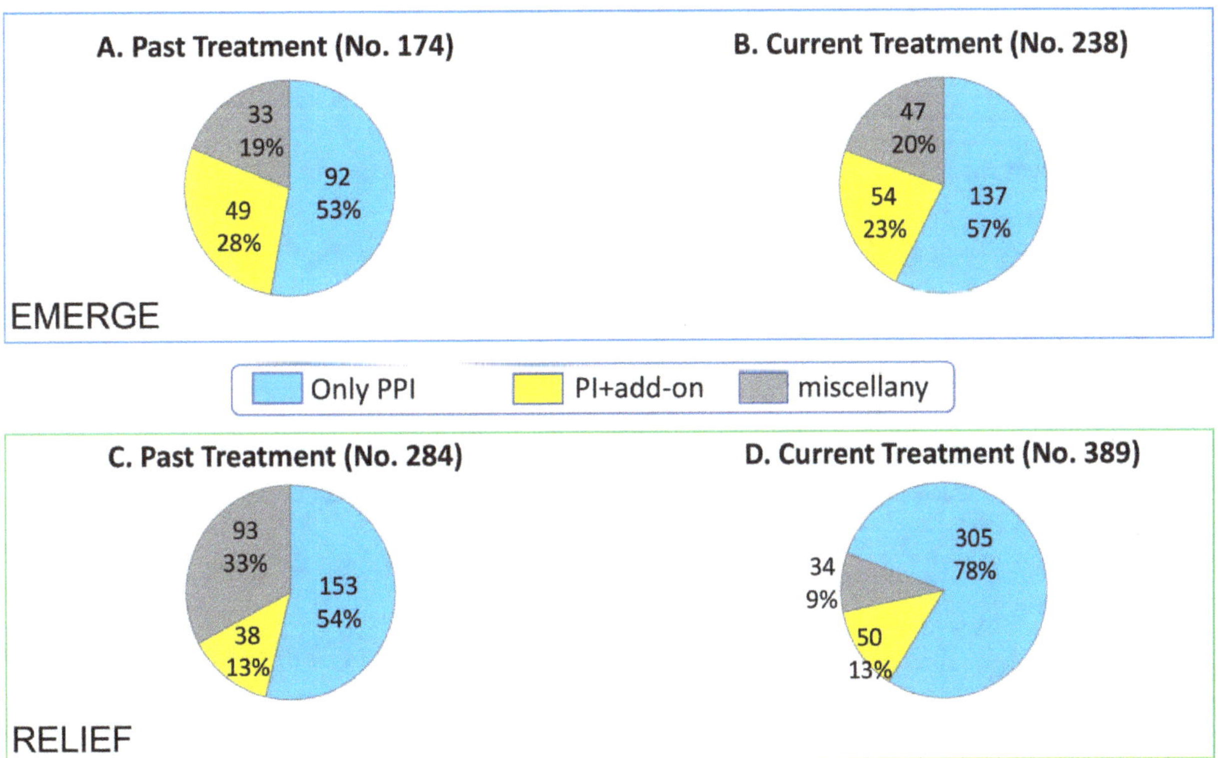

Figure 3. Distribution of different types of treatments prescribed in the past (panel A, C) or currently used (panel B, D): monotherapy with PPI, PPI in add-on, and miscellany in EMERGE (panel A, B) and RELIEF (panel C, D) patients.

treatments (i.e., prescriptions made during the visits) and specifically of Marial® as monotherapy, PPI as monotherapy or PPI in add-on, there was difference in EMERGE (**Figure 4A**) and in RELIEF (**Figure 4B**) patients ($p < 0.0001$): LPR patients were preferentially treated with Marial® alone, whereas GERD patients were treated essentially with PPI plus add-on.

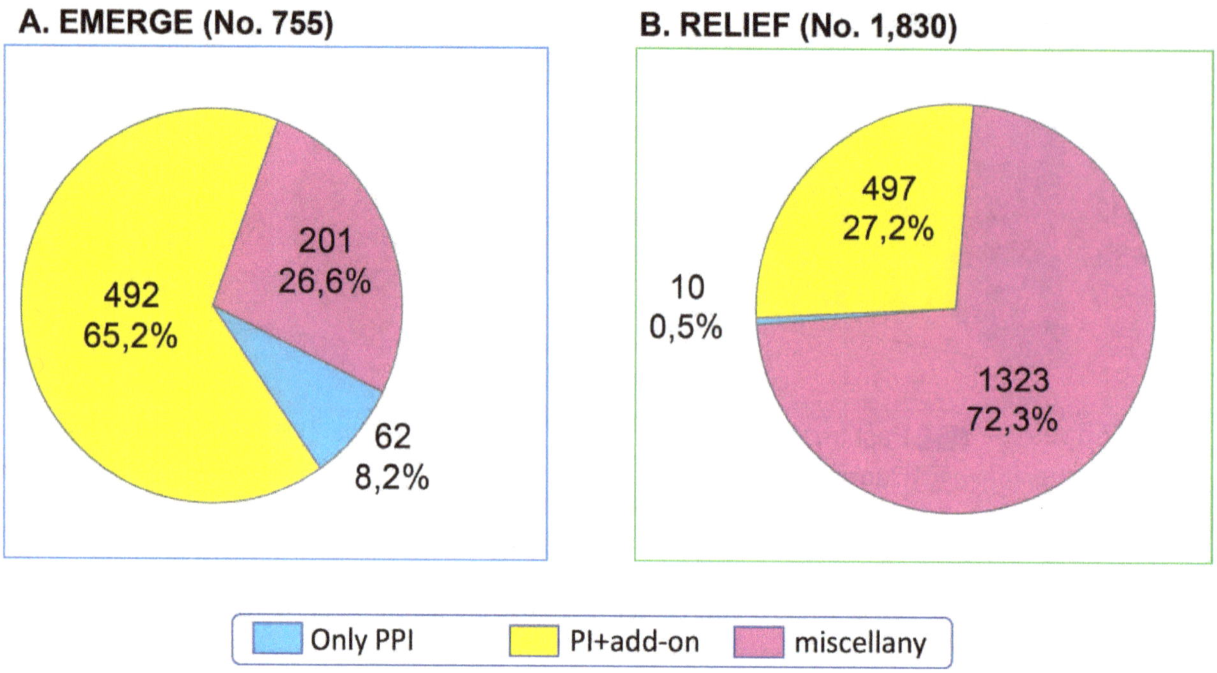

Figure 4. Distribution of the Marial® as monotherapy, PPI as monotherapy or PPI in add-on in new prescribed treatments (i.e., prescription during the visit) in EMERGE (panel A) and RELIEF (panel B) patients.

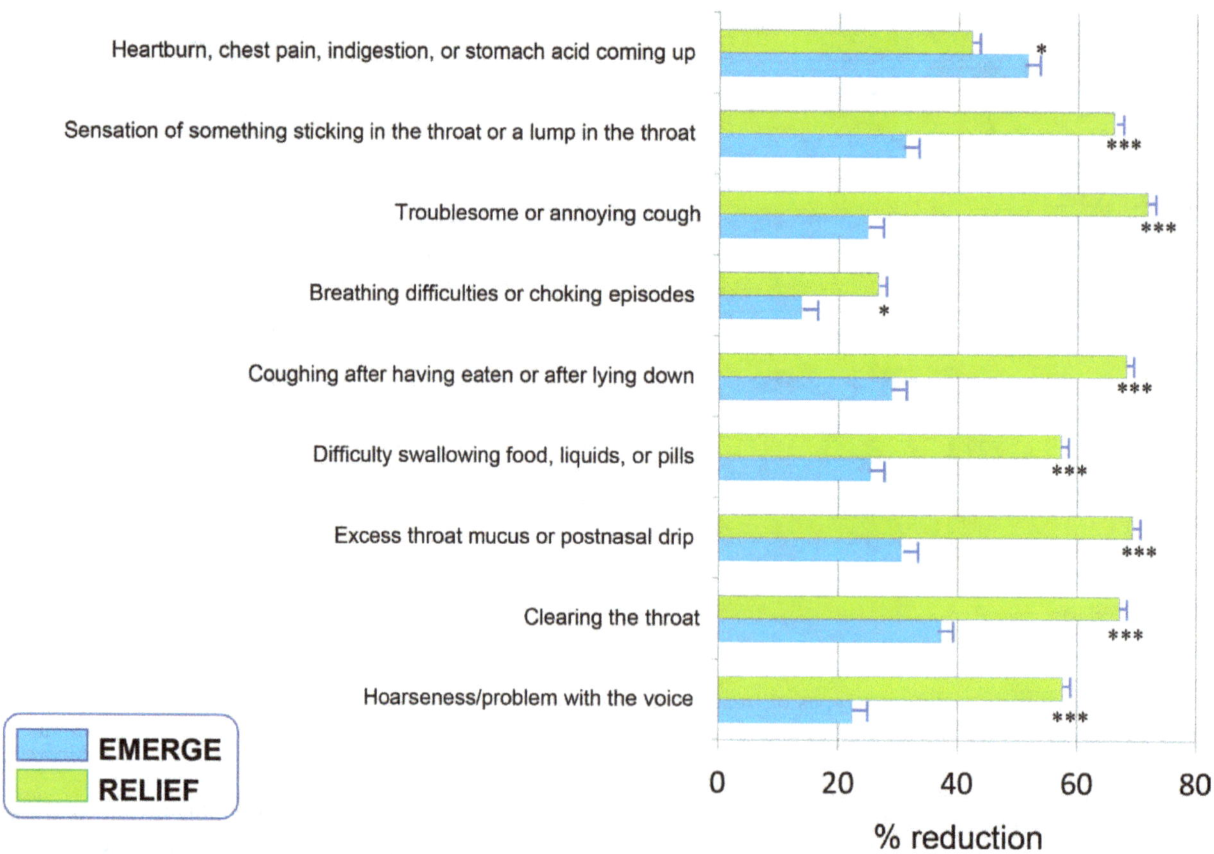

Figure 5. Reduction in RSI values for each single symptom before and after a 4 week-treatment with Marial® as monotherapy in EMERGE and in RELIEF patients.

Comparing the patients' perception of treatment efficacy, reduction in RSI values for each single symptom before and after a 4 week-treatment with Marial® alone or with PPI in add-on in EMERGE and RELIEF patients are reported in **Figures 5** and **6**. Marial® alone treatment induced a statistically significant higher reduction in each single symptom in RELIEF patients than in EMERGE patients, with the exception of heartburn, chest pain, indigestion, or stomach acid coming up (**Figure 5**). Similar results were obtained evaluating the reduction in RSI values in patients treated with PPI in add-on that was able to determine a higher statistically significant decrease in RELIEF than in EMERGE patients in each single symptom, with the exception of heartburn, chest pain, indigestion, or stomach acid coming up (**Figure 6**).

In conclusion, these two surveys provided some interesting outcomes: (i) diagnostic questionnaires (RSI, RFS, and GIS) are reliable and useful both during the visit and to orient the treatment decision; (ii) GERD and LPR present different clinical features; (iii) as consequence the treatments (both previous and actual) are different; (iv) the introduction of Marial® significantly affected the otolaryngologist approach and partially the gastroenterologist orientation; (v) Marial® was effective both in LPR and GERD patients; (vi) Marial® showed more effectiveness than conventional therapy (PPI plus add-on); and (vii) LPR patients were more responsive to medical treatments than GERD patients. Therefore, these outcomes may give a pragmatic usefulness to both otolaryngologists and gastroenterologists in clinical practice.

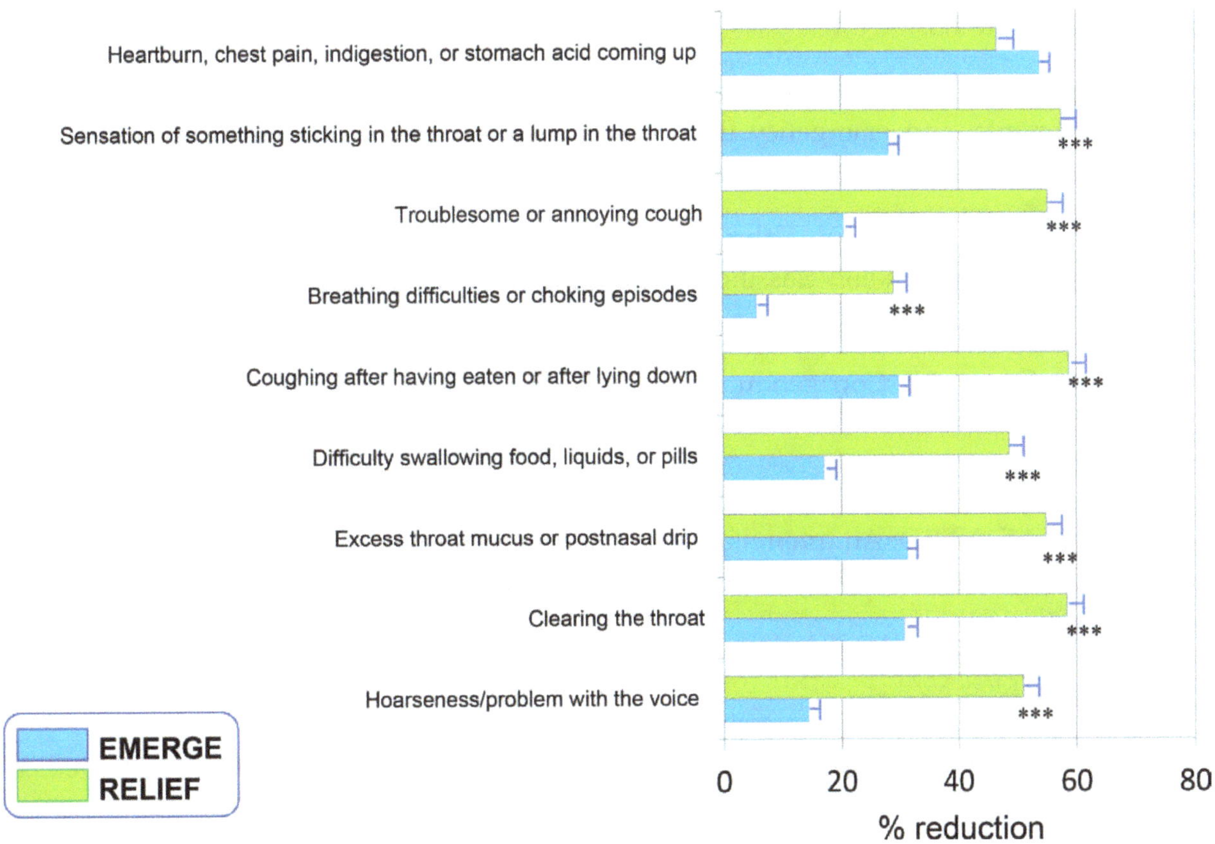

Figure 6. Reduction in RSI values for each single symptom before and after a 4 week-treatment with PPI + add-on in EMERGE and in RELIEF patients.

Author details

Aragona Salvatore Emanuele[1], Mereghetti Giada[1] and Giorgio Ciprandi[2*]

*Address all correspondence to: gio.cip@libero.it

1 Center of Regenerative Medicine, Humanitas Mater Domini, Castellanza (VA), Italy

2 Ospedale Policlinico San Martino, Genoa, Italy

References

[1] Sidhwa F, Moore A, Alligood E, Fisichella PM. Diagnosis and treatment of the extra-esophageal manifestations of gastroesophageal reflux disease. Annals of Surgery. 2017; **265**:63-67

[2] Rubenstein JH, Chen JW. Epidemiology of gastroesophageal reflux disease. Gastroenterology Clinics of North America. 2014;**43**:1-14

[3] Francis DO, Rymer JA, Slaughter JC, et al. High economic burden of caring for patients with suspected extraesophageal reflux. The American Journal of Gastroenterology. 2013;**108**:905-911

[4] Schappert SM, Burt CW. Ambulatory care visits to physician offices, hospital outpatient departments, and emergency departments: United States, 2001-02. Vital and Health Statistics. 2006:1-66

[5] Vakil N, van Zanten SV, Kahrilas P, Dent J, Jones R, Global Consensus Group. The Montreal definition and classification of gastroesophageal reflux disease: A global evidence-based consensus. The American Journal of Gastroenterology. 2006;**101**:1900-1920

[6] Katz P, Gerson LB. Corrigendum: Guidelines for the diagnosis and management of the gastroesophageal reflux disease. The American Journal of Gastroenterology. 2013;**108**: 308-328

[7] Savarino E. NERD: An umbrella term including heterogenous subpopulations. Nature Reviews. Gastroenterology & Hepatology. 2013;**10**:371-380

[8] Quasim A. Section II FGIDs: Diagnostic groups. Esophageal disorders. Gastroenterology. 2016;**150**:1368-1379

[9] Salihefendic N, Zidzic M, Cabric E. Laryngopharyngeal reflux disease—LPRD. Medical Archives. 2017;**71**:215-218

[10] Capagnolo AM, Priston J, Heidrichthoen R, Medeiros T, Assuncao RA. Laryngopharyngeal reflux: Diagnosis, treatment and latest research. International Archives of Otorhinolaryngology. 2014;**18**:184-191

[11] Dent J, El-Serag HB, Wallander MA, Johansson S. Epidemiology of gastroesophageal reflux disease: A systematic review. Gut. 2005;**54**:710-717

[12] Koufman JA. Laryngopharyngeal reflux 2002: A new paradigm of airway disease. Ear, Nose, & Throat Journal 2004; (Suppl. 1):10-29

[13] Saritas Yuksel E, Vaezi MF. New developments in extraesophageal reflux disease. Gastroenterología y Hepatología. 2012;**8**:590-599

[14] Barry DW, Vaezi MF. Laryngopharyngeal reflux: More questions than answers. Cleveland Clinic Journal of Medicine. 2010;**77**:327-334

[15] Belafsky PC, Postma GN, Amin MR, Koufman JA. Symptoms and findings of laryngopharyngeal reflux. Ear, Nose, & Throat Journal 2004; (Suppl. 1):30-39

[16] Abou-Ismail A, Vaezi MF. Evaluation of patients withsuspected laryngopharyngeal reflux: A practical approach. Current Gastroenterology Reports. 2011;**13**:213-218

[17] Martinucci I, de Bortoli N, Savarino E, Nacci A, Romeo SO, Bellini M, Savarino V, Fattori B, Marchi S. Optimal treatment of laryngopharyngeal reflux disease. Therapeutic Advances in Chronic Disease. 2013;**4**:287-301

[18] Kung YM, Hsu WH, Wu MC, Wang JW, Liu CJ, Su YC, et al. Recent advances in the pharmacological management of gastroesophageal reflux disease. Digestive Diseases and Sciences. 2017;**62**:3298-3316

[19] Sigterman KE, van Pinxteren B, Bonis PA, Lau J, Numans ME. Short-term treatment with proton pump inhibitors, H2-receptor antagonists and prokinetics for gastroesophageal reflux disease-like symptoms and endoscopy negative reflux disease. Cochrane Database of Systematic Reviews. 2013:CD002095

[20] Sifrim D, Zerbib F. Diagnosis and management of patients with reflux symptoms refractory to proton pump inhibitors. Gut. 2012;**61**:1340-1354

[21] Fass R, Shapiro M, Dekel R, Sewell J. Systematic review: Proton-pump inhibitor failure in gastro-oesophageal reflux disease—Where next? Alimentary Pharmacology & Therapeutics. 2005;**22**:79-94

[22] Fass R. Proton-pump inhibitor therapy in patients with gastrooesophageal reflux disease: Putative mechanisms of failure. Drugs. 2007;**67**:1521-1530

[23] Fass R, Gasiorowska A. Refractory GERD: What is it? Current Gastroenterology Reports. 2008;**10**:252-257

[24] Scarpellini E, Ang D, Pauwels A, et al. Management of refractory typical GERD symptoms. Nature Reviews. Gastroenterology & Hepatology. 2016;**13**:281-294

[25] Kahrilas PJ, McColl K, Fox M, et al. The acid pocket: A target for treatment in reflux disease? The American Journal of Gastroenterology. 2013;**108**:1058-1064

[26] Mitchell DR, Derakhshan MH, Robertson EV, McColl KE. The role of the acid pocket in gastroesophageal reflux disease. Journal of Clinical Gastroenterology. 2016;**50**:111-119

[27] Strugala V, Avis J, Jolliffe IG, Johnstone LM, Dettmar PW. The role of an alginate suspension on pepsin and bile acids–key aggressors in the gastric refluxate. Does this have implications for the treatment of gastro-oesophageal reflux disease? The Journal of Pharmacy and Pharmacology. 2009;**61**:1021-1028

[28] Kwiatek MA, Roman S, Fareeduddin A, Pandolfino JE, Kahrilas PJ. An alginate-antacid formulation (Gaviscon double action liquid) can eliminate or displace the postprandial 'acid pocket' in symptomatic GERD patients. Alimentary Pharmacology & Therapeutics. 2011;**34**:59-66

[29] Rohof WO, Bennink RJ, Smout AJ, Thomas E, Boeckxstaens GE. An alginate-antacid formulation localizes to the acid pocket to reduce acid reflux in patients with gastroesophageal reflux disease. Clinical Gastroenterology and Hepatology. 2013;**11**:1585-1591

[30] Sweis R, Kaufman E, Anggiansah A, et al. Post-prandial reflux suppression by a raft-forming alginate (Gaviscon advance) compared to a simple antacid documented by magnetic resonance imaging and pH-impedance monitoring: Mechanistic assessment in healthy volunteers and randomised, controlled, double-blind study in reflux patients. Alimentary Pharmacology & Therapeutics. 2013;**37**:1093-1102

[31] Dettmar PW, Sykes J, Little SL, Bryan J. Rapid onset of effect of sodium alginate on gastro-oesophageal reflux compared with ranitidine and omeprazole, and relationship between symptoms and reflux episodes. International Journal of Clinical Practice. 2006;**60**:275-283

[32] De Ruigh A, Roman S, Chen J, Pandolfino JE, Kahrilas PJ. Gaviscon double action liquid (antacid & alginate) is more effective than antacid in controlling post-prandial oesophageal acid exposure in GERD patients: A double-blind crossover study. Alimentary Pharmacology & Therapeutics. 2014;**40**:531-537

[33] Mandel KG, Daggy BP, Brodie DA, Jacoby HI. Review article: Alginate-raft formulations in the treatment of heartburn and acid reflux. Alimentary Pharmacology & Therapeutics. 2000;**14**:669-690

[34] Lai IR, Wu MS, Lin JT. Prospective, randomized, and active controlled study of the efficacy of alginic acid and antacid in the treatment of patients with endoscopy-negative reflux disease. World Journal of Gastroenterology. 2006;**12**:747-754

[35] Pouchain D, Bigard MA, Liard F, et al. Gaviscon(R) vs. omeprazole in symptomatic treatment of moderate gastroesophageal reflux. A direct comparative randomised trial. BMC Gastroenterology. 2012;**12**:18

[36] Woodland P, Lee C, Duraisamy Y, et al. Assessment and protection of esophageal mucosal integrity in patients with heartburn without esophagitis. The American Journal of Gastroenterology. 2013;**108**:535-543

[37] Sun J, Yang C, Zhao H, et al. Randomised clinical trial: The clinical efficacy and safety of an alginate-antacid (Gaviscon double action) versus placebo, for decreasing upper gastrointestinal symptoms in symptomatic gastroesophageal reflux disease (GERD) in China. Alimentary Pharmacology & Therapeutics. 2015;**42**:845-854

[38] Chiu CT, Hsu CM, Wang CC, et al. Randomised clinical trial: Sodium alginate oral suspension is non-inferior to omeprazole in the treatment of patients with non-erosive gastroesophageal disease. Alimentary Pharmacology & Therapeutics. 2013;**38**:1054-1064

[39] Manabe N, Haruma K, Ito M, et al. Efficacy of adding sodium alginate to omeprazole in patients with nonerosive reflux disease: A randomized clinical trial. Diseases of the Esophagus. 2012;**25**:373-380

[40] Glicksman JT, Mick PT, Fung K, Carroll TL. Prokinetic agents and laryngopharyngeal reflux disease: A systematic review. Laryngoscope. 2014;**124**:2375-2379

[41] McGlashan JA, Johnstone LM, Sykes J, Strugala V, Dettmar PW. The value of a liquid alginate suspension (Gaviscon advance) in the management of laryngopharyngeal reflux. European Archives of Oto-Rhino-Laryngology. 2009;**266**:243-251

[42] Zerbib F, Dulery C. Facts and fantasies on extraesophageal reflux. A gastroenterologist perspective. Journal of Clinical Gastroenterology. 2017;**51**:769-776

[43] Vertigan AE, Bone SL, Gibson PG. Laryngeal sensory dysfunction in laryngeal hypersensitivity syndrome. Respirology. 2013;**18**:948-956

[44] Aziz Q, Fass R, Gyawali CP. Functional esophageal disorders. Gastroenterology. In press. DOI: 10.1053/j.gastro.2016.02.012. [Epub ahead of print]

[45] Miller TA, Jacobson ED. Gastrointestinal cytoprotection by prostaglandins. Gut. 1979; **20**:75-87

[46] Johansson C, Bergström S. Prostaglandin and protection of the gastroduodenal mucosa. Scandinavian Journal of Gastroenterology. 1982;**77**:21-46

[47] Tasman-Jones C. Pathogenesis of peptic ulcer disease and gastritis: Importance of aggressive and cytoprotective factors. Scandinavian Journal of Gastroenterology. 1986: **122**:1-122:5

[48] Orlando RC. Cytoprotection by sucralfate in acid-exposed esophagus: A review. Scandinavian Journal of Gastroenterology. 1987;**127**:97-100

[49] Lauritsen K, Rask-Madsen J. Peptic ulcer disease, cytoprotection, and prostaglandins. Archives of Internal Medicine. 1990;**150**:695-701

[50] Chater PI, Wilcox MD, Brownlee IA. Alginate as a protease inhibitor in vitro and in a model gut system: Selective inhibition of pepsin but not trypsin. Carbohydrate Polymers. 2015;**131**:142-151

[51] Internal Clinical Guidelines Team (UK). Dyspepsia and Gastro-Oesophageal Reflux Disease: Investigation and Management of Dyspepsia, Symptoms Suggestive of Gastro-Oesophageal Reflux Disease, or Both. London: National Institute for Health and Care Excellence (UK); 2014 Sep

[52] Davies I, Burman-Roy S, Murphy MS, Guideline Development Group. Gastro-oesophageal reflux disease in children: NICE guidance. BMJ. 2015;**350**:7703

[53] Aragona SE, Mereghetti G, Ciprandi G. The gastric reflux: the therapeutical role of Marial. Journal of Biological Regulators and Homeostatic Agents. 2018 Apr 26;**32**(4). [Epub ahead of print]

[54] Bianchetti M, Peralta S, Nicita R, Aragona SE, Ciprandi G. The EMERGE (emerging from Gastroesophageal Reflux): an Italian survey—I. The viewpoint of the Gastroenterologist. Journal of Biological Regulators and Homeostatic Agents. 2018 Apr 26;**32**(4). [Epub ahead of print]

[55] Bianchetti M, Peralta S, Nicita R, Aragona SE, Ciprandi G. The EMERGE (emerging from Gastroesophageal Reflux): an Italian survey—II. The viewpoint of the patient. Journal of Biological Regulators and Homeostatic Agents. 2018 Apr 26;**32**(4). [Epub ahead of print]

[56] Bianchetti M, Peralta S, Nicita R, Aragona SE, Ciprandi G. Correlation between the Reflux Finding Score and the GERD Impact Scale in patients with Gastroesophageal Reflux Disease. Journal of Biological Regulators and Homeostatic Agents. 2018 Apr 26;**32**(4). [Epub ahead of print]

9

Chemotherapy for Gastric Cancer — What Comes Next?

Shouji Shimoyama

1. Introduction

Gastric cancer (GC) is the fourth (in men) and fifth (in women) most commonly newly diagnosed cancer worldwide and the third (in men) and fifth (in women) leading cause of cancer death [1]. Radical resection remains the only way cure, but cure rates following surgery for resectable GC in the West lag behind those in Japan. In addition, many GC patients will suffer recurrence even after curative resection in approximately 50% of cases [2], which eventually results in a still poor 5-year survival rate of <30% both in the USA [3] and in Europe [4]. Although the 5-year survival rate in Japan is much better than that in the West, there is a global consensus that advanced GC patients need further anticancer therapy.

Currently, five classes of cytotoxic agents (fluoropyrimidines, platinums, taxanes, topoisomerase inhibitors, and anthracyclines) and new molecular targeting agents have been used in GC. Recent randomized controlled trials (RCTs) in the field of treatment for advanced GC have established first-line chemotherapy, although the approach and management for advanced GC varies from region to region so that there is no worldwide consensus on this matter. The most promising regimens are ECF (epirubicin, cisplatin, and 5-fluorouracil) in Europe [5], DCF (docetaxel, cisplatin, and 5-fluorouracil) in the USA (V325 trial) [6], and SP (S-1 and cisplatin) in Japan (SPIRITS trial) [7]. Strikingly, however, the global RCT conducted in the USA (FLAGS trial) failed to exhibit any survival advantage of the SP regimen over the FP (5-fluorouracil plus cisplatin) regimen [8]. Very recently, trastuzumab combined with cisplatin and fluoropyrimidines has been found to be active for human epidermal growth factor receptor-2 (HER2 or ERBB2)-positive GC (ToGA trial) [9]. Although these regimens are active, the treatment progress is painfully slow [4]. The median time to progression (TTP) or progression free survival (PFS) was 7.4 months by ECF [5], 5.6 months by DCF [6], 6.0 months by Japanese style SP [7], 4.8 months by global style SP [8], and 6.7 months even by adding trastuzumab [9], suggesting that many advanced GC patients experience failure after first-line chemotherapy.

Interestingly, the median TTP or PFS of these regimens are almost equivalent (5.6-7.4 months) [5-7] while median overall survival times (OS) differ between the studies (Figure 1). The 13 months of median OS by the Japanese SP regimen [7] was apparently longer than those (8.7-9.2 months) by ECF and DCF regimens [5,6] (Figure 1). In addition, even by the use of the SP regimen, the post-progression survival –the survival length difference between median PFS and median OS– differed considerably, being 7 months in the SPIRITS trial [7] and 3.8 months in the FLAGS trial [8] (Figure 1). Such inter-trial differences in post-progression survival are partly attributable to different proportions of subsequent second-line therapy after the failure of first-line chemotherapy, being over 70% in the SPIRITS trial while 30-45% in other trials [6, 8,9]. In this regard, patients who retain good performance status at the time of first-line treatment failure are candidates for second-line therapy. Currently, however, no standard regimens for any second-line therapy hitherto determined suggest an urgent need for the establishment of second-line therapy. Reflecting this urgency, clinical research concerning second-line therapy has been recently commenced. In the era of post first-line chemotherapy, this chapter reviews the next research issues deserving of focus in the field of advanced GC treatment.

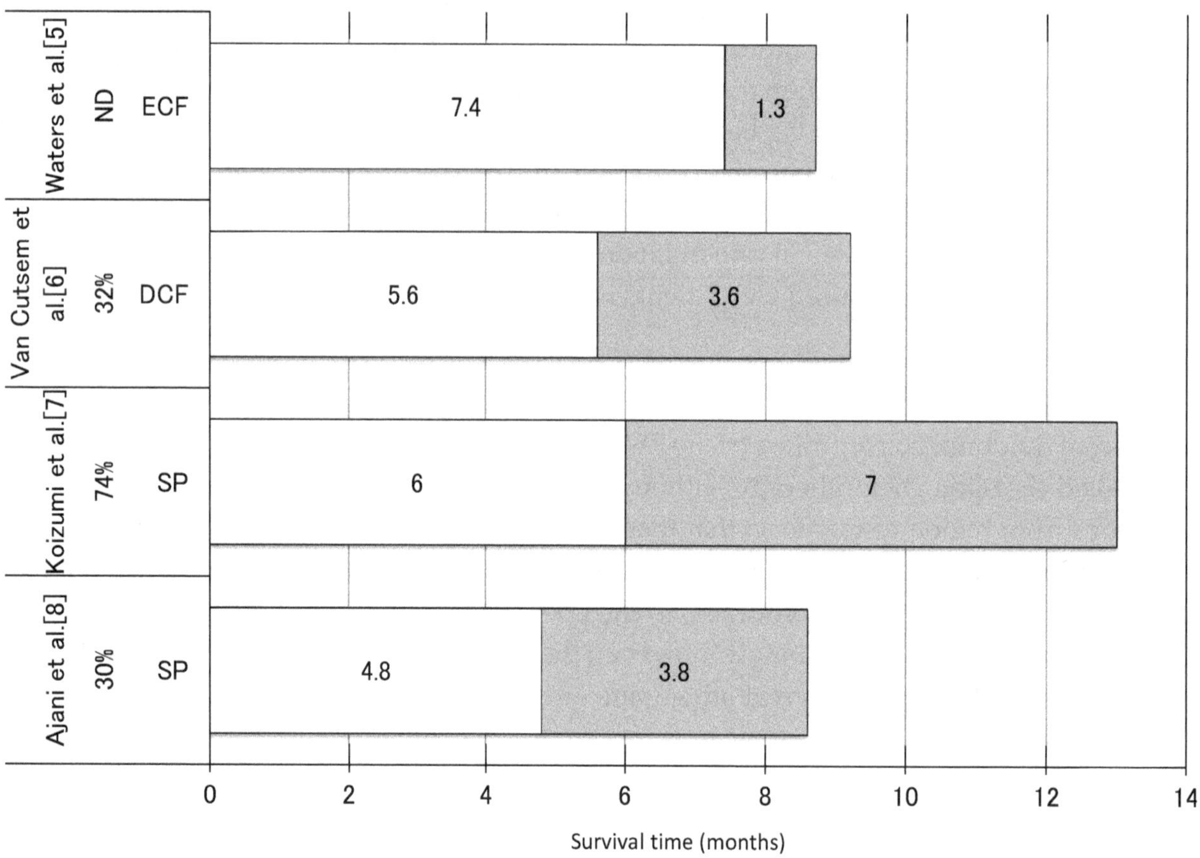

Figure 1. Median TTP or PFS (white bar) and post-progression free survivals (gray bar) of the previous first-line RCTs. The sum of the white and gray bars indicates median OS. Percentages indicate the proportion of patients receiving further therapy. The reference numbers are expressed in brackets. ECF; epirubicin, cisplatin, and 5-fluorouracil, DCF; docetaxel, cisplatin, and 5-fluorouracil, SP; S-1 and cisplatin. ND; not described.

2. Rationale for second-line therapy

The significance of second-line therapy after disease progression by first-line chemotherapy has been evaluated by several randomized comparisons of survival times between second-line therapy and best supportive care (BSC) or placebos. Various kinds of agents have been investigated in the RCTs of second-line therapy, such as chemotherapy drugs [10-12] and molecular targeting agents [13-15]. Some of these trials have demonstrated significantly improved survival times by second-line therapies as compared with BSC or a placebo (Table 1).

The AIO conducted a RCT to compare irinotecan (21 patients) with BSC (19 patients) [10]. Although this study was closed prematurely due to poor patient accrual, irinotecan could significantly (p=0.012) prolong median OS (4.0 months) as compared to those by BSC (2.4 months). The second RCT conducted in Korea [11] assigned patients in a ratio of 2:1 to chemotherapy (docetaxel or irinotecan) plus BSC (133 patients) or BSC alone (69 patients). Choice of chemotherapy drugs was left to the discretion of the investigators. Median OS of the chemotherapy arm (5.3 months) was significantly (p=0.007) longer than those of the BSC arm (3.8 months). This survival difference may be partly ascribed to the significantly (p=0.02) greater number of patients receiving further chemotherapy (third-line chemotherapy) in the chemotherapy arm (40%) than in the BSC arm (22%) because median OS was longer (8.0 months) for patients who received subsequent treatment than those who did not (3.76 months), regardless of treatment arm. Of note, the lack of any difference in median OS between docetaxel use (5.2 months) and irinotecan use (6.5 months) implies that both agents are equally active, although bias for patient allocation can not be denied. In the third RCT conducted in the UK [12], 168 patients were allocated to either docetaxel plus active symptom control or active symptom control alone (84 patients each). The median OS in the docetaxel group (5.2 months) was significantly longer (p=0.01) than that in the active symptom control alone group (3.6 months). Measurements of disease specific quality of life showed benefits for docetaxel in reducing dysphagia and abdominal pain.

The efficacy of molecular targeting agents as a second-line setting has been investigated by three other RCTs [13-15]. First, a GRANITE-1 trial [13] randomly assigned 656 patients at a 2:1 schedule either to everolimus (n=439) or a matching placebo (n=217). Significantly longer median PFS by everolimus (1.7 months, p<0.0001) than that by placebo (1.4 months) did not reflect a difference in median OS (5.4 months in the everolimus arm versus 4.3 months in the placebo arm, p=0.12). Such a discrepancy, namely a significant PFS difference and nonsignificant OS difference, could be ascribed to the fact of the similar or even longer median OS (4.3 months) in the placebo arm in this study as compared to those (2.4-3.8 months) of BSC arms in other second-line RCTs [10-12]. Therefore, one should remember that the longer survival length in the control arm might diminish any statistical significance even when the experimental regimen is effective. Subsequently, a global REGARD trial [14] was able for the first time to demonstrate that ramucirumab, a monoclonal antibody of vascular endothelial growth factor receptor (VEGFR)-2, was significantly superior to placebo with regard to median OS (5.2 months versus 3.8 months, p=0.047) and median PFS (2.1 months versus 1.3 months, p<0.0001), respectively. In addition, more patients receiving ramucirumab experienced stable or improved QOL than those in the placebo arm. Finally, apatinib, a tyrosine-inhibitor agent targeting VEGFR with an anticipated anti-angiogenesis effect, has been now tested in a clinical trial (NCT 01512745) [15]. This study aims to determine whether apatinib can improve PFS or OS compared to placebos.

Subsequently, a metaanalysis has very recently elucidated a 36% reduction in the risk of death (p<0.0001) by second-line therapy [16], suggesting that second-line therapy is effective and should be considered in some segments of GC patients refractory to first-line therapy.

3. Seeking the best regimen of second-line therapy

Several randomized trials have been released to explore the optimal combination and doses for second-line therapy using the currently active agents or those deemed active. The agents investigated by these trials include chemotherapeutic drugs [17-20], a molecular targeting agent [21], and their combinations [22-26].

The efficacy of chemotherapy as a second-line setting has been investigated in several RCTs. In the TCOG GI-0801 trial [17], median PFS was significantly longer (3.8 months, n=64) by biweekly irinotecan plus cisplatin than by irinotecan alone (2.8 months, n=63), but median OS did not differ between the arms (10.7 months versus 10.1 months). Notably, the proportion of patients receiving third-line therapy was the same (75%) in both groups. The results of another randomized trial (ECRIN) have been reported in the abstract form [18], in which irinotecan plus cisplatin (n=84) was compared with irinotecan alone (n=84) in patients refractory to an S-1 containing regimen. WJOG 4007 [19] is a RCT comparing weekly paclitaxel (n=108) with biweekly irinotecan (n=111) in GC patients refractory to fluoropyrimidines plus cisplatin. Although there are no statistically significant differences between weekly paclitaxel and biweekly irinotecan for median OS (9.5 months vs 8.4 months, p=0.38), median PFS (3.6 months vs 2.3 months, p=0.33), or response rate (20.9% vs 13.6%, p=0.24), the median OS of both arms are equally longer than those of the previous second-line studies (Table 1, Figure 2). Several explanations are possible for the longer median OS in this study. One explanation is the lower proportion of patients with severe peritoneal metastasis in this study (25.6%) as compared with those in the AIO [10] (45%) and Kang [11] (45%) studies. Another explanation is that the proportion of patients receiving third-line therapy in this study was substantial, being 89.8% in the paclitaxel arm and 72.1% in the irinotecan arm. Interestingly, the third-line therapy was an irinotecan-containing regimen in 75% of patients of the paclitaxel arm and a taxane-containing regimen in 60% of the irinotecan arm. Including later lines, 81% patients in the paclitaxel arm received irinotecan and 68% of patients in the irinotecan arm received paclitaxel. The more prolonged median OS in both arms of the WJOG 4007 than those of the previous studies implies that both irinotecan and paclitaxel in second- and further-line settings could potentially contribute to prolonged survival. The ongoing fourth RCT (JACCRO GC05) [20] has been comparing irinotecan plus S-1 with irinotecan alone to GC patients refractory to S-1. Since the standard regimen in adjuvant and advanced settings in Japan is respectively S-1 and S-1 plus cisplatin, this study will provide one answer to the clinically important question of whether the prolonged use of S-1 is effective even to the S-1 resistant patients whom the clinicians face.

	Study drug	Dose and schedule	Number of patients		median OS		median PFS	
			Study arm	Control arm	Study arm	Control arm	Study arm	Control arm
Thuss-Patience [10]	Iriontecan	250-350mg/m2, q3w	21	19	4 p=0.012	2.4	2.5	ND
Kang [11]	Iriontecan or Docetaxel	150mg/m2, q2w or 60mg/m2, q3w	133	69	5.3 p=0.007	3.8	ND	ND
COUGAR-02 [12]	Docetaxel	75mg/m2, q3w	84	84	5.2 p=0.01	3.6	ND	ND
GRANITE-1 [13]	Evelorimus	10mg/day	439	217	5.4 p=0.12	4.3	1.7 p<0.001	1.4
REGARD [14]	Ramucirumab	8mg/kg, q2w	238	117	5.2 p=0.047	3.8	2.1 p<0.0001	1.3

OS; overall survival, PFS; progression free survival, ND; not described

Table 1. Published results of randomized controlled trials of second-line therapy versus best supportive care or placebo.

The RCT comparing a molecular targeting agent with a chemotherapeutic agent has been ongoing. HER2-positive advanced GC patients have been allocated to either trastuzumab emtansine or taxane (GATSBY, NCT01641939) [21].

A combination of molecular targeting agents and chemotherapy agents has been investigated in several RCTs. First, paclitaxel with or without lapatinib, which binds to the intracellular tyrosine kinase domains of ERBB1 and ERBB2 (HER2), was compared in HER2-positive advanced GC (TYTAN) [22]. Neither median OS nor median PFS were prolonged by lapatinib plus paclitaxel (n=132) as compared to paclitaxel alone (n=129). Second, the results of the RAINBOW trial [23,24], which compared ramucirumab plus paclitaxel with placebo plus paclitaxel, have been very recently reported in the abstract form. Sixty hundred and sixty-five GC patients, who were refractory to cisplatin and fluoropyrimidine-containing regimens, were randomized in a 1:1 ratio to receive paclitaxel plus ramucirumab or paclitaxel plus a placebo. The paclitaxel and ramucirumab arm showed a significant benefit in median OS (HR=0.807, p=0.0169) and median PFS (HR=0.635, p<0.0001). The subsequent geographical region-stratified analysis elucidated that the advantage of median PFS and median OS was more evident in Western patients than in Japanese patients (Figure 2). Such a regional difference could partly explained by a higher use of post-discontinuation treatment in Japan (75% of patients) than in Western countries (36-38% of patients), which may eventually mask any potential OS benefit of ramucirumab plus paclitaxel in Japan. Two other RCT trials [25,26] are now ongoing. Paclitaxel with or without everolimus has been compared in patients with advanced GC refractory to fluoropyrimidine containing regimens [25]. Patients will be randomized in a 1:1 ratio for a total of 240 patients per treatment arm. Nimotuzumab plus irinotecan versus irinotecan monotherapy as second-line therapy has been investigated in

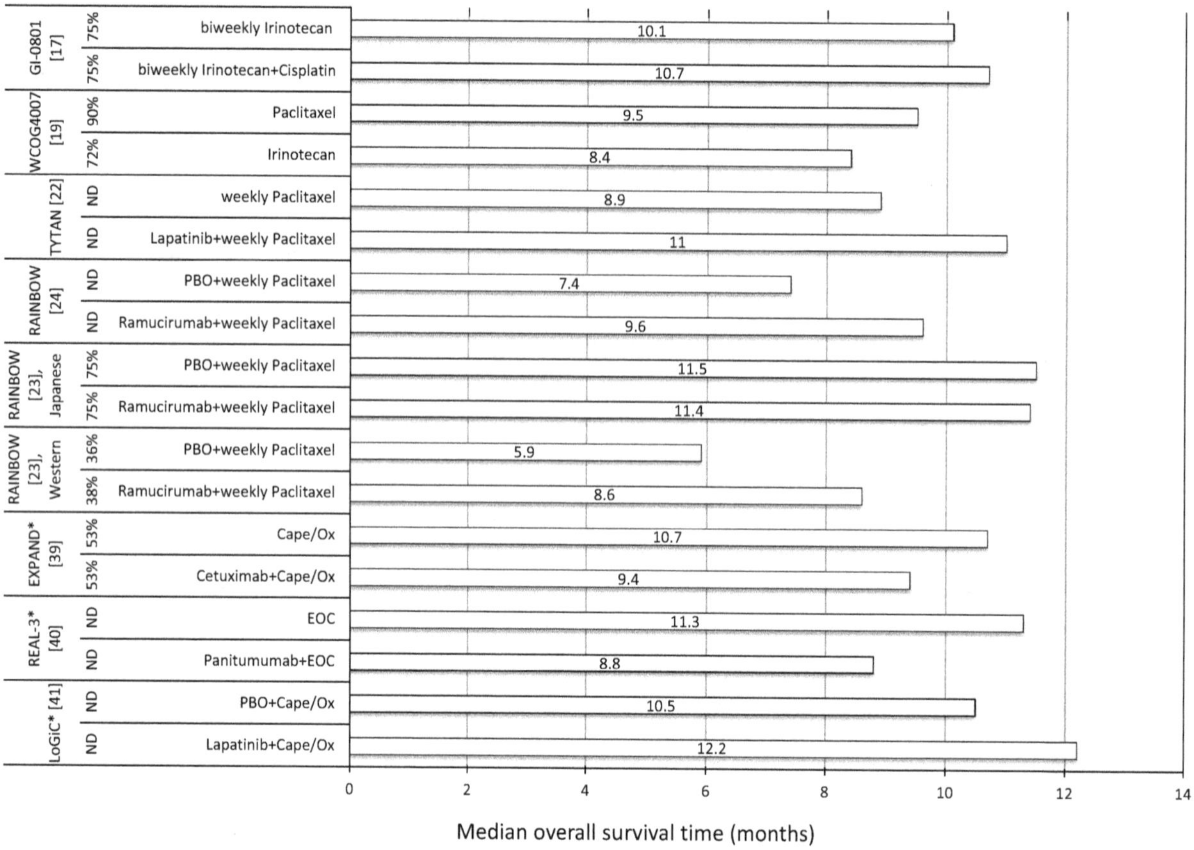

Figure 2. Comparisons of median OS between the previous RCTs. The percentage indicates the proportion of patients receiving further therapy in each trial. The reference numbers are expressed in brackets. *; first-line trials, BSC; best supportive care, PBO; placebo, Cape; capecitabine, Ox; oxaliplatin, EOC; epirubicin, oxaliplatin, and capecitabine, ND; not described.

patients with ERBB1 overexpressed advanced GC [26]. This is a Japan and Korea collaborative RCT allocating patients at 1:1 ratio for a total of approximately 400 patients per arm.

The results of some trials have been published; however, at present, trials in which the primary endpoint has been met have been unfortunately very limited. The positive results hitherto obtained include a prolonged PFS by a combination of irinotecan and cisplatin after the failure of S-1 based first-line chemotherapy, and prolonged PFS and OS by ramucirumab in combination with weekly paclitaxel. The results of other studies, especially using molecular targeting agents, are awaited.

4. Consideration of adverse events

When considering second-line therapy, clinicians must be aware that, by definition, patients receiving second-line therapy are not chemonaive and experience treatment failure; thus, they are more likely to be resistant to therapy than first-line treatment. Furthermore, patient performance status is more likely to deteriorate due to a recurrent cancer burden and treatment against it. Indeed, widely ranging grades of gastrointestinal symptoms-related adverse events occurred in a substantial proportion of patients in the BSC arms of clinical trials, suggesting a poor quality of life even by the BSC. In addition, a more intensive regimen aiming at a prolonged OS may cause a higher likelihood of severe adverse events that may result in treatment discontinuation and limitation. For example, the DCF regimen caused 82% of grade 3-4 neutropenia and 29% of febrile neutropenia. Therefore, balancing efficacy and adverse events should be taken into account when developing second-line therapy. The development of more intensive while less toxic second-line regimens could be positioned as a breakthrough marker of GC treatment, which can then ultimately achieve further survival prolongation without treatment withdrawal.

In this context, another direction for research is to establish less toxic regimens with preserved anticancer activity. As described earlier, the conventional first-line treatment comprises 5-fluorouracil and emetogenic/nephrotoxic cisplatin. Therefore, the challenges for a less toxic regimen are the substitution of oxaliplatin for nephrotoxic cisplatin [27,28] or substitution of oral capecitabine for intravenous 5-fluorouracil [29]. Such substitutions aim to reduce toxicity and maintain organ function, thus avoiding treatment withdrawal and prolonged treatment duration.

Fluorouracil, leucovorin, and oxaliplatin (FLO) were associated with significantly less anemia, nausea, vomiting, fatigue, renal toxicity, and serious adverse events related to the treatment as compared with fluorouracil, leucovorin, and cisplatin (FLP) [27]. In addition, there was a better trend toward improved median PFS by FLO than FLP. Similarly, as compared to SP, S-1 plus oxaliplatin (SOX) resulted in a reduced risk of grade 3/4 neutropenia (41.5% vs 19.5%) and febrile neutropenia (6.9% vs 0.9%) while median PFS was similar between the two regimens (5.4 months versus 5.5 months) [28]. These findings further support the possibility that the substitution of oxaliplatin for cisplatin reduced toxicity while maintaining efficacy. Accordingly, length of hospital stay per cycle of SOX regimen (0.85 day) was significantly shorter than that for the SP regimen (6 days) [28]. Furthermore, capecitabine and cisplatin (XP) versus 5-fluorouracil and cisplatin (FP) proved similar median OS (10.5 months versus 9.3 months), suggesting that the inconvenience of infusional 5-fluorouracil could be replaced by oral capecitabine, thus realizing a more simplified dosing schedule [29]. Whether this concept can be applied to second-line therapy warrants further investigation.

5. Future perspectives

With the development of a new generation of cytotoxic agents and molecular targeting agents, the research field of GC treatment appears to be transitioning into a new era with a focus on the targetable molecules in GC. Several molecular targeting agents are currently being evaluated both in first- and second-line settings. The pending results of ongoing clinical trials motivates researchers to continue the challenge of establishing the best second-line regimens or less toxic combinations for the treatment of advanced GC.

a. Clarifying the genetic alterations of targeted molecules and their interactions.

Unfortunately, in sharp contrast to colorectal cancer in which there has been a significant achievement in treatment by the use of molecular targeting agents, only one agent (ramucirumab) has been currently proved to be an agent for second-line therapy presumably due to the genetic complexity and molecular heterogeneity of the disease.

Recent findings have highlighted the mechanisms of the actions of molecular targeting agents or patterns of expression of targetable molecules in several tumors. For example, genetic alterations that are critical for cell growth occur with considerably different frequencies, being 60%, 33%, and 32% in cancers of the pancreas, biliary tract, and colon, respectively [30]. Furthermore, certain combinations of targets are expressed in a mutually exclusive or co-occurring manner in the same tumor. A mutually exclusive fashion would be a case being KRAS and BRAF in colorectal cancer, or ERBB1 and KRAS in lung cancer [31]. The co-occurring expression of targets is a case of being ERBB2 and PIK3CA in breast cancer [32]. With regard to GC, although KRAS mutations are initially recognized as an infrequent phenomenon in GC [33], the alterations and amplifications of other genes --both known or previously unreported-- have been subsequently found in a substantial number of GC patients in a mutually exclusive manner [34,35] or co-amplified manner [36]. These findings create a challenge in the treatment regimen with either a use of each blockade of each targetable molecule or a use of dual- or pan-inhibitors of kinases [37]. In addition, elucidation of the roles of each domain in ERBB2 that plays a role in resistance to anti-HER2 therapy further provides the theoretical basis to modify therapeutic strategies to circumvent this resistance [38]. These advances may expand therapeutic options, thereby making larger proportions of GC patients possible candidates for molecular targeting therapies than previously appreciated. Accordingly, there may be a desperate need for multiple gene profiling which could help establish rational molecular criteria for patient inclusion and exclusion in clinical trials. Patient selection by gene profiling may allow better patient recruitment for those most likely to respond to targeted therapies.

b. Positive and negative interactions between chemotherapy and molecular targeting therapies.

It should be noted that the recent clinical trials of first-line molecular targeting therapies regrettably resulted in some negative results [39-41] (Figure 2). The addition of cetuximab to cisplatin plus capecitabine had a similar median PFS (4.4 months) and median OS (9.4 months) compared to cisplatin plus capecitabine alone (5.6 months and 10.7 months, respectively) [39] (EXPAND). Surprisingly, the addition of panitumumab to epirubicin, oxaliplatin, and capecitabine (EOC) resulted in a significantly shorter (p=0.013) median OS (8.8 months) compared to EOC (11.3 months) (REAL-3) [40]. Furthermore, lapatinib in combination with capecitabine and oxaliplatin could not show any significant survival benefit (LoGiC) [41]. These negative results lead to speculation that there may be ideal combinations or compatibility between chemotherapy and molecular targeting therapy. In addition, even the addition of panitumumab to EOC achieved only similar median OS to those of the WCOG 4007 trial (Figure 2) [19,40]. Therefore, a certain combination, such as anti-EGFR antibody and capecitabine or oxaliplatin, may be ineffective or even interfere with the other. This speculation can be supported by the observation that addition of cetuximab to oxaliplatin plus fluoropyrimidine-based chemotherapy failed to demonstrate survival benefits for advanced colorectal cancer [42].

c. Need to evaluate the updated molecular profile.

Another obstacle for the progression of second-line treatment lies in the possibility that the molecular profile of GC is likely to change under the stress of treatment. Generally, lower response rates and shorter survival times in patients receiving second-line therapy than chemonaive patients may partly be explained by such molecular changes that lead to a resistance to therapy. Ideally, the on-demand tissue samples from tumor sites currently of interest are needed to assess the updated genetic and molecular patterns and to predict whether the planned second-line therapy is really effective. However, direct tumor tissue sampling and subsequent gene analysis are often hampered by virtually inaccesible tumor localization and by overly small sample volumes to perform gene analysis. It is necessary to discover novel markers which can be alternatives for those obtained only by direct tumor tissue sampling as well as to improvise new methods to assess them in order to select the right patients for the right second-line regimen.

Motivated by the first promising results of trastuzumab use in the ToGA trial, several molecular targeting therapies have been challenged in clinical trials. Continuous efforts should be necessary to clarify the mutation and amplification of targeted molecules, and novel methods for their genetic profiling should probably become part of clinical routines. Ultimately, GC patients harboring unique genetic profiles of targeted molecules should be allocated into specific, suitable trials. Targeted therapies tailored to individual genetic profiles maximize treatment efficacy because this allows the recruitment of selected, most suitable patients rather than unselected ones [43].

6. Conclusions

Against the background of survival advantages of second-line therapy over BSC in GC patients refractory to first-line treatment, efforts to establish the most effective regimens have been just begun. Parallel to the development of molecular targeting agents, the investigated regimens comprise doublet or triplet chemotherapeutic agents, molecular targeting agents, and their combinations. In addition, the minimization of adverse events should be taken into account to avoid treatment discontinuation. There is a desperate need to explore genetic mutations of targeted molecules and the interactions between them, to establish novel methods to assess them, to clarify the positive or negative interactions between chemotherapy and molecular targeting agents, and to find regimens in which adverse events are least likely to occur for avoiding treatment discontinuation. These could help determine rational molecular criteria for patient inclusion and exclusion in clinical trials, realize the most efficient patient recruitment for those most likely to respond to therapies, and accelerate the establishment of the most effective second-line therapy that could achieve greater survival prolongation.

Author details

Shouji Shimoyama

Address all correspondence to: shimoyama@apost.plala.or.jp

Gastrointestinal Unit, Settlement Clinic, Towa, Adachi-ku, Tokyo, Japan

References

[1] Jemal A, Bray F, Center MM, Ferlay J, Ward E, Forman D. Global cancer statistics. CA Cancer J Clin. 2011; 61(2): 69-90.

[2] Buzzoni R, Bajetta E, Di Bartolomeo M, Miceli R, Beretta E, Ferrario E, Mariani L. Pathological features as predictors of recurrence after radical resection of gastric cancer. Br J Surg. 2006; 93(2): 205-9.

[3] Siegel R, Ma J, Zou Z, Jemal A. Cancer statistics, 2014. CA Cancer J Clin. 2014; 64(1): 9-29. doi: 10.3322/caac.21208.

[4] De Angelis R, Sant M, Coleman MP, Francisci S, Baili P, Pierannunzio D, Trama A, Visser O, Brenner H, Ardanaz E, Bielska-Lasota M, Engholm G, Nennecke A, Siesling S, Berrino F, Capocaccia R; EUROCARE-5 Working Group. Cancer survival in Europe 1999-2007 by country and age: results of EUROCARE--5-a population-based study. Lancet Oncol. 2014; 15(1): 23-34. doi: 10.1016/S1470-2045(13)70546-1.

[5] Waters JS, Norman A, Cunningham D, Scarffe JH, Webb A, Harper P, Joffe JK, Mackean M, Mansi J, Leahy M, Hill A, Oates J, Rao S, Nicolson M, Hickish T. Long-term survival after epirubicin, cisplatin and fluorouracil for gastric cancer: results of a randomized trial. Br J Cancer. 1999; 80: 269-72.

[6] Van Cutsem E, Moiseyenko VM, Tjulandin S, Majlis A, Constenla M, Boni C, Rodrigues A, Fodor M, Chao Y, Voznyi E, Risse ML, Ajani JA; V325 Study Group. Phase III study of docetaxel and cisplatin plus fluorouracil compared with cisplatin and fluorouracil as first-line therapy for advanced gastric cancer: a report of the V325 Study Group. J Clin Oncol. 2006; 24: 4991-7.

[7] Koizumi W, Narahara H, Hara T, Takagane A, Akiya T, Takagi M, Miyashita K, Nishizaki T, Kobayashi O, Takiyama W, Toh Y, Nagaie T, Takagi S, Yamamura Y, Yanaoka K, Orita H, Takeuchi M. S-1 plus cisplatin versus S-1 alone for first-line treatment of advanced gastric cancer (SPIRITS trial): a phase III trial. Lancet Oncol. 2008; 9(3): 215-21. doi: 10.1016/S1470-2045(08)70035-4.

[8] Ajani JA, Rodriguez W, Bodoky G, Moiseyenko V, Lichinitser M, Gorbunova V, Vynnychenko I, Garin A, Lang I, Falcon S. Multicenter phase III comparison of cisplatin/S-1 with cisplatin/infusional fluorouracil in advanced gastric or gastroeso-

phageal adenocarcinoma study: the FLAGS trial. J Clin Oncol. 2010; 28(9): 1547-53. doi: 10.1200/JCO.2009.25.4706.

[9] Bang YJ, Van Cutsem E, Feyereislova A, Chung HC, Shen L, Sawaki A, Lordick F, Ohtsu A, Omuro Y, Satoh T, Aprile G, Kulikov E, Hill J, Lehle M, Rüschoff J, Kang YK; ToGA Trial Investigators. Trastuzumab in combination with chemotherapy versus chemotherapy alone for treatment of HER2-positive advanced gastric or gastro-oesophageal junction cancer (ToGA): a phase 3, open-label, randomised controlled trial. Lancet. 2010; 376(9742): 687-97. doi: 10.1016/S0140-6736(10)61121-X.

[10] Thuss-Patience PC, Kretzschmar A, Bichev D, Deist T, Hinke A, Breithaupt K, Dogan Y, Gebauer B, Schumacher G, Reichardt P. Survival advantage for irinotecan versus best supportive care as second-line chemotherapy in gastric cancer--a randomised phase III study of the Arbeitsgemeinschaft Internistische Onkologie (AIO). Eur J Cancer. 2011; 47(15): 2306-14. doi: 10.1016/j.ejca.2011.06.002.

[11] Kang JH, Lee SI, Lim do H, Park KW, Oh SY, Kwon HC, Hwang IG, Lee SC, Nam E, Shin DB, Lee J, Park JO, Park YS, Lim HY, Kang WK, Park SH. Salvage chemotherapy for pretreated gastric cancer: a randomized phase III trial comparing chemotherapy plus best supportive care with best supportive care alone. J Clin Oncol. 2012; 30(13): 1513-8. doi: 10.1200/JCO.2011.39.4585.

[12] Ford HE, Marshall A, Bridgewater JA, Janowitz T, Coxon FY, Wadsley J, Mansoor W, Fyfe D, Madhusudan S, Middleton GW, Swinson D, Falk S, Chau I, Cunningham D, Kareclas P, Cook N, Blazeby JM, Dunn JA; COUGAR-02 Investigators. Docetaxel versus active symptom control for refractory oesophagogastric adenocarcinoma (COUGAR-02): an open-label, phase 3 randomised controlled trial. Lancet Oncol. 2014; 15(1): 78-86. doi: 10.1016/S1470-2045(13)70549-7.

[13] Ohtsu A, Ajani JA, Bai YX, Bang YJ, Chung HC, Pan HM, Sahmoud T, Shen L, Yeh KH, Chin K, Muro K, Kim YH, Ferry D, Tebbutt NC, Al-Batran SE, Smith H, Costantini C, Rizvi S, Lebwohl D, Van Cutsem E. Everolimus for previously treated advanced gastric cancer: results of the randomized, double-blind, phase III GRANITE-1 study. J Clin Oncol. 2013; 31(31): 3935-43. doi: 10.1200/JCO.2012.48.3552.

[14] Fuchs CS, Tomasek J, Yong CJ, Dumitru F, Passalacqua R, Goswami C, Safran H, dos Santos LV, Aprile G, Ferry DR, Melichar B, Tehfe M, Topuzov E, Zalcberg JR, Chau I, Campbell W, Sivanandan C, Pikiel J, Koshiji M, Hsu Y, Liepa AM, Gao L, Schwartz JD, Tabernero J; REGARD Trial Investigators. Ramucirumab monotherapy for previously treated advanced gastric or gastro-oesophageal junction adenocarcinoma (REGARD): an international, randomised, multicentre, placebo-controlled, phase 3 trial. Lancet. 2014; 383(9911): 31-9. doi: 10.1016/S0140-6736(13)61719-5.

[15] http://www.ClinicalTrial.gov. NCT 01512745

[16] Kim HS, Kim HJ, Kim SY, Kim TY, Lee KW, Baek SK, Kim TY, Ryu MH, Nam BH, Zang DY. Second-line chemotherapy versus supportive cancer treatment in ad-

vanced gastric cancer: a meta-analysis. Ann Oncol. 2013; 24(11): 2850-4. doi: 10.1093/annonc/mdt351.

[17] Higuchi K, Tanabe S, Shimada K, Hosaka H, Sasaki E, Nakayama N, Takeda Y, Moriwaki T, Amagai K, Sekikawa T, Sakuyama T, Kanda T, Sasaki T, Azuma M, Takahashi F, Takeuchi M, Koizumi W; Tokyo Cooperative Oncology Group, Tokyo, Japan. Biweekly irinotecan plus cisplatin versus irinotecan alone as second-line treatment for advanced gastric cancer: a randomised phase III trial (TCOG GI-0801/BIRIP trial). Eur J Cancer. 2014; 50(8): 1437-45. doi: 10.1016/j.ejca.2014.01.020.

[18] Inagaki H, Nishikawa K, Fujitani K, Sugimoto N, Shigematsu T, Ishiguro T, Tsuburaya A, Nakamura M, Nashimoto A, Yamane T, Yamada M, Imano M, Iijima S, Oka Y, Kataoka M, Hironaka S, Andoh H, Morita S, Sakamoto J, Tsujinaka T. Efficacy analyses of a randomized phase III clinical trial of combined therapy with CPT-11/CDDP versus CPT-11 alone in patients with advanced or recurrent gastric cancer refractory to prior S-1 chemotherapy. Proc ASCO 2013; abstr 69.

[19] Hironaka S, Ueda S, Yasui H, Nishina T, Tsuda M, Tsumura T, Sugimoto N, Shimodaira H, Tokunaga S, Moriwaki T, Esaki T, Nagase M, Fujitani K, Yamaguchi K, Ura T, Hamamoto Y, Morita S, Okamoto I, Boku N, Hyodo I. Randomized, open-label, phase III study comparing irinotecan with paclitaxel in patients with advanced gastric cancer without severe peritoneal metastasis after failure of prior combination chemotherapy using fluoropyrimidine plus platinum: WJOG 4007 trial. J Clin Oncol. 2013; 31(35): 4438-44. doi: 10.1200/JCO.2012.48.5805.

[20] http://www.ClinicalTrial.gov. NCT 00639327

[21] http://www.ClinicalTrial.gov. NCT 01641939

[22] Satoh T, Xu RH, Chung HC, Sun GP, Doi T, Xu JM, Tsuji A, Omuro Y, Li J, Wang JW, Miwa H, Qin SK, Chung IJ, Yeh KH, Feng JF, Mukaiyama A, Kobayashi M, Ohtsu A, Bang YJ. Lapatinib plus paclitaxel versus paclitaxel alone in the second-line treatment of HER2-amplified advanced gastric cancer in Asian populations: TyTAN--a randomized, phase III study. J Clin Oncol. 2014; 32(19): 2039-49. doi: 10.1200/JCO.2013.53.6136.

[23] Hironaka S, Shimada Y, Sugimoto N, Komatsu Y, Nishina T, Yamaguchi K, Segawa Y, Omuro Y, Tamura T, Doi T, Yukisawa S, Yasui H, Nagashima F, Gotoh M, Esaki T, Emig M, Chandrawansa K, Muro K, Wilke H, Ohtsu A. RAINBOW: A global, phase III, randomized, double-blind study of ramucirumab (RAM) plus paclitaxel (PTX) versus placebo (PL) plus PTX in the treatment of metastatic gastroesophageal junction and gastric adenocarcinoma (mGC) following disease progression on first-line platinum- and fluoropyrimidine-containing combination therapy—Efficacy analysis in Japanese and Western patients. Proc ASCO 2014; abstr 4005

[24] Wilke H, Van Cutsem E, Oh SC, Bodoky G, Shimada Y, Hironaka S, Sugimoto N, Lipatov ON, Kim T-Y, Cunningham D, Ohtsu A, Rougier P, Emig M, Carlesi R, Chandrawansa K, Muro K. RAINBOW: A global, phase III, randomized, double-blind

study of ramucirumab plus paclitaxel versus placebo plus paclitaxel in the treatment of metastatic gastroesophageal junction (GEJ) and gastric adenocarcinoma following disease progression on first-line platinum- and fluoropyrimidine-containing combination therapy rainbow IMCL CP12-0922 (I4T-IE-JVBE). Proc ASCO 2014; abstr LBA7

[25] http://www.ClinicalTrial.gov. NCT 01248403

[26] http://www.ClinicalTrial.gov. NCT 01813253

[27] Al-Batran SE, Hartmann JT, Probst S, Schmalenberg H, Hollerbach S, Hofheinz R, Rethwisch V, Seipelt G, Homann N, Wilhelm G, Schuch G, Stoehlmacher J, Derigs HG, Hegewisch-Becker S, Grossmann J, Pauligk C, Atmaca A, Bokemeyer C, Knuth A, Jäger E; Arbeitsgemeinschaft Internistische Onkologie. Phase III trial in metastatic gastroesophageal adenocarcinoma with fluorouracil, leucovorin plus either oxaliplatin or cisplatin: a study of the Arbeitsgemeinschaft Internistische Onkologie. J Clin Oncol. 2008; 26(9): 1435-42. doi: 10.1200/JCO.2007.13.9378.

[28] Higuchi K, Koizumi W, Yamada Y, Nishikawa K, Gotoh M, Fuse N, Sugimoto N, Nishina T, Amagai K, Chin K, Niwa Y, Negoro Y, Imamura H, Tsuda M, Yasui H, Fujii H, Yamaguchi K, Yasui H, Hamada C, Hyodo I. Randomized phase III study of S-1 plus oxaliplatin versus S-1 plus cisplatin for first-line treatment of advanced gastric cancer. Proc ASCO 2013; abstr 60

[29] Kang YK, Kang WK, Shin DB, Chen J, Xiong J, Wang J, Lichinitser M, Guan Z, Khasanov R, Zheng L, Philco-Salas M, Suarez T, Santamaria J, Forster G, McCloud PI. Capecitabine/cisplatin versus 5-fluorouracil/cisplatin as first-line therapy in patients with advanced gastric cancer: a randomised phase III noninferiority trial. Ann Oncol. 2009; 20(4): 666-73. doi: 10.1093/annonc/mdn717.

[30] Schubbert S, Shannon K, Bollag G. Hyperactive Ras in developmental disorders and cancer. Nat Rev Cancer. 2007; 7(4): 295-308.

[31] Ding L, Getz G, Wheeler DA, Mardis ER, McLellan MD, Cibulskis K, Sougnez C, Greulich H, Muzny DM, Morgan MB, Fulton L, Fulton RS, Zhang Q, Wendl MC, Lawrence MS, Larson DE, Chen K, Dooling DJ, Sabo A, Hawes AC, Shen H, Jhangiani SN, Lewis LR, Hall O, Zhu Y, Mathew T, Ren Y, Yao J, Scherer SE, Clerc K, Metcalf GA, Ng B, Milosavljevic A, Gonzalez-Garay ML, Osborne JR, Meyer R, Shi X, Tang Y, Koboldt DC, Lin L, Abbott R, Miner TL, Pohl C, Fewell G, Haipek C, Schmidt H, Dunford-Shore BH, Kraja A, Crosby SD, Sawyer CS, Vickery T, Sander S, Robinson J, Winckler W, Baldwin J, Chirieac LR, Dutt A, Fennell T, Hanna M, Johnson BE, Onofrio RC, Thomas RK, Tonon G, Weir BA, Zhao X, Ziaugra L, Zody MC, Giordano T, Orringer MB, Roth JA, Spitz MR, Wistuba II, Ozenberger B, Good PJ, Chang AC, Beer DG, Watson MA, Ladanyi M, Broderick S, Yoshizawa A, Travis WD, Pao W, Province MA, Weinstock GM, Varmus HE, Gabriel SB, Lander ES, Gibbs RA, Meyerson M, Wilson RK. Somatic mutations affect key pathways in lung adenocarcinoma. Nature. 2008; 455(7216): 1069-75. doi: 10.1038/nature07423.

[32] Saal LH, Holm K, Maurer M, Memeo L, Su T, Wang X, Yu JS, Malmström PO, Mansukhani M, Enoksson J, Hibshoosh H, Borg A, Parsons R. PIK3CA mutations correlate with hormone receptors, node metastasis, and ERBB2, and are mutually exclusive with PTEN loss in human breast carcinoma. Cancer Res. 2005; 65(7): 2554-9.

[33] Lee SH, Lee JW, Soung YH, Kim HS, Park WS, Kim SY, Lee JH, Park JY, Cho YG, Kim CJ, Nam SW, Kim SH, Lee JY, Yoo NJ. BRAF and KRAS mutations in stomach cancer. Oncogene. 2003; 22(44): 6942-5.

[34] Shimoyama S. BRAF mutations and their implications in molecular targeting therapies for gastrointestinal cancers. J Pharmacogenom Pharmacoproteomics 2011; 2: e102. doi: 10.4172/2153-0645.1000e102

[35] Deng N, Goh LK, Wang H, Das K, Tao J, Tan IB, Zhang S, Lee M, Wu J, Lim KH, Lei Z, Goh G, Lim QY, Tan AL, Sin Poh DY, Riahi S, Bell S, Shi MM, Linnartz R, Zhu F, Yeoh KG, Toh HC, Yong WP, Cheong HC, Rha SY, Boussioutas A, Grabsch H, Rozen S, Tan P. A comprehensive survey of genomic alterations in gastric cancer reveals systematic patterns of molecular exclusivity and co-occurrence among distinct therapeutic targets. Gut. 2012; 61(5): 673-84. doi: 10.1136/gutjnl-2011-301839.

[36] Kiyose S, Nagura K, Tao H, Igarashi H, Yamada H, Goto M, Maeda M, Kurabe N, Suzuki M, Tsuboi M, Kahyo T, Shinmura K, Hattori N, Sugimura H. Detection of kinase amplifications in gastric cancer archives using fluorescence in situ hybridization. Pathol Int. 2012; 62(7): 477-84. doi: 10.1111/j.1440-1827.2012.02832.x.

[37] Prahallad A, Sun C, Huang S, Di Nicolantonio F, Salazar R, Zecchin D, Beijersbergen RL, Bardelli A, Bernards R. Unresponsiveness of colon cancer to BRAF(V600E) inhibition through feedback activation of EGFR. Nature. 2012; 483(7387): 100-3. doi: 10.1038/nature10868.

[38] Shimoyama S. Unraveling trastuzumab and lapatinib in gastric cancer. Future steps. Mol Clin Oncol 2014; 2 (2): 175-181. DOI: 10.3892/mco.2013.218

[39] Lordick F, Kang YK, Chung HC, Salman P, Oh SC, Bodoky G, Kurteva G, Volovat C, Moiseyenko VM, Gorbunova V, Park JO, Sawaki A, Celik I, Götte H, Melezínková H, Moehler M; Arbeitsgemeinschaft Internistische Onkologie and EXPAND Investigators. Capecitabine and cisplatin with or without cetuximab for patients with previously untreated advanced gastric cancer (EXPAND): a randomised, open-label phase 3 trial. Lancet Oncol. 2013; 14(6): 490-9. doi: 10.1016/S1470-2045(13)70102-5.

[40] Waddell TS, Chau I, Barbachano Y, de Castro DG, Wotherspoon A, Saffery C, Middleton GW, Wadsley J, Ferry DR, Mansoor W, Crosby TDL, Coxon FY, Smith D, Waters JS, Iveson T, Falk S, Slater S, Okines AFC, Cunningham D. A randomized multicenter trial of epirubicin, oxaliplatin, and capecitabine (EOC) plus panitumumab in advanced esophagogastric cancer (REAL3). Proc ASCO 2012; abstr LBA4000

[41] Hecht JR, Bang Y-J, Qin S, Chung H-C, Xu J-M, Park JO, Jeziorski K, Shparyk Y, Hoff PM, Sobrero AF, Salman P, Li J, Protsenko S, Buyse ME, Afenjar K, Kaneko T, Kemn-

er A, Santillana S, Press MF, Slamon DJ. Lapatinib in combination with capecitabine plus oxaliplatin (CapeOx) in HER2-positive advanced or metastatic gastric, esophageal, or gastroesophageal adenocarcinoma (AC): The TRIO-013/LOGiC Trial. Proc ASCO, 2013; abstr LBA4001

[42] Maughan TS, Adams RA, Smith CG, Meade AM, Seymour MT, Wilson RH, Idziaszczyk S, Harris R, Fisher D, Kenny SL, Kay E, Mitchell JK, Madi A, Jasani B, James MD, Bridgewater J, Kennedy MJ, Claes B, Lambrechts D, Kaplan R, Cheadle JP; MRC COIN Trial Investigators. Addition of cetuximab to oxaliplatin-based first-line combination chemotherapy for treatment of advanced colorectal cancer: results of the randomised phase 3 MRC COIN trial. Lancet. 2011; 377(9783): 2103-14. doi: 10.1016/S0140-6736(11)60613-2.

[43] Asaoka Y, Ikenoue T, Koike K. New targeted therapies for gastric cancer. Expert Opin Investig Drugs. 2011; 20(5): 595-604. doi: 10.1517/13543784.2011.566863.

10

Reconstructive Procedures after Total Gastrectomy for Gastric Cancer

Nebojsa S. Ignjatovic, Tomislav D. Randjelovic, Miroslav P. Stojanovic, Goran Z. Stanojevic and Miodrag N. Djordjevic

Abstract

Till this day, there are more than 60 described surgical procedures of the intestinal reconstructions after a total gastrectomy. In 1897, Schlatter reconstructed the digestive tract by creating a termino-lateral esophagojejunostomies that was the first successful total gastrectomy. Many of the total gastrectomy pioneers did the reconstruction by esophagoduodenostomy or by forming a loop esophagojejunostomy. The main reconstruction modalities after a total gastrectomy are a restitution of the intestinal continuity, without a preservation of the duodenal food passage (esophagojejunostomy with a Roux-en-Y configuration) and a restitution of the intestinal continuity with a preservation of the duodenal passage (esophagojejunostomy with Roux-en-Y configuration and forming of the lateral-terminal jejunoduodenal anastomosis double tract and jejunal interposition by Longmire). The surgeries in these categories can be combined with forming of an enteral pouch or a stomach reservoir which would simulate a reservoir of a normal intact stomach. The ideal reconstruction procedure after total gastrectomy should replace all lost functions of the stomach. Preservation of duodenal transit with replacement of the jejunal segment, the so-called physiological route, is now believed to be preferential for postoperative nutritional condition, prevents persistent postgastrectomy syndrome, and improves the quality of life. Reconstructive procedures which allow duodenal passage should be regarded as a key to physiological reconstruction.

Keywords: gastric cancer, total gastrectomy, reconstructive procedures, nutritive status, quality of life

1. Introduction

1.1. Background and history

The development of stomach surgery is one of the most fascinating chapters in the history of surgery. The era of surgical treatment of gastric cancer (GC) began with the first successfully performed distal subtotal gastrectomy in 1881 by Theodor Billroth. The first total gastrectomy (TG) was probably carried out by Conner in 1887 in Cincinnati, but the patient died [1]. The first successful TG due to GC was performed by Carl Schlatter in Switzerland in 1897 [2]. The patient was a 56-year-old woman who lived less than 14 months and died from secondary metastatic deposits in the liver. Krönlein first introduced the term TG in 1898. Charles Brigham of San Francisco in the same year performed the first successful TG in the United States to create an esophagoduodenal anastomosis, using the Murphy button [3]. The high postoperative mortality in TG performed in the 1940s, was reduced by the introduction of antibiotics, the use of blood transfusions, and the improvement of anesthetics and surgical techniques. During this period TG was proposed as a routine surgical treatment for all resectable GC. This approach was later abandoned due to inability to improve the survival rate, high operative mortality, and increased incidence of undesirable postoperative effects after TG [4]. By 1980, TG was rarely performed and was only applied in highly selective cases [5]. The contribution of these and many other authors during the nineteenth century provided a basis for modern surgical treatment of patients with GC. From the beginning of the 1940s, radical resection, including regional lymphadenectomy for all GC, was recommended [6]. Operations of such extensions, at that time, were burdened with unacceptable morbidity and mortality. To date, efforts have been made to define the optimal extent of resection, lymphadenectomy, and reconstruction.

Digestive tract reconstruction after TG was mostly performed initially by creating a direct anastomosis of the esophagus with a duodenum or with a jejunum loop. The inevitable problem of billiard regurgitation was solved in 1909 by adopting the creation of the Roux-en-Y (RY) type of esophagojejunostomy configuration [7]. A large number of surgeons continued to perform jejunum loop reconstruction until 1947, when Orr promoted the concept of end-to-end anastomosis using the RY-type configuration of esophagojejunostomy, which is now a standard procedure for reconstruction after TG [8].

2. Reconstructive procedures after total gastrectomy

2.1. Concept of reconstructive procedures after total gastrectomy

During the first successful TG in 1897, Schlatter reconstructed the digestive tract by creating end-to-side esophagojejunostomy [2]. Many of the pioneers of TG performed reconstruction with esophagoduodenostomy or formed loop esophagojejunostomy [7, 9]. High operational risk and frequent malnutrition observed during the postoperative period gave TG an unfavorable reputation. The loop esophagojejunostomy technique was modified by Hoffman in 1922.

He added a small side-to-side jejunojejunostomy between two ends of the jejunum loop [10]. This provided partial bypass to the duodenal content and reduced the frequency of alkaline reflux esophagitis. The major immediate postoperative problem after TG concerned the integrity of anastomosis on the esophagus. Later postoperative problems were associated with reconstruction and nutritional status and quality of life that is more affected by the aspects of reconstruction than the anastomosis on the esophagus itself.

To date, more than 60 different reconstructive procedures (RP) of intestinal reconstructions have been described after TG which were, and are now, in use in surgical institutions [11, 12]. The main modalities of reconstruction after TG are restoration of intestinal continuity, without preserving duodenal passage (DP) of food (esophagojejunostomy with RY configuration) and restoration of intestinal continuity with the preservation of DP (esophagojejunostomy with RY configuration and formation of side-to-end jejunoduodenostomy double tract (DT) and Longmire's longitudinal interposition). Operations in these categories can be combined with the formation of an enteral pouch or a gastric reservoir that simulates the function of the reservoir of the normal intact stomach. The RP with pouch and neo-stomach formation have been developed to provide food tanks, with the goal of preserving duodenal transit and providing the anatomy and physiology of the digestive tract. Advantages and disadvantages of these RP continue to be the subject of discussion due to the existence of contradictory results from various studies.

2.2. Reconstructive procedures without duodenal passage preservation after total gastrectomy

2.2.1. *Esophagojejunostomy Roux-en-Y configuration*

The RY configuration of esophagojejunostomy has become the most widely used method of reconstructing intestinal continuity around the world [13, 14]. This precious intestinal configuration is now used in reconstruction and drainage of the stomach, esophagus, and pancreatic-biliary tree, as well as in bariatric surgery [15].

The procedure was inaugurated by César Roux (1857–1934), a Swiss surgeon and professor, in 1893 [16]. Initially, after TG, the jejunum loop was placed in a retrocolonic fashion. RY configuration of esophagojejunostomy immediately became objectionable due to a recurrent complication, that is, the potential formation of ulceration on the jejunal anastomosis [7]. The idea of using the RY configuration for reconstruction after TG was introduced early, in 1909 [9]. Despite Reid's 1925 report on the use of this RP, most of the surgeons of that time continued to prefer loop esophagojejunostomy with an anastomosis between two jejunum loops, thereby preventing the alkaline reflux of duodenal content and consecutive esophagitis [17]. In 1940, several papers again drew attention to the Roux-en-Y intestinal configuration, and in 1947, Orr reintroduces end-to-side esophagojejunostomy in creating a RY configuration (**Figures 1–3**) [8].

The primary factor in creating RY is the preservation of adequate vascularization. Jejunum vascularization comes from superior mesenteric artery, aorte abdominalis' branch. Superior mesenteric artery branches for vascularization of the intestinum are formed on its left side, and their number is variable 13–21, for vascularization of jejunum 3–7 (average 5) and 8–17 (average 11) for the ileum. Intestinal arteries branch in the mesenterium, and through the

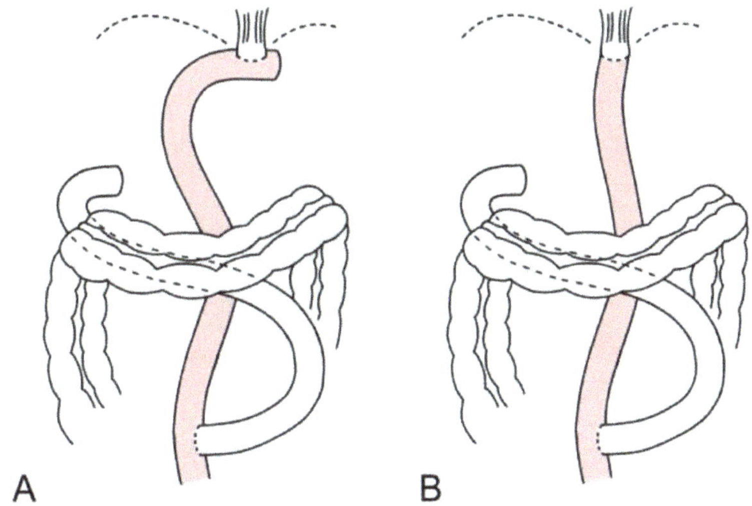

Figure 1. Schematic representation of reconstruction after TG without DP with a standard RY configuration with the creation of (A) end-to-side or (B) end-to-end esophagojejunostomy.

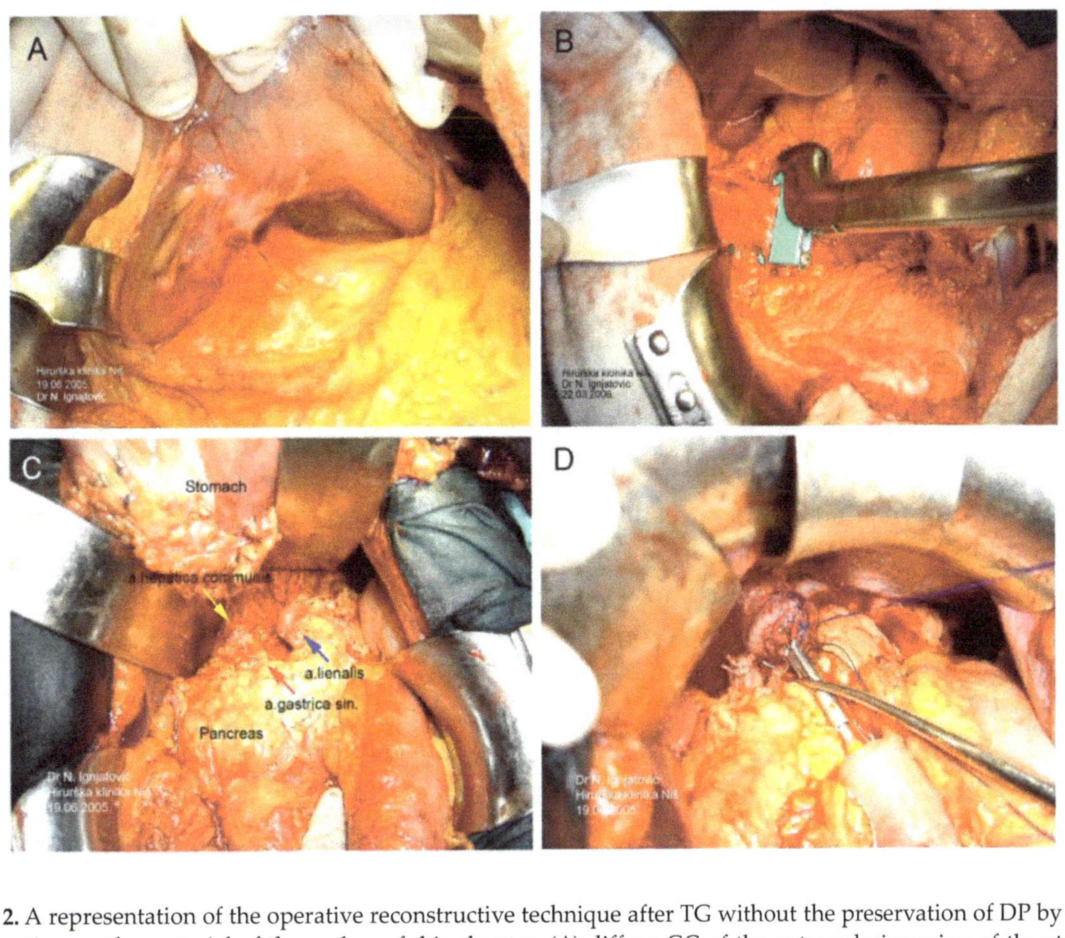

Figure 2. A representation of the operative reconstructive technique after TG without the preservation of DP by the RY configuration on the material of the author of this chapter: (A) diffuse GC of the antropyloric region of the stomach; (B) closure of the duodenal residue using a linear stapler TA 30; (C) lymphovascular dissection of the plexus coeliacus, a.hepaticae communis (yellow arrow), a.gastricae sin. (red arrow), and a.lienalis (blue arrow); (D) bringing the jejunum loop to the approximation with distal esophagus and forming end-to-end esophagojejunostomy with circular stapler CEEA Ø25 mm.

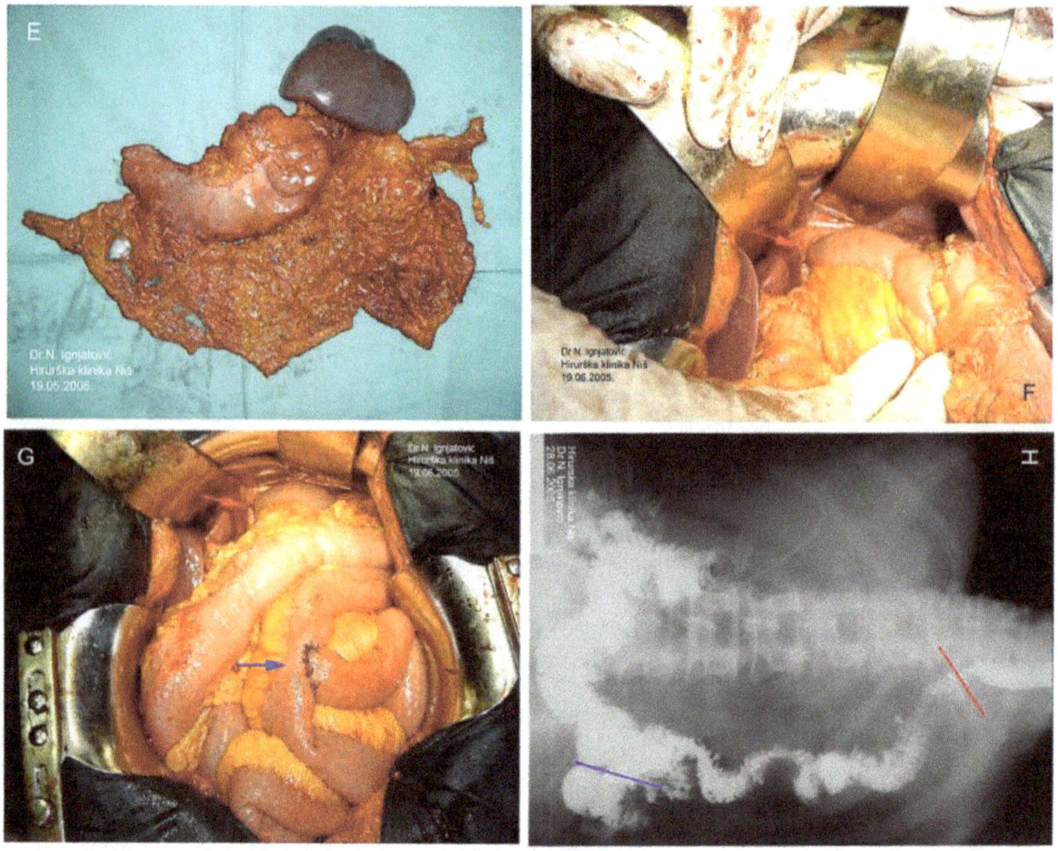

Figure 3. A representation of the operative reconstructive technique after TG without the preservation of DP by the RY configuration on the material of the author of this chapter: (E) specimen of the stomach, spleen, and large omentum, (F) formed end-to-end esophagojejunostomy (red arrow), (G) formed end-to-side jejunojejunostomy with Roux Y anastomosis (blue arrow), (H) contrast radiography: sufficient anastomosis of esophagojejunostomy (red line) and end-to-side jejunojejunostomy with Roux-en-Y anastomosis (blue line).

vascular arcades of the I–IV orders, they connect to one another before the separation of terminal vasa recta entering the small intestine on the mesenteric edge. Arcades are more developed in the proximal part of the intestinum. They are arranged in three rows, so that arcades allow good vascularization and formation of isolated segments. Vasa recta are terminal type, and each such blood vessel vascularizes about 0.5 cm of the intestinal wall [18]. There are long and short arteriolae rectae. The long arteriole recta are divided into two branches, anterior and posterior. Entering the jejunum wall, each of those branches vascularizes specific area of the jejunum wall and they anastomose on the antimesenteric edge. The antimesenteric edge has the weakest vascularization and therefore is susceptible to the occurrence of dehiscence after the creation of anastomosis. Short arteriolae rectae, which can directly originate from the paraintestinal arterial arcades, or from other arterioles, are intended for the vascularization of the mesenteric intestine [19]. The regularly firmed distal end of the RY jejunum loop was mobilized by dividing two vasa recta [7].

The main goal in choosing the reconstruction of the esophago-intestinal continuity RY configuration after TG without preserving DP is to prevent the formation of biliary reflux into the esophagus. Biliary contents can cause damage to the esophagus mucous membranes, or alkaline esophagitis [20]. In 1924, the proposed RY loop length was only 7.5 cm, but it increased steadily and significantly over time. Wells proposed in 1956 a length of 20–25 cm. The smallest length of the RY loop of 35 cm proved to be capable of preventing the formation of alkaline biliary reflux [21]. The vast majority of experienced surgeons today use RY loop length of 40–60 cm. The wide application of the RP RY configuration is attributed to its simplicity because it uses a minimum number of anastomosis.

In order to adequately replace the stomach and increase the reservoir of the jejunal substituent, the RP RY configuration was modified by Hunt and later by Lawrence by creating a jejunal pouch [22, 23]. Several modalities of the reconstruction of the jejunal pouch include forming formations J-pouch, Ω-pouch, S-pouch, and an aboral pouch [22–25].

Forming the Hunt-Lawrence pouch, the jejunum in length is brought up posterior to the transverse colon. The distal portion of the divided afferent limb, with approximate length of 15–20 cm, is placed posterior to the transverse colon, plicated to the proximal efferent limb and retained by traction sutures. A small stab wound is formed at the midportion of each limb of plicated loops, and a linear stapler is introduced through it, while side-to-side anastomoses are created upward and down along the antimesenteric borders. Following the inspection of the anastomotic lines for complete hemostasis, a circular stapler (stapler CEEA) is introduced through the central hole of the pouch for the esophagojejunostomy.

The hole is closed transversely with a running suture following the withdrawal of the circular stapler. Intestinal continuity is then reestablished by hand in RY fashion, about 20–30 cm below the pouch (**Figures 4** and **5**) [26–28].

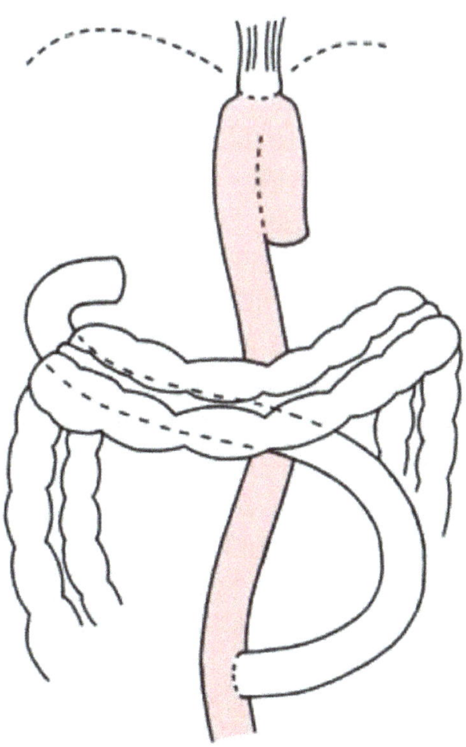

Figure 4. Schematic representation of reconstruction after TG without DP with a the Hunt-Lawrence pouch.

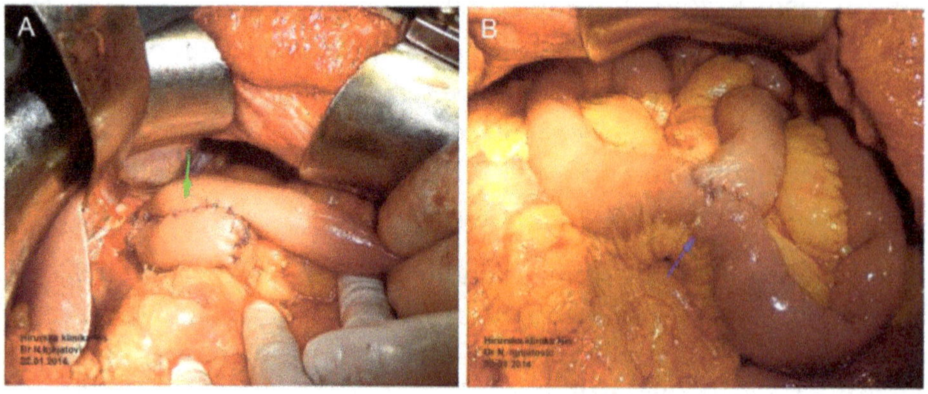

Figure 5. A representation of operative reconstructive technique after TG without DP preservation by the pouch configuration on the material of the author of this chapter: (A) end-to-side esophagojejunostomy is formed (red arrow) and longitudinal side-to-side jejunojejunostomy (green arrow); (B) end-to-side jejunojejunostomy is created with Roux-en-Y anastomosis (blue arrow).

The use of pouch reconstruction provides a reduction in the occurrence of dumping syndrome, postoperative weight development, regurgitation of bile, and insufficient size of indigested meals [27].

2.3. Reconstructive procedure with duodenal passage preservation after total gastrectomy

2.3.1. Esophagojejunostomy Roux-en-Y double tract configuration

The RP using the jejunum after TG with the preservation of DP is the esophagus RY configuration of the DT in the establishment of esophagoduodenal continuity. The description of operational technique was first provided in 1965 by Japanese authors Kajitani and Sato [29]. In this RP after TG, the duodenum in the first act remains open, and after the creation of an esophagojejunal anastomosis according to the principles of the operational technique of carrying RY configurations with a duodenum duct, an additional distal end-to-side jejunoduodenal anastomosis is established at about 20 cm distal from created esophagojejunal anastomosis [30]. Today's modification of the originally described technique is the creation of end-to-end duodenal anastomosis at 35–40 cm distal from esophagojejunal anastomosis [31]. Creation of distal termino-lateral jejunojejunal anastomosis is performed according to the principles of the original RY configuration of esophagojejunostomy at about 60 cm from end-to-side or end-to-end esophagojejunal anastomosis (**Figure 6**). Creation of esophagojejunal anastomosis is performed by a manual two-layer suture technique or the use of the CEEA circular surgical stapler, while the creation of jejunoduodenal and jejunojejunal anastomosis is performed by a manual two-layer suture technique (**Figure 7**) [31, 32]. The RY configuration of the DT is now applied in some institutions in Japan.

2.3.2. Esophagojejunostomy with the interposition of the jejunal segment by Longmire

RP using the jejunum after TG with the preservation of DP is the interposition to isoperistaltics free jejunal segment according to the Longmire method in establishing esophagoduodenal

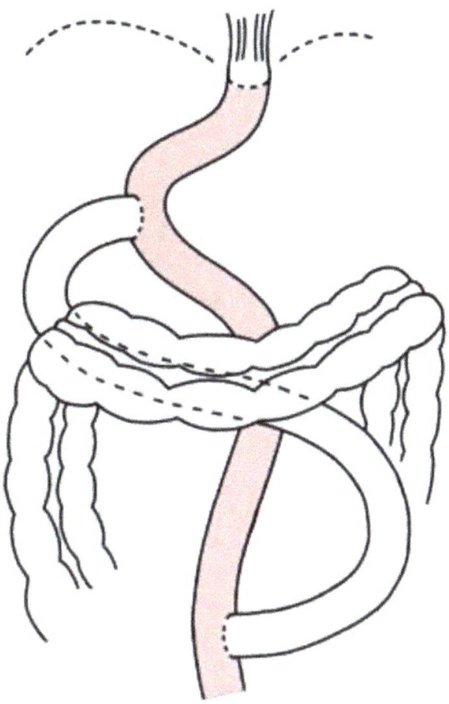

Figure 6. Schematic representation of reconstruction after TG with DP with a RY configuration of DT with the creation of end-to-end esophagojejunostomy and side-to-end jejunoduodenostomy.

continuity. After Seo's first attempt in 1941, the inauguration of this RP after TG was performed by Longmire in 1951, even though the idea was proposed 3 years earlier by Saccharow [33–36].

Hays interposed a triple jejunal pouch between the esophagus and duodenum in 1953 [37]. Gütgemann recommended the interposition of a very long jejunum loop of at least 30 cm in length to increase the reservoir function of the inserted jejunal pouch [38]. Poth in 1966 favored the interposition of an antiperistaltic jejunal pouch in various combinations [39]. In 1972, Schrader and Koslowski interposed an additional 10 cm shorter antiperistaltic jejuna segment, which anastomosed distally from Longmire's reconstruction [40]. They favored the view that a short anisoperistaltic interposition of the neuromuscular segment could slow down the gastric emptying and simulate neopylorus [40, 41]. In 1982, Cuschieri created a large jejunum pouch interposed between the esophagus and the duodenum [42]. Nakane and Schwarz recommended Hunt-Lawrence Shaped pouch in 1990, interposed between the esophagus and duodenum [27, 43]. The reconstruction of the ileocecal interposition described by Lee and Hunnicutt is also in use with the basic idea of replacing the ileocecal valve as a substitute for the cardiac sphincter [44, 45]. This reconstruction provides anatomic barrier between the neo-stomach and the esophagus to prevent biliopancreatic reflux.

The original RP after TG by Longmire implies the establishment of an esophagoduodenal continuity using a previously fully mobilized intestinal segment on a free vascular sponge ante- or in a retrocolonic fashion by using an isolated first jejunal segment of 15 cm in length (**Figure 8**) [34].

This type of reconstruction is also known as the Beal-Longmire operation. Today, after the mobilization of the first segment of the jejunum in the length of at least 25–35 cm and with a longer

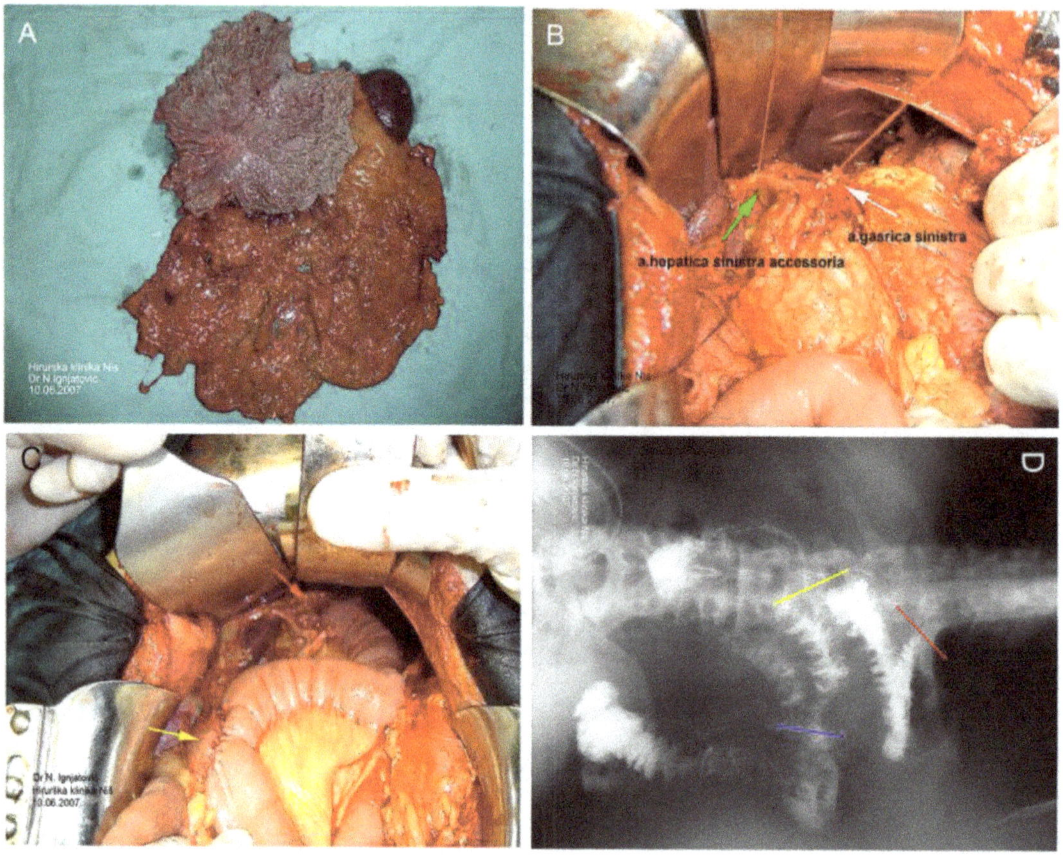

Figure 7. A representation of the operative reconstructive technique after TG with the preservation of DP by the RY configuration on the material of the author of this chapter: (A) specimen of the stomach (stomach open by large curvature), spleen, and large omentum, (B) arterial variation of branching a.hepaticae sinistrae accessoriae (yellow arrow) from a.gastricae sinistrae (white arrow), (C) formed end-to-end esophagojejunostomy (red arrow) and side-to-end jejunoduodenostomy (yellow arrow), (D) contrast radiography: sufficient anastomosis of esophagojejunostomy (red line), jejunoduodenostomy (yellow line), and jejunojejunostomy with Roux-en-Y anastomosis (blue line).

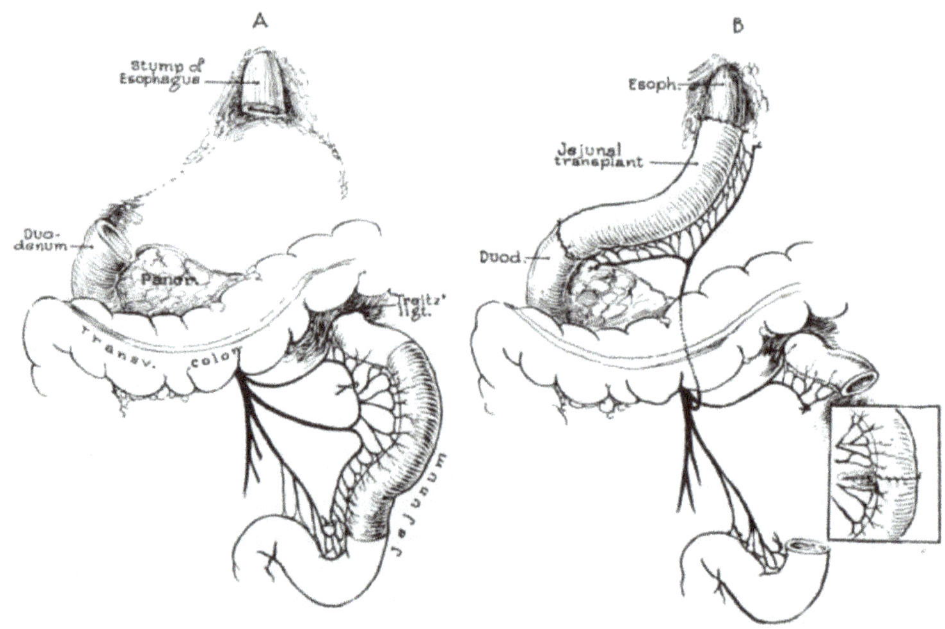

Figure 8. Original schematic representation of reconstruction after TG with DP by Longmire [34].

mesentery, both of these structures have retrocolonic transmesocolic position and they make anastomosis with the esophagus and duodenum in the isoperistaltic position. Modification by Schreiber and Gütgemann uses the jejunum segment in a length of 40 cm [38, 46]. Creating a proximal termino-lateral or end-to-end esophagojejunostomy is performed by a manual dual-layer technique or the use of a circular stapler (stapler CEEA), while a distal end-to-end jejuno-duodenostomy is performed by a manual two-layer mint technique. It is very important that the torsion and tension of the mesenterium be avoided in creating an isolated jejunum segment. The continuity of the resected proximal end of the first segment and the second segment of the jejunum with the application of a two-layer manual knot tying technique is established with end-to-end jejunojejunostomy (**Figures 9** and **10**).

In 1952, Longmire and Beal stated that all patients with reconstructed isolated jejunal segment after 4 months of follow-up were able to restore regular nutrition and preoperative body weight. In all patients, there was no early onset of pyrosis and epigastric pain [34]. Longmire also states that after adequate mobilization of the duodenum and avoidance of tension on the esophageal and jejunoduodenal anastomosis itself and the normalization of food passage through the duodenal segment, the benefits of interposition with the jejunal segment have been achieved: increasing the capacity of the isolated jejunal segment with the dilatation of the intestinal wall itself and the smaller regurgitation of biliary and intestinal contents [34]. Longmire points out that with this RP, there was no significant increase in operative risk during the performance of total gastrectomy, that is, the risks of vascular ischemia that are present in the transposition of the ileum and ascendant colon were eliminated. The reconstruction

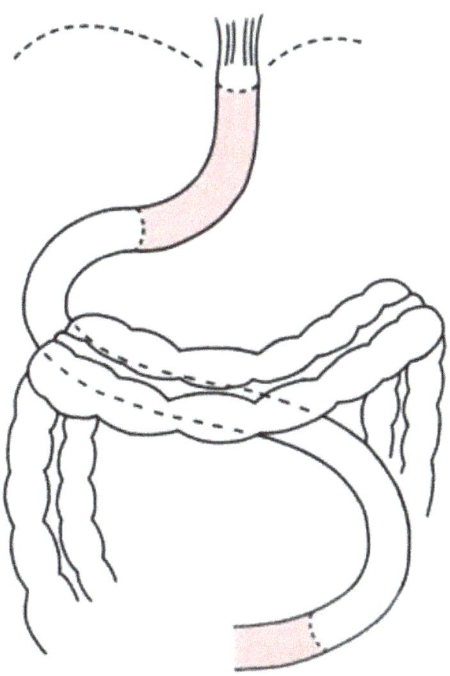

Figure 9. Schematic representation of reconstruction after TG with DP by Longmire, by interposition of jejunal segment with the creation of end-to-end esophagojejunostomy and end-to-end jejunoduodenostomy.

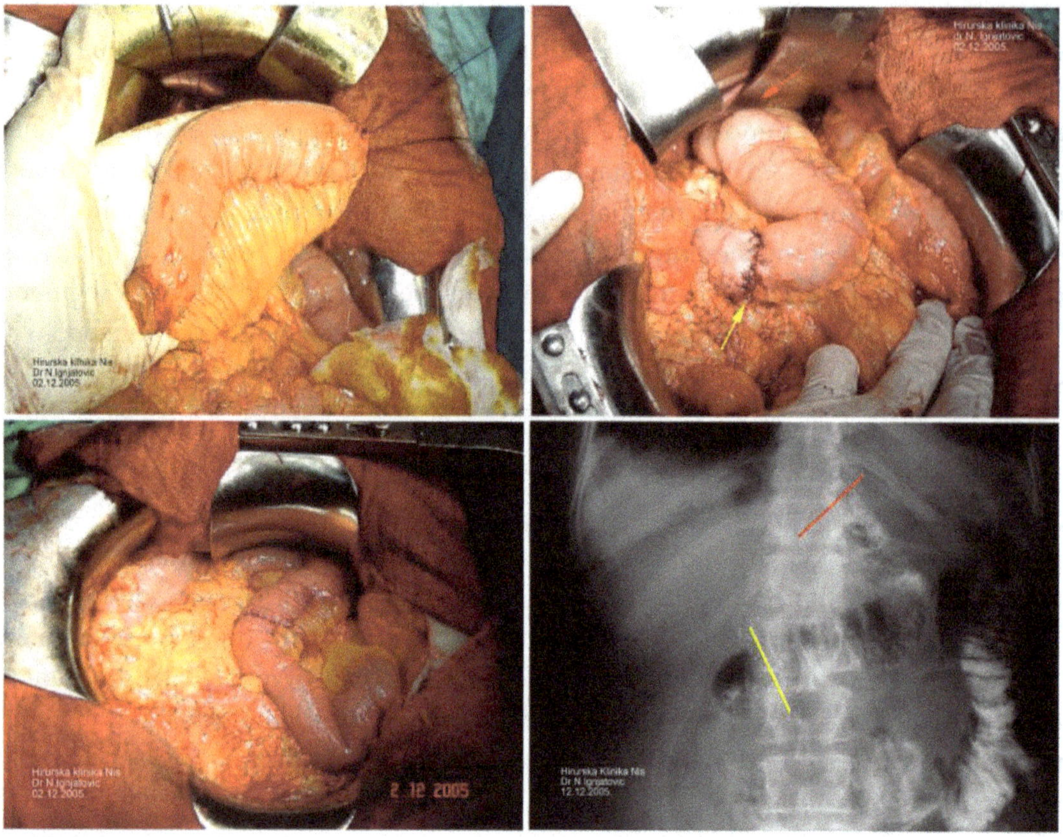

Figure 10. A representation of the operative reconstructive technique after TG with the preservation of DP by Longmire on the material of the author of this chapter: (A) isolated free jejunal segment on the vascular retina placed in a retrocolonic fashion, (B) formed end-to-end esophagojejunostomy (red arrow) and end-to-end jejunoduodenostomy (yellow arrow), (C) formed end-to-end jejunojejunostomy, (D) contrast radiography: sufficient anastomosis of esophagojejunostomy (red line) and jejunoduodenal anastomosis (yellow line).

of the intestinal continuity with the Longmire's jejunal interposition provides theoretical advantages over the reconstruction of the RY configuration [31].

3. Advantages of reconstructive procedures with preservation duodenal passage after total gastrectomy

The survival rate after TG in GC has been improved thanks to early diagnostics and advanced operating techniques. Many reconstructive techniques after TG have been developed in efforts to prevent postgastrectomy syndrome and preserve the physiological nutritional status of patients and rapid return to normal daily preoperative activities [47]. At the same time, the procedure for gastric reconstruction should be technically easily performed with minimal postoperative complications. RP that meet these requirements are those with the preservation of DP RY configuration of DT, Longmire procedure for the esophagus interposition of the jejunal segment, as well as the procedure of interposition with the jejunal pouch (e.g., Hunt-Lawrence pouch) [31].

Following a RP, the RY configuration of DT, food on the intestinal digestive pathway passes the duodenum and makes the intestinal wall distension by stimulating the ganglion cells of the myenteric and submucosal plexus, thereby leading to an adequate regulation of intestinal motility. This physical contact with the intestinal mucosa stimulates a large number of cells to produce peptides with hormonal, paracrine, and neurocrine effects. Chymus entering the duodenum primarily stimulates secretion: secretin, cholecystokinin, cholecystokinin-pancreozymin, enteroglucagon, vasoesthetic peptide, motilin, somatostatin, gastric inhibitory peptide, intestinal gastrin, serotonin, insulin, insulin glucagon, P substance, neurotensin, and enkephalin. These numerous polypeptides have a complex initial and stimulating regulatory role in the food digestion phase: bile release, gallbladder contact stimulation, Oddi sphincter relaxation, pancreatic juice secretion, vasodilation of the blood vessels of the mesentery of the intestinum and portal vein, intestinal secretion and peristalsis, absorption of food, secretion of insulin, and inhibitory effects in the interdigestive phase [48]. Kelly and authors suggest an explanation of the cause of the secondary deficiency of pancreatic secretion, inadequate stimulation, insufficient microvasculus of the heme and pancreatic enzymes, and weakened dietary fat assimilation in the new conditions of the absence of DP after TG [49]. Some non-randomized, retrospective studies have demonstrated the superiority of the performance of the jejunal interposition on the RY configuration of esophagojejunostomy when it comes to nutrition and the ability of postoperative rehabilitation [50–52]. However, due to a terminal vascular stem, the interposition of the jejunal segment as a free intestinal transplant between the esophagus and the duodenum is considered a high-risk procedure compared to other RP [53].

The nutritional status of patients after TG is changed. In many patients, calorie intake is inadequate, thus making it impossible to regain preoperative body weight. The causes of nutritional status disorders are the lack of appetite or problems caused by abnormal food passage. In order to maintain an ideal nutritional status, i.e., to preserve the integrity of the tissue and the function of the cells of the organism, nutrition requires essential nutrients and energy materials, regularity of food intake, regularity of passage and digestion, adequate resorption, and utilization of nutrients. Loss of body weight after TG is temporary and represents a significant postoperative problem in asthenic patients with GC. The mechanism of body weight loss includes malabsorption, malnutrition, and the consumption of material elements due to tissue restitution. It is known that the state of nutrition of the patient correlates with morbidity and mortality. Malnutrition usually manifests itself as a weight loss (15–24% of preoperative weight), which many authors cite in their studies in patients after TG [54]. If ingested food does not pass through the duodenum, an adequate mixture of the chymus with gallbladder and pancreatic enzymes is not formed. Therefore, the mixing of chymus and gallbladder and pancreatic contents is delayed beyond the time required for proper digestion in the distal parts of the jejunal Roux loop beneath the anastomosis with a jejunum in reconstruction without DP. Relative pancreatic insufficiency may also lead to malabsorption of patients in whom reconstruction excludes the passage of food through the duodenum [54]. Studies have shown that patients with TG who have undergone DP prevention have less loss of body weight and body mass index and have fewer symptoms as consequences of RP [55–58]. Fat and protein malabsorption occurs in over 50% of patients after total gastrectomy. In most patients, malabsorption of fat after TG is of doubtful clinical significance. The cause of steatorrhea after gastrectomy is most likely multifactorial: loss of digestive enzymes of the stomach, reduced stimulation of pancreatic and bile secretions, inappropriate or inadequate mixing of food with bile and pancreatic juice, increased bowel motility, and excessive bacterial colonization of the small intestine. Carbohydrate absorption can be reduced by excessive bacterial colonization and the use of nonmalignant carbohydrates [57].

Postgastrectomy sideropenia anemia is caused by iron-induced malabsorption that occurs after reconstruction with the circumvention of the duodenal segment in which its resorption normally occurs. The iron resorption disorder in patients following TG is due to gastric acid deficiencies that allow the passage of nonabsorptive Fe^{2+} into the absorbent Fe^{3+} form and the removal of the duodenum as the main site of absorption of iron from the passage of the chymus [55].

In a study by Bae and authors, there were very serious deficiencies of vitamin B_{12} in patients after TG. This indicates that parenteral substitution of vitamin B_{12} in gastrectomized patients is necessary due to inadequate absorption in the intestines. The serum level of vitamin B_{12} was significantly reduced after TG and is believed to be due to its deficiency in absorption. Bae also pointed out that anemia due to deficiency of vitamin B_{12} is a process that develops within a few years [54].

The term postgastrectomy bone disease describes bone disease after TG. It can occur as an osteomalacia or osteoporosis that is more pronounced than in normal physiological aging. Postgastrectomy bone disease is probably due to RP after TG in which the duodenum and proximal jejunum from food passage are excluded, since they are the major sites for the absorption of calcium in physiological conditions [59]. Calcium absorption is primarily performed in the duodenum and jejunum and depends on the level of vitamin D [60]. Accelerated transit of food through the intestinum also reduces calcium absorption time, while the presence of steatorrhea leads to the formation of insoluble calcium soaps that can contribute to calcium malabsorption [59].

Liedman reported in his study that a significant increase in alkaline phosphatase levels in patients after 3–10 years after TG, in a group of patients with a RY RP [61]. Heiskanen and authors have reported that the serum level of alkaline phosphatase has been used to detect postgastrectomic osteomalacia. In other prospective studies after partial gastrectomy and TG, normal and elevated serum levels of alkaline phosphatase were observed [62]. In a group of patients with reconstructed RY configurations in the study of Iivonen and authors, serum alkaline phosphatase activity increased significantly over the course of 3 postoperative years with a tendency to be higher than the group of patients with DP preservation [63].

Bassotti and authors were probably the first to examine the intestinal motility of the Roux loop after a complete gastrectomy by manometric route and concluded that patients with reconstruction of the Roux-en-Y configuration had significant motor abnormality in the Roux loop [64]. Sun and authors in their study claimed that the continuity of the gastrointestinal tract plays a key role in the coordination of intestinal motility [65]. Studies have shown that surgical manipulation of the gastrointestinal tract, in the form of resection followed by reanastomosis, results in intestinal motility disturbance [47, 64]. In support of this assertion, several studies suggest that the interruption of motility due to gastrointestinal resection is actually due to damage to the pacemaker for the gastrointestinal tract, i.e., interstitial cell of Cajal (ICC). The ICC is responsible for the creation and propagation of slow electrical waves that coordinate the stages of contraction of the intestine [65]. The entire problem of postgastrectomy symptoms may be attributed to accelerated intestinal transit. Fast transit results in accelerated glucose uptake, which causes increased insulin secretion. Accelerated transport of peptides and lipids gives an unusually large incentive to the secretion of cholecystokinin and stimulation of feedback regulation. In the end, there are abnormally high levels of gastrointestinal hormones and increased production of somatostatin. Excreted somatostatin has an inhibitory effect on GUT hormones, but this further reduces bowel motility and digestive juice production. This entire phenomenon becomes less significant in time due to the adaptation of the intestine [66].

Several studies have shown that the presence of postprandial hyperglycemia following TG reconstruction can indicate an abnormal glucose metabolism, possibly representing intolerance to glucose or diabetes at an early stage [43]. In relation to the type of RP, Schwarz and authors have found significantly higher levels of glucose in a patient with RY reconstruction, when there was no DP preservation in patients with pouch, as opposed to patients undergoing a RP in which DP was preserved. There was no development of pathological glucose tolerance in patients with established DP prevention [43]. Kalmár and authors have published significantly higher levels of postprandial glucose in patients with exclusion of DP RY reconstruction than the control group, thus supporting the hypothesis that the exclusion of DP disrupts homeostasis of glucose more than reconstruction with the preservation of DP [66]. Observing duodenal preservation, the glucose homeostasis disorder was significantly higher in patients with RY procedure [65].

With the standardization of TG performance due to GC, the survival period of operative patients has significantly increased and hence the possibility of postgastrectomy syndrome. The causes of the postgastrectomy syndrome can be hypocaloric food intake, exclusion of duodenal passage, loss of absorption surface, lack of peptic digestion, excessive bacterial colonization, and the occurrence of exocrine and endocrine pancreatic insufficiency [57]. Symptoms related to food intake due to abnormal transit reported in several studies relate to the onset of early and late dumping syndrome, alkaline reflux, pyrosis, loss of appetite, feeling of satiety and fullness, epigastric pain, meteorism, dysphagia, and diarrhea [67]. Schwarz and authors, as well as Zherlov and authors, have shown in their studies that reconstruction in which DP is preserved has a lower incidence of postgastrectomy symptoms [43, 68]. Persistent postprandial discomfort and fullness may be to some extent due to poor receptive adaptation of the proximal part of the small intestine. In addition to poor receptive adaptation of the proximal part of the small intestine, the distal end of the Roux loop can also act as a functional obstruction, which leads to Roux-stasis syndrome, which is characterized by epigastric pain, nausea, and vomiting, and is most likely due to the lack of motor function in the distal region Roux loop [57, 69].

The lack of gastric acid after TG and altered intestinal motility in reconstruction with RY configuration with or without pouch seems to lead to bacterial colonization, which may be one of the main causes of malnutrition after TG. Excessive bacterial growth leads to the formation of damage to the mycelium and decongestion of bile salts. Several mechanisms blame for malabsorption of fat: loss of gastric emulsification of triglycerides, rapid food passage, and pancreatic stimulation disorder [63].

The overall impact of many symptoms after a RP can be summarized in the health quality of life. The quality of life is a multidimensional approach that consists of functional, emotional, physical, and social aspects, as well as from subjective disease symptoms and adverse effects of therapy. Controlling gastrointestinal symptoms seems important in an attempt to reduce damage to quality of life [70]. In their study, Hoksch and authors confirmed that reconstruction with the preservation of DP is the most optimal procedure in improving the quality of life of patients after TG [58].

4. Conclusion

TG is widely used as a major surgical treatment for GC. TG results in risk of postgastrectomy syndrome, such as weight loss, dumping syndrome, biliary reflux esophagitis, and a reduction in the quality of life [3, 4]. The ideal RP after TG should replace all lost functions of the stomach, provide an optimal enough reservoir that can accommodate to the size of the meal, prevent reflux, ensure strong propulsion of equal-sized boluses of chyme entering the duodenum, and respond properly to the changing levels of gastrointestinal hormones and neural information [7]. The choice of RP should ensure good digestive function to prevent persistent postgastrectomy syndrome. Preservation of duodenal transit with replacement of the jejunal segment, the so-called physiological route, is now believed to be preferential for postoperative nutritional condition. RP which allow DP should be regarded as a key to physiological reconstruction.

Acknowledgements

The author would like to thank Professor Dr. Dobrila Stanković Djordjević, Dean of the Faculty of the Medicine and Professor Dr. Nebojsa Djordjević, Chairman of Department of Surgery, Faculty of the Medicine, University of Nis, Nis, Serbia for constructive support; his teacher of surgery Professor Dr. Miroslav Jeremic for helping generously.

Author details

Nebojsa S. Ignjatovic[1]*, Tomislav D. Randjelovic[2], Miroslav P. Stojanovic[1], Goran Z. Stanojevic[1] and Miodrag N. Djordjevic[1]

*Address all correspondence to: n.ignjat@gmail.com

1 Department of Surgery, School of Medicine, University of Nis, Nis, Serbia

2 Department of Surgery, School of Medicine, University of Belgrade, Belgrade, Serbia

References

[1] Conner PS. Report of a case of complete extirpation of the stomach. Medical Newsletter. 1887;**45**:587

[2] Schlatter CA. A unique case of complete removal of the stomach– Successful esophago-enterostomy recovery. Le Médecin de Réserve. 1897;**52**:909-914

[3] Herrington Jr JL. Various types of pouch replacement following total gastrectomy: Historical data and current thoughts regarding total gastrectomy. The American Surgeon. 1968;**34**:879-887

[4] ReMine WH, Priestley JT. Late results after total gastrectomy. Surgery, Gynecology & Obstetrics. 1952;**94**:519-525

[5] Inberg MV, Heinonen R, Laurén P. Total and proximal gastrectomy in the treatment of gastric carcinoma: A series of 305 cases. World Journal of Surgery. 1981;**5**:249-257. DOI: 10.1007/bf01658304

[6] Lemmon WT, Paschal GW. Total gastrectomy for carcinoma of the stomach. Annals of Surgery. 1940;**112**:31-36. DOI: 10.1097/00000658-194007000-00004

[7] Ikard RW. Collective reviews. The Y anastomoses of César Roux. Surgery, Gynecology & Obstetrics. 1989;**169**:559-567

[8] Orr TG. A modified technique for total gastrectomy. Archives of Surgery. 1947;**54**:279-286. DOI: 10.1001/archsurg.1947.01230070285003

[9] Waugh JM, Hood RTJ. Gastric operations: A historical review I. Quarterly Review of Surgery, Obstetrics and Gynecology. 1953;**10**:201-214

[10] Hoffman V. Eine Methode des plastischen Magenersatzes. Zentralblatt für Chirurgie. 1922;**4**:1477-1482

[11] Lygidakis NJ. Total gastrectomy for gastric carcinoma: A retrospective study of different procedures and assessment of a new technique of gastric reconstruction. The British Journal of Surgery. 1981;**68**:649-655. DOI: 10.1002/bjs.1800680913

[12] Lawrence WJ. Reconstruction after total gastrectomy: What is preferred technique? Journal of Surgical Oncology. 1996;**63**:215-220. DOI: 10.1002/(sici)1096-9098(199612)63:4<215::aid-jso1>3.0.co;2-f

[13] Herfarth C, Schlag P, Buhl K. Surgical procedures for gastric substitution. World Journal of Surgery. 1987;**11**:689-698. DOI: 10.1007/bf01656591

[14] Piessen G, Triboulet JP, Mariette C. Reconstruction after gastrectomy: Which technique is best? Journal of Visceral Surgery. 2010;**147**:273-283. DOI: 10.1016/j.jviscsurg.2010.09.004

[15] Hutchison RL, Hutchison AL. César Roux and his original 1893 paper. Obesity Surgery. 2010;**20**:953-956. DOI: 10.1007/s11695-010-0141-z

[16] Roux C. De la gastroenterostomie. Revue de Chirurgie. 1893;**13**:402-403

[17] Reid MR. Total gastrectomy. Surgery, Gynecology & Obstetrics. 1925;**41**:667-672

[18] Netter FH. Atlas of Human Anatomy, Professional Edition. 4th ed. Philadelphia: WB Saunders Co; 2006. DOI: 10.1186/1477-7800-4-28

[19] Hansen JT. Netter's Clinical Anatomy. 3rd ed. Philadelphia: Elsevier; 2006. DOI: 10.1002/ca.20339

[20] Liedman B, Andersson H, Berglund B. Food intake after gastrectomy for gastric carcinoma: The role of a gastric reservoir. The British Journal of Surgery. 1996;**83**:1138-1143. DOI: 10.1002/bjs.1800830835

[21] Wells C, Johnston JH. Revision to the Roux-en-Y anastomosis for post-gastrectomy syndromes. Lancet. 1956;**2**:479-481. DOI: 10.1016/s0140-6736(56)91969-9

[22] Hunt CJ. Construction of food pouch from segment of jejunum as substitute for stomach in total gastrectomy. A.M.A. Archives of Surgery. 1952;**64**:601-608. DOI: 10.1001/archsurg.1952.01260010619009

[23] Lawrence WJ. Reservoir construction after total gastrectomy: An instructive case. Annals of Surgery. 1962;**155**:191-198. DOI: 10.1097/00000658-196200000-00004

[24] Liedman B, Bosaeus I, Hugosson I. Long-term beneficial effects of a gastric reservoir on weight control after total gastrectomy: A study of potential mechanisms. The British Journal of Surgery. 1998;**85**:542-547. DOI: 10.1046/j.1365-2168.1998.00747.x

[25] Horvath OP, Kalmar K, Cseke L. Nutritional and life-quality consequences of aboral pouch construction after total gastrectomy: A randomized, controlled study. European Journal of Surgical Oncology. 2001;**27**:558-563. DOI: 10.1053/ejso.2001.1172

[26] Nakane Y, Okumura S, Akehira K. Jejunal pouch reconstruction after total gastrectomy for cancer. A randomized controlled trial. Annals of Surgery. 1995;**222**:27-35. DOI: 10.1097/00000658-199507000-00005

[27] Nakane Y, Michiura T, Inoue K. A randomized clinical trial of pouch reconstruction after total gastrectomy for cancer: Which is the better technique, Roux-en-y or interposition? Hepato-Gastroenterology. 2001;**48**:903-907

[28] Largiader F, Sauberli H. Rekonstruktion nach Gastrektomie, insbesondere mit Jejunumersatzmagen. Helvetica Chirurgica Acta. 1972;**39**:883-886

[29] Kajitani K, Sato J. Evaluation of the procedures of total gastrectomy and proximal gastrectomy. Japan Surgical Society. 1965;**66**:1285-1287

[30] Iwahashi M, Nakamori M, Nakamura M. Evaluation of double tract reconstruction after total gastrectomy in patients with gastric cancer: Prospective randomized controlled trial. World Journal of Surgery. 2009;**33**:1882-1888. DOI: 10.1007/s00268-009-0109-0

[31] Bandurski R, Gryko M, Kamocki Z. Double tract reconstruction (DTR)– An alternative type of digestive tract reconstructive procedure after total gastrectomy—own experience. Polski Przeglad Chirurgiczny. 2011;**83**:70-75. DOI: 10.2478/v10035-011-0011-y

[32] Fujiwara Y, Kusunoki M, Nakagawa K, Tanaka T, Hatada T, Yamamura T. Evaluation of J-pouch reconstruction after total gastrectomy: ϱ-double tract vs. J-pouch double tract. Digestive Surgery. 2000;**17**:475-482. DOI: 10.1159/000051943

[33] Seo S. Stomach resection transplanting jejunum. Japan Surgical Society. 1941;**42**:1004

[34] Longmire WP, Beal JM. Construction of a substitute gastric reservoir following total gastrectomy. Annals of Surgery. 1952;**135**:637-645. DOI: 10.1097/00000658-195205000-00007

[35] Traverso LW. The Longmire I, II, and III operations. American Journal of Surgery. 2003; **185**:399-406. DOI: 10.1016/s0002-9610(03)00045-x

[36] Sharma D. Choice of digestive tract reconstructive procedure following total gastrectomy: A critical reappraisal. The Indian Journal of Surgery. 2004;**66**:270-276

[37] Hays RP. Anatomic and physiologic reconstruction following total gastrectomy by the use of a jejunal food pouch. Surgical Forum. 1953;**4**:291-296

[38] Gütgemann A, Schreiber HW, Bernhard A. Erfahrungen mit der totalen Gastrektomie. Langenbecks Arch Klin Chir Ver Dtsch Z Chir. 1963;**303**:73-93. DOI: 10.1007/bf01440407

[39] Poth EJ, Smith LB. Gastric pouches: Their evaluation. American Journal of Surgery. 1966; **112**:721-727. DOI: 10.1016/0002-9610(66)90112-7

[40] Kieninger G, Koslowski L, Kummer D. Stomach replacement by iso-anisoperistaltic jejunum interposition (Tübinger replacement stomach). Chirurg. 1981;**52**:505-510

[41] Herbington JL. Remedial operations for severe postgastrectomy symptoms (dumping): Emphasis on an antiperistaltic (reversed) jejunal segment interpolated between gastric remnant and duodenum and role of vagotomy. Annals of Surgery. 1965;**162**:789-862. DOI: 10.1097/00000658-196511000-00001

[42] Cuschieri A. Long term evaluation of a reservoir jejunal interposition with an isoperistaltic conduit in the management of patients with the small stomach syndrome. The British Journal of Surgery. 1982;**69**:386-388. DOI: 10.1002/bjs.1800690710

[43] Schwarz A, Büchler M, Usinger K. Importance of the duodenal passage and pouch volume after total gastrectomy and reconstruction with the Ulm pouch: Prospective randomized clinical study. World Journal of Surgery. 1996;**20**:60-66; discussion 66-67. DOI: 10.1007/s002689900011

[44] Lee CMJ. Transposition of a colon segment as a gastric reservoir after total gastrectomy. Surgery, Gynecology & Obstetrics. 1951;**92**:456-465

[45] Hunnicutt AJ. Replacing stomach after total gastrectomy with right ileocolon. A.M.A. Archives of Surgery. 1952;**65**:1-11. DOI: 10.1001/archsurg.1952.01260020013001

[46] Baumgartl F, Kremer K, Schreiber HW. Spezielle Chirurgie für die Praxis. Stuttgart: Georg Thieme Verlag; 1973. 738 p. DOI: 10.1002/bjs.1800610431

[47] Adachi S, Inagawa S, Enomoto T. Subjective and functional results after total gastrectomy: Prospective study for long-term comparison of reconstruction procedures. Gastric Cancer. 2003;**6**:24-29. DOI: 10.1007/s101200300003

[48] Johnson LR. Physiology of the Gastrointestinal Tract. 5th ed. Vol. 1. Amsterdam, Boston, Heidelberg, London, New York, Oxford, Paris, San Diego, San Francisco, Singapore, Sydney, Tokyo: Academic Press, Elsevier; 2012. DOI: 10.1016/c2009 1 64521-4

[49] Kelly WD, MacLean LD, Perry JF. A study of patients following total or near-total gastrectomy. Surgery. 1954;**35**:964-982

[50] Heil T, Etzrodt H, Mattes P. Gastrectomy with and without duodenal transit: Release of glucagon, insulin and somatostatin. Scandinavian Journal of Gastroenterology. 1981; **67**(Suppl):83-87

[51] Miholic J, Meyer HJ, Muller MJR. Nutritional consequences of total gastrectomy: The relationship between mode of reconstruction, postprandial symptoms, and body composition. Surgery. 1990;**108**:488-494

[52] Henley FA. Gastrectomy with replacement. A preliminary communication with an introduction. The British Journal of Surgery. 1952;**40**:118-128. DOI: 10.1002/bjs.18004016006

[53] Moreno-Gonzales E, Carboni M. A safe and rapid esophagojejunoduodenostomy after total gastrectomy. Surgery, Gynecology & Obstetrics. 1988;**167**:73-74

[54] Bae JM, Park JW, Yang HK, Kim JP. Nutritional status of gastric cancer patients after total gastrectomy. World Journal of Surgery. 1998;**22**:254-260; discussion 260-261. DOI: 10.1007/s002689900379

[55] Schölmerich J. Postgastrectomy syndromes—Diagnosis and treatment. Best Practice & Research. Clinical Gastroenterology. 2004;**18**:917-933. DOI: 10.1016/j.bpg.2004.08.003

[56] Ignjatovic N, Stanojevic G, Ignjatovic J. Impact of reconstructive procedures with and without preserving the duodenal passage on body weight in patients after total gastrectomy for gastric cancer. Srpski Arhiv za Celokupno Lekarstvo. 2017;**145**:26-31. DOI: 10.2298/sarh151123004i

[57] Olbe L, Lundell L. Intestinal function after total gastrectomy and possible consequences of gastric replacement. World Journal of Surgery. 1987;**11**:713-719. DOI: 10.1007/bf01656593

[58] Hoksch B, Ablassmaier B, Zieren J. Quality of life after gastrectomy: Longmire's reconstruction alone compared with additional pouch reconstruction. World Journal of Surgery. 2002;**26**:335-341. DOI: 10.1007/s00268-001-0229-7

[59] Tovey FI, Hall ML, Ell PJ. A review of postgastrectomy bone disease. Journal of Gastroenterology and Hepatology. 1992;**7**:639. DOI: 10.1111/j.1440-1746.1992.tb01498.x

[60] Mahlay NF, Verka LG, Thomsen K. Vitamin D status before Roux-en-Y and efficacy of prophylactic and therapeutic doses of vitamin D in patients after Roux-en-Y gastric bypass surgery. Obesity Surgery. 2009;**19**:590-594. DOI: 10.1007/s11695-008-9698-1

[61] Liedman B, Andersson H, Bosaeus I, Hugosson I, Lundell L. Changes in body composition after gastrectomy: Results of a controlled, prospective clinical trial. World Journal of Surgery. 1997;**21**:416-421

[62] Heiskanen JT, Kröger H, Pääkkönen M, Parviainen MT, Lamberg-Allardt C, Alhava E. Bone mineral metabolism after total gastrectomy. Bone. 2001;**28**:123-127. DOI: 10.1016/s8756-3282(00)00404-x

[63] Iivonen MK, Ahola TO, Matikainen MJ. Bacterial overgrowth, intestinal transit, and nutrition after total gastrectomy. Comparison of a jejunal pouch with Roux-en-Y reconstruction in a prospective random study. Scandinavian Journal of Gastroenterology. 1998;**33**:63-70. DOI: 10.1080/00365529850166220

[64] Bassotti G, Gulla P, Betti C. Manometric evaluation of jejunal limb after total gastrectomy and Roux-Orr anastomosis for gastric cancer. The British Journal of Surgery. 1990;**77**:1025-1029. DOI: 10.1002/bjs.1800770924

[65] Sun YS, Ye ZY, Zhang Q. Beneficial effects of continual jejunal interposition after subtotal gastrectomy. Medizinhistorisches Journal. 2012;**125**:2846-2852

[66] Kalmár K, Németh J, Kelemen D. Postprandial gastrointestinal hormone production is different, depending on the type of reconstruction following total gastrectomy. Annals of Surgery. 2006;**243**:465-471. DOI: 10.1097/01.sla.0000205740.12893

[67] Tyrväinen T, Sand J, Sintonen H. Quality of life in the long-term survivors after total gastrectomy for gastric carcinoma. Journal of Surgical Oncology. 2008;**97**:121-124. DOI: 10.1002/jso.20925

[68] Zherlov G, Koshel A, Orlova Y. New type of jejunal interposition method after gastrectomy. World Journal of Surgery. 2006;**30**:1475-1480. DOI: 10.1007/s00268-005-7980-0

[69] Ignjatovic NS, Jeremic MM, Ranđelović TD. Gastric and duodenal surgery. In: Jermic MM, editor. Abdominal Surgery. Vol. I. Nis: University of Nis, School of Medicine, Pelikan print; 2009. pp. 547-656

[70] Bradley EL. Postoperative syndrome nach totaler gastrektomie. In: Siewert JR, Blum AL, editors. Postoperative Syndrome. Berlin: Springer; 1980. pp. 153-175. DOI: 10.1007/978-3-642-95341-5_8

11

Gastric GIST

Tamer Saafan

Abstract

Gastrointestinal stromal tumor (GIST) is the most common mesenchymal tumor of the gastrointestinal tract. The stomach is considered the most common site of GIST, and the most common histopathological type of GISTs is spindle cell. Mutational analysis may help in defining the management of GIST. Multiple stratification modules are available for the estimation of GISTs' prognosis. Surgery is considered the only curative option for GISTs. The discovery of KIT protein has allowed better identification of GISTs and has allowed creation of selective tyrosine kinase inhibitors which dramatically affected GIST management. Results of trials on neoadjuvant imatinib therapy are promising. Adjuvant imatinib therapy is recommended for 3 years and has proven to improve outcome in high-risk GISTs. New therapeutic agents are now available in case of imatinib resistance. Follow-up of patients with GISTs depends on the type of GIST.

Keywords: GIST, gastric GIST, imatinib, tyrosine kinase inhibitors, primary GIST, metastatic GIST, recurrent GIST, imatinib resistance, KIT, PDGFRA

1. Introduction

Gastrointestinal stromal tumor (GIST) is the most common mesenchymal tumor of the gastrointestinal tract (GIT) [1, 2]. All GISTs are considered to have some degree of malignant potential [3]. The most common site of GISTs is the stomach (60%) [4]. Other common sites are jejunum and ileum (30%), duodenum (5%), rectum (2–3%), colon (1–2%), and esophagus (<1%) [4].

It has been estimated that GISTs comprise about 18% of all sarcomas and 80% of mesenchymal tumors found in the GIT [5]. GIST's true incidence has been underestimated as they were usually misdiagnosed as leiomyomas, leiomyosarcomas, and leiomyoblastomas [6]. A study which used the Surveillance, Epidemiology and End Results (SEER) data from the National Cancer Institute, reported that the incidence of GIST has increased from 0.028 cases per 100,000 in 1992 to 0.688 cases per 100,000 in 2002, which is a 25-fold increase in incidence. This increase occurred after the availability of diagnostic criteria, especially after the year 2000 [7]. In 1992, 93% of mesenchymal tumors of GIT were identified as smooth muscle neoplasm and 6% as GISTs. In 1995, Miettinen et al. [8] discovered that 70% of GIST are positive for CD34, a myeloid progenitor cell antigen. Furthermore, CD34 were also found in Schwann cell tumors and some smooth muscle tumors [6]. In the late 1990s, Hirota et al. [9] discovered that GIST expresses KIT (CD117), a receptor tyrosine kinase encoded by the proto-oncogene c-kit. Subsequent studies showed that mutations in c-KIT are present in 85–100% of GIST cases, but not in leiomyomas or leiomyosarcomas. These findings made a breakthrough in identifications and management of GISTs. In the SEER data published by Perez et al. [7], 82% of mesenchymal tumors of GIST were classified as GIST and 17% were classified as smooth muscle neoplasms in 2002, which shows how GISTs were poorly identified and were under-diagnosed [7]. GISTs appear to be more common in African Americans, Asians, and Pacific Islanders than in Caucasian patients, and men appear to have a slightly increased incidence [7, 10]. GISTs tend to be infrequent before the age of 30 and are most common after the age of 60 [7]. The median age of diagnosis is between 58 and 65 years [7, 10–13]. Two studies from Europe have shown that GIST incidence is about 1.1 cases/100,000/year [11, 14].

Though rare, GISTs can also affect the pediatric population. A study carried out by Miettinen et al. which included 1782 patients with gastric GIST, reported 44 cases under the age of 21 (2.6%) [15] with an age range from 5 to 21 and a median age of 14.5 years [15]. Prakash et al. [16] reported six cases of gastric GIST with a mean age of 12.8 and an age range from 10 to 18. Pediatric GISTs are commonly of epithelioid type, occur more in females, and have a higher incidence of multifocal presentation and lymph node metastasis. Pediatric GISTs also tend to lack a KIT or a platelet-derived growth factor receptor-α (PDGFRA) mutation [17, 18].

2. Risk factors

There are no known risk factors for GIST. Though most of GISTs are sporadic, the minority occur as part of hereditary syndrome.

Familial GIST syndrome: several family members with hereditary mutations in either the KIR or PDGFRA genes have been reported in the study [19–28]. These families have a higher risk to develop multiple gastric and small bowel GISTs. Some patients may have skin hyperpigmentation, dysphagia, gastrointestinal autonomic nerve tumors, intestinal fibromatosis, and inflammatory fibroid polyps [19–28].

Carney-Stratakis syndrome is an autosomal-dominant disease which is characterized by dyad of multifocal GISTs and paragangliomas [29]. Patients do not have KIT or PDGFRA mutations, but do have mutations of succinate dehydrogenase subunits (SDH) A, B, C, or D [30].

Carney's triad: a very rare non-heritable syndrome characterized by gastric GIST, paraganglioma and pulmonary chondromas. These patients are characterized by mutations succinate dehydrogenase subunit (SDH) C [29] but lack mutations of KIT and PDGFRA.

Neurofibromatosis type 1: patients with NF1 are more predisposed for multifocal GISTs that mainly affect the small intestine [31].

3. Molecular biology

GISTs are characterized by mutations in KIT and PDGFRA genes that encode tyrosine kinase receptor type III [32].

3.1. KIT-mutant GIST

Though 95% of GISTs are positive for KIT, only 60–85% have mutations in KIT. The most common mutations encountered are mutations of exon 11 (juxtamembrane domain) [4] which is found in about two-thirds of GISTs. Exon 9 (extracellular domain) is less common (9–20%) and is principally correlated with GIST of the small bowel and has a greater malignant potential [4, 33].

3.2. PDGFRA-mutant GIST

About 5–10% of GISTs have PDGFRA mutations which have a tendency for localized gastric GIST and epithelioid type [4]. The most common type of mutation is the PDGFRA exon 18 mutation D842V, which is associated with imatinib resistance and has a lower risk of recurrence than GIST with KIT mutations as well as a more benign course 9 [34].

3.3. Wild-type GIST

Approximately 12–15% of adult GIST and 90% of pediatric GIST do not have KIT and PDGFRA mutations [33]. Wild-type (WT) GISTs comprise GISTs that arise in NF1, Carney-Stratakis syndrome, and Carney triad [4]. WT GISTs may have other forms of mutations. BRAF V600E substitution has been described in 7–13% of WT GISTs [35, 36]. About 30% of WT GISTs are SDH deficient and occur solely in the stomach. They mainly affect children and young adults and have a variation in their nature from being indolent to progressive [4].

4. Histopathology

The three main histopathologic subtypes of GIST are spindle cell, epithelioid, and mixed types, with spindle cell type being the most common constituting about 70% of GISTs, while the other two subtypes, epithelioid and mixed, are less common, accounting for 20 and 10% of all GISTS, respectively [6]. Epithelioid GIST is commonly observed in the stomach and omentum [6]. About 95% of GIST will be immunohistochemical positive for CD117(c-KIT) [4]. Epithelioid type has a weaker KIT positivity than spindle cell type [37]. In addition, 70–90% are positive for CD34, 20–30% for actin, 8–10% for S-100, and 2–4% for desmin [38]. DOG1 marker, also known as ANO1, has more than 95% sensitivity for GIST and is expressed in more than 35% of GISTs negative for c-kit [39, 40].

5. Clinical picture

About 60% of GISTs occur in the stomach, 30% in the jejunum and ileum, 5% in the duodenum, 2–3% in the rectum, 1–2% in the colon, and < 1% in the esophagus [4]. About 70% of GISTs are symptomatic, 20% are asymptomatic, and 10% are discovered at autopsy [41]. The main symptoms of GIST are GI bleeding, abdominal discomfort, and abdominal mass. GISTs are highly vascular tumors and may grow quickly and cause massive gastrointestinal or intraperitoneal hemorrhage [42]. Obstruction symptoms such as dysphagia, obstructive jaundice, and small bowel obstruction may also occur [42].

Extragastrointestinal GISTs occur in less than 10% of GISTs and mainly occur intra-abdominally and affect omentum and mesentery. Such tumors are considered more aggressive than gastric GIST and have a poorer prognosis similar to small bowel GISTs [43, 44].

About 50% of patients will present with metastatic disease with the most common site of metastasis being liver at about 65%. Other common metastatic sites are omentum and peritoneum. Extra-abdominal metastasis, lung bone, and lymph node metastasis are not common [13].

6. Prognosis

Various risk stratification models (**Table 1**) have been proposed that are based on site, size, mitotic index, and tumor rupture. Gastric GISTs are known to have better prognosis than non-gastric GIST [46].

Tumor rupture is known to be associated with a very high risk of GIST recurrence [47]. TNM staging is also available for GIST staging [48]. However, these stratification systems are not commonly used in clinical practice.

As an alternative to the risk classification systems that stratify patients into distinct groups, others have quantified the risk of disease recurrence after complete resection as a continuous variable through the use of a GIST nomogram that includes the disease site [49]. Different nomograms have been developed by others as well.

GIST nomograms [49, 50] have been used to assess the risk of disease recurrence after complete resection as a continuous variable instead of the risk stratification systems that stratify patients into separate groups. Recently, a new risk stratification system has been developed in which tumor size and mitotic counts were assessed as continuous, nonlinear variables, and prognostic contour maps were then generated based upon these data plus site and tumor rupture [51]. These prognostic contour maps resulting from nonlinear modeling are used for the assessment of individualized outcomes.

Deletion type of mutations affecting codons 557 and 558 in KIT gene is considered a risk factor for recurrence regardless of different classification systems [4].

Pfetin is a prognostic biomarker which is still under investigation with promising results. Lack of Pfetin expression seems to be associated with a higher GIST recurrence [52]. Orita et al. [52]

Classification system	Prognostic criteria	Risk definition	Risk groups	Comments
NIH [6]	Tumor size Mitotic index	Aggressive behaviors of GISTs	Very low risk Low risk Intermediate risk High risk	Does not differentiate between malignant and benign tumors knowing the fact that even small-size tumors with a low mitotic count may metastasize Does not take GIST site into consideration
Modified NIH [45]	Tumor size Mitotic index Primary tumor site Tumor rupture	Risk of recurrence	Very low risk Low risk Intermediate risk High risk	Tumor location outside the stomach is a prognostic factor for survival independent of the mitotic count and tumor size
AFIP [46]	Tumor size Mitotic index location	Risk of recurrence	Very low risk Low risk Intermediate risk High risk	This classification considered a total area of 5 mm^2 in 50 fields HPF characterized by the use of different optical components, while in practice, 50 HPF typically corresponds to a total area of 10 mm^2 This classification is recommended by GEIS guidelines

Table 1. Different stratification systems for GISTs.

had 45 GIST cases, of which 37 were in the stomach. All GIST patients had R0 resection. There were seven recurrences with five recurrences being gastric GIST recurrences. Thirteen GIST patients were Pfetin negative and 5/13 Pfetin negative GISTs had recurrences [52].

7. Diagnostic evaluation

A computed tomography (CT) scan (**Figure 1a** and **b**) is considered the first imaging to be done to evaluate anatomic location, extension, and metastasis of GISTs. Oral and IV contrast should be given to delineate bowel margins. GISTs can display endophytic and exophytic growth, and large GISTs may appear heterogeneous due to focal areas of hemorrhage or necrosis [53]. Magnetic resonance imaging (MRI) is used to further evaluate liver metastasis or rectal GIST [54]. Fluorodeoxyglucose-positron emission tomography (FDG-PET) is highly sensitive but not specific for GIST, and it is mainly useful to monitor response to tyrosine kinase inhibitors [55, 56].

Upper GI endoscopy may be useful for gastric GIST. Both GISTs and leiomyomas will appear as a submucosal mass with normal overlying mucosa and bulging into gastric lumen. Mucosal ulceration may occur. Endoscopic ultrasound (**Figure 2**) may not be useful, however, when combined with FNA sensitivity, and accuracy may reach 82 and 86%, respectively [57]. Routine biopsy is not needed routinely for local resectable gastric GISTs proved by imaging studies.

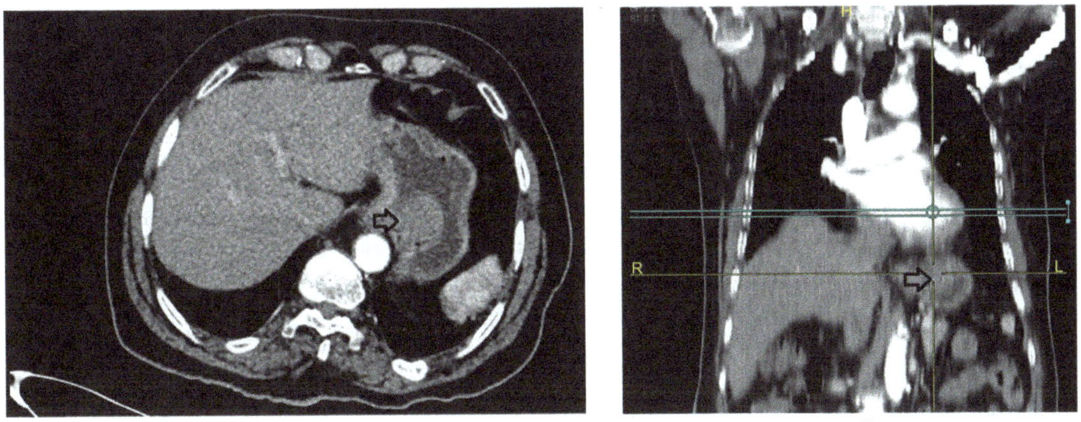

(A) (B)

Figure 1. An axial (A) and coronal (B) CT image showing a well-defined mass lesion (arrow) in the anterior gastric wall in the proximal stomach measuring 2.9x2.5x2.7.

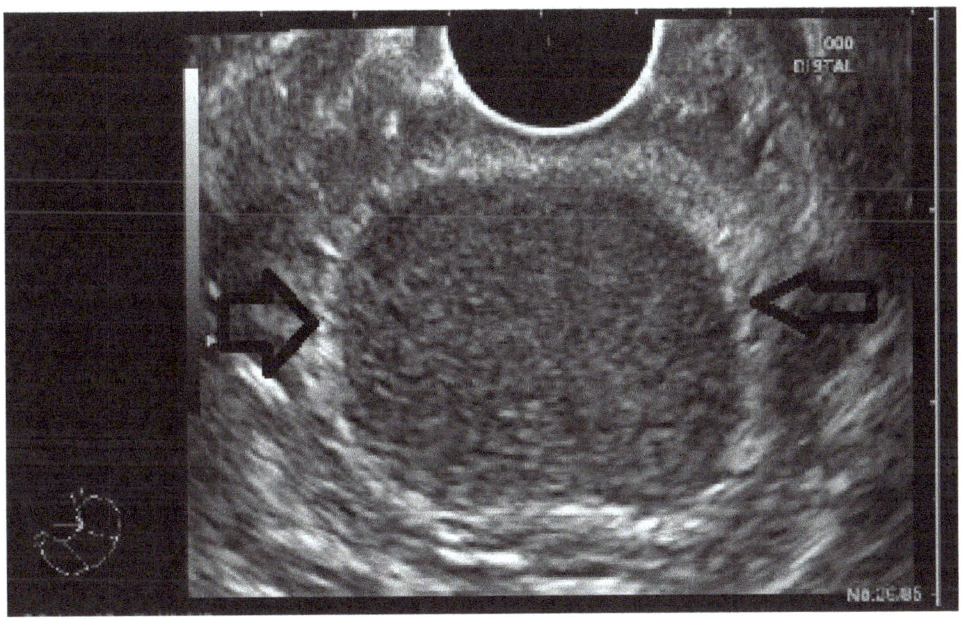

Figure 2. Gastric EUS showing a well-defined hypoechoic gastric submucosal lesion (between the two arrows) from the fourth layer of the stomach wall suggestive of GIST.

8. Management

Complete surgical resection is the recommendation of choice for localized GIST with a target of R0 resection with complete surgical removal of the tumor without disturbing the capsule [4]. Though surgery is considered the only curative option for GISTs, a multidisciplinary approach is needed for best medical and surgical management. Segmental resection of the stomach as wedge resection is accepted, and extensive resection is usually not needed. Lymphadenectomy is also not required as GISTs rarely metastasize to lymph nodes [4]. The discovery of KIT(CD117) (receptor tyrosine kinase) in GISTs has revolutionized GISTs management. Imatinib mesylate is a selective tyrosine kinase inhibitor that selectively inhibits KIT and had a significant impact on the prognosis of GISTs as will be discussed subsequently.

8.1. Management of primary resectable disease

8.1.1. Preoperative therapy for primary GISTs

There is still no consensus on the role of neoadjuvant imatinib therapy in resectable GISTs [4]. However, imatinib therapy might be considered for advanced or borderline resectable tumors. Multiple prospective and randomized trials have shown that neoadjuvant imatinib therapy (with a dose of 400 mg/day) in cases of advanced GIST will cause a reduction in tumor size and enable an R0 resection with an increased chance of organ preservation (**Table 2**). However, if KIT exon 9 mutation is detected and neoadjuvant therapy is planned, the dose may be increased to 800 mg per day as recommended by the European Society for Medical Oncology (ESMO) guidelines.

Study	Published year	Type of study	Type of patients assessed	Dose of imatinib given	Median follow-up	Primary end point	Results
RTOG (Radiation Therapy Oncology Group) 0132 [1, 116]	2009	Phase II prospective	1. Advanced primary GIST of >5 cm (Group A, 30 p) 2. Recurrent or metastatic tumors of ≥2 cm (group B, 22 p)	Neoadjuvant 600 mg/day for 8–12 weeks of treatment with a median of 65 days then 600 mg/day adjuvant therapy for 2 years	1. Group A 4.9 y 2. Group B 5.5 y	RFS	1. The 2-y estimated overall survival was 93.3 and 90.9% in Group A and Group B, respectively, with a median follow-up of 3 y 2. The 5-y PFS and OS were 57% in group A, 30% in group B, and 77% in group A, 68% in group B, respectively
McAufliffe et al. [117]	2009	Phase II randomized	Primary GIST Metastatic GIST of ≥1 cm 3. 19 patients involved	Neoadjuvant 600 mg/day given at 3, 5, or 7 days; then adjuvant 600 mg/day for 2 years	32 m	Tumor cell apoptosis	All patients had a radiographic response with 1 week of imatinib therapy. In addition, the rate of tumor cell apoptosis had a positive correlation duration of imatinib therapy where the maximum tumor cell apoptosis was seen with 7 days neoadjuvant imatinib therapy
APOLLON [118]	2012	Prospective open-label phase II	1. KIT or PDFRA positive GIST. Tumors had to be locally advanced, potentially resectable, and no metastasis 2. 45 patients involved	Neoadjuvant for 6 months 400 mg/day with no postoperative adjuvant therapy	36 m	Overall tumor response	1. R0 resection was achieved in 30/34 patients and PFS at 3 years was 85.2%. 2. Predicted operation was downsized with imatinib therapy

Study	Published year	Type of study	Type of patients assessed	Dose of imatinib given	Median follow-up	Primary end point	Results
Kurokawa et al. [59]	2017	Phase II prospective	1. Primary GISTs in the stomach with tumor size of ≥10 cm with no metastasis 2. 53 patients enrolled	1. Neoadjuvant 400 mg/day for 6 months 2. Adjuvant 400 mg/day for at least 1 year	32 m	R0 resection rate	1. The R0 resection was achieved in 91% of patients (48/53) and at least half of the stomach was spared in 42/48 patients who had R0 resection. 2. After R0 resection, all patients received imatinib 400 mg/day for at least 1 year. The 2-year OS and PFS were 98 and 89%, respectively

RFS, recurrence-free survival; OS, overall survival; y, years; m, months.

Table 2. Summary of studies assessing the role of neoadjuvant imatinib in treatment of GIST.

8.1.2. Surgery for primary GISTs

Surgical resection with negative margins is the recommended treatment for localized primary GISTs and is the only curative treatment for GIST [58, 59]. A published study that contained 200 GIST patients [13] with 46.5% of the cases being primary local GISTs and 39% of the cases gastric GIST, which was the most common type, reported that complete resection was achieved in 80 patients (86%) with primary disease, and those patients had a 54% of a 5-year survival rate with a median survival of 66 months, while patients with incompletely resected or unresectable disease had a median survival of 22 months. Complete resection of even a locally advanced disease is associated with improved survival [60].

Surgical resection is recommended for GISTs with a size of 2 cm or more [61]. However, there is still no consensus on the management of GIST less than 2 cm [62, 63]. Multiple studies have reported the occurrence of microscopic gastric GIST [64–67]. Agaimy et al. [68] discovered microscopic GISTs in 22.5% of consecutive autopsies for adults of >50 years old with all lesions detected in cardia, fundus, and proximal body. Kawanowa et al. [67] reported 35% of microscopic GISTs in patients who had gastric resection for stomach cancer. Ninety percent of these microscopic GISTs were in the upper body.

GISTs have been reported as an incidental finding discovered by routine OGDs and in gastric specimens post sleeve gastrectomy [69, 70] and have caused a dilemma about whether routine preoperative gastroscopy should be done before each bariatric procedure to avoid missing such incidental tumors [70]. Sepe et al. [71] had developed an algorithmic approach for gastric GIST which was adopted by The National Comprehensive Cancer Network (NCCN). They proposed that GISTs with no high-risk EUS features (irregular border, cystic spaces, ulceration, echogenic foci, and heterogeneity) can be followed up by EUS. NCCN adopted this approach and suggested that EUS surveillance every 6–12 months may be done for GISTs of <2 cm with no high-risk features [72].

Endoscopic resection of gastric small submucosal tumors is a promising technique with a favorable outcome. Andalib et al. [73] described endoscopic resection of 12 cases with gastric GISTs arising from muscularis propria with an average size of 2.4 cm and no complications of bleeding or perforation. However, 50% of cases had positive microscopic margins but there is no evidence that a positive microscopic margin after macroscopic resection requires re-excision [74], and with an average follow-up of 12 months, none of the patients had recurrence. Zhou et al. [75] described endoscopic resection of 26 cases of gastric submucosal tumors, out of which 16 were gastric GISTs. The mean tumor size was 2.8 cm and all of the tumors were resected completely without interruption of capsule. None of the patients had severe complications as bleeding perforation or abdominal abscess [75]. No recurrence was found with a mean follow-up of 8 months. Nevertheless, tumor spillage and perforation after endoscopic resection had been described [76], and the technique needs to be validated by prospective multicenter trials and cannot be routinely recommended.

As mentioned before, surgery is the main and only curative option for primary localized resectable GISTs [77]. The primary technical goal of surgery is complete macroscopic resection with an intact pseudocapsule and a negative microscopic margin (R0 resection) [77]. Routine lymphadenectomy is not needed as adult GISTs rarely metastasize to lymph nodes [78]. Pediatric GISTs, however, have a higher incidence of lymph node metastasis [78] and lymphadenectomy may be needed for this population [79, 80].

Wedge resection with negative margins is the usual treatment for gastric GISTs [81] unless the tumor is found invading the surrounding tissues where en bloc resection of involved surrounding organs may be appropriate [81]. Patients with low-grade tumors may have a 5-year survival up to 80%. It is still important to avoid tumor rupture and spillage, as this is associated with an increased risk of recurrence and low survival rates [47, 60]. The role of laparoscopy in gastric GISTs is developing with promising outcomes. Two meta-analysis studies have concluded that, when compared to open, laparoscopy seems to result in shorter hospital stays with no difference in operative time, adverse events, estimated blood loss, margin positivity, or overall survival (OS) and recurrence rates [82, 83]. Current NCCN guidelines [84] recommend that a laparoscopic wedge resection for gastric GISTs of 5 cm or less is appropriate and tumor resection may be done using a laparoscopic or a laparoscopic-assisted technique with hand port for GISTs more than 5 cm.

8.1.3. Adjuvant therapy for primary GISTs

Unlike neoadjuvant imatinib therapy, the role of adjuvant imatinib therapy is better established. Recurrence rates of 50% have been reported in localized GISTs that have been completely resected [4]. Multiple randomized trials have proven the efficacy of adjuvant imatinib.

The first randomized phase II trial done on the role of adjuvant imatinib was The American College of Surgeons Oncology Group (ACOSOG) trial Z9000 [85] which assessed the role of adjuvant imatinib dose of 400 mg/day for 1 year for patients with a high-risk GIST. High risk was defined in this study as a tumor diameter of >10 cm, intraperitoneal tumor rupture, or up to four peritoneal implants. The study involved 106 patients with GISTs, 50% of the cases were gastric GISTs. After a median follow-up of 7.7 years, the 1-, 3-, and 5-year overall survivals (OS) were 99, 97, and 83%, respectively, which is much better than historical controls (35%) [85]. The 1-, 3-, and 5-year RFS rates were 96, 60, and 40%, respectively. Recurrence free survival (RFS) was lower with a larger tumor size, KIT exon 9 mutation, a high mitotic rate, and older age. They concluded that adjuvant imatinib for 1 year prolongs RFS and OS, but the optimal duration of adjuvant imatinib was still to be decided.

Three phase III trials have assessed the efficacy of adjuvant imatinib, ACOSOG Z9001 [86], SSG XVIII trials [87], and EORTC 62024 [88]. Only ACOSOG Z9001and EORTC 62024 had no treatment control arm. The American College of Surgeons Oncology Group (ACOSOG) trial Z9001 [86] is the first randomized phase III, double-blinded, placebo-controlled, multicenter trial done regarding the role of adjuvant imatinib therapy. A total of 359 patients were randomized to receive imatinib 400 mg/day for 1 year, and 354 patients were randomized to receive placebo for 1 year following surgical resection of the tumor. The trial reported that imatinib therapy significantly prolonged RFS when compared to placebo (98 versus 83%) in all risk categories (based upon size, mitotic rate, and location in the GI tract) [86]. Overall survival was similar at 1 year with 99.2 versus 99.7%, and imatinib therapy was tolerated with low side effects. The trial planned a minimum follow-up of 3 years for the patients but it was stopped early with a shorter median follow-up of 19.7 months. The lack of difference in overall survival in this trial may be explained by a short duration follow-up, a limited number of relapses, and a high degree of efficacy of imatinib in relapsed disease [89]. As a result of this study, The U.S. Food and Drug Administration approved adjuvant imatinib in the adjuvant setting by the U.S. Food and Drug Administration for GISTs of ≥3 cm, without guidance as to the optimal duration of treatment or which patients are most likely to benefit. The long-term results of this study were published with a median follow-up of 74 months with no difference in the 5-year RFS and OS.

Another phase III prospective, randomized, open-label trial was done by The Scandinavian Sarcoma Group (SSG) XVIII [87]. This trial compared 36 versus 12 months therapy of adjuvant imatinib (400 mg daily) in 400 patients with a high-risk-resected GIST with a median follow-up of 54 months. A high-risk GIST was defined as a tumor size of >10 cm, a mitotic count of >10/50 high-power fields (HPF), a tumor size of >5 cm with a mitotic rate of >5/HPF, or a tumor rupture. About 50% of the patients had gastric GIST in this study. The study reported prolonged 5-year RFS and OS rates for patients assigned for 36 months imatinib adjuvant therapy compared with patients assigned for the 12-month group, 65.6 versus 47.9% and 92% versus 81.7%, respectively. The results of this trial resulted in NCCN guidelines recommending adjuvant imatinib for at least 3 years for patients with intermediate or high risk of GIST recurrence [90]. In a latter follow-up report for the Scandinavian trial with a median follow-up of 90 months, patients assigned to a 3-year group had a persistent favorable outcome with significantly greater RFS (71 versus 52% and overall survival (92 versus 85%) [91].

The EORTC 62024 trial [88] is a phase III open-label randomized trial which assessed the efficacy of adjuvant imatinib for 2 years in localized surgically resected high- or intermediate-risk GISTs [88]. After surgical resection, 908 patients were randomized to either receive 2 years of imatinib 400 mg/day or observation alone. After a median follow-up of 4.7 years, RFS at 3 years was 84% in imatinib group versus 66% in control group and 69 versus 63% at 5 years ($P < 0.001$). No difference was detected in a 5-year OS. The 5-year imatinib failure-free survival (IFFS, the time to death or starting a TKI other than imatinib) was 87% in imatinib group and 84% in control group ($P = 0.23$). Among patients with a high-risk GIST (528 patients), there was a trend favoring adjuvant imatinib ($P = 0.087$).

As a result of the findings of the previous trials, both NCCN and ESMO guidelines as well as consensus of the scientific community recommend 3 years of adjuvant treatment with imatinib in high-risk patients [4]. By contrast, adjuvant therapy is not needed in low-risk patients, and there are no sufficient data to support adjuvant imatinib therapy in intermediate-risk patients [4]. Whether doses higher than 400 mg/day should be used is still questionable. Moreover, whether the imatinib dose should be continued more than 3 years is not known. A single-arm phase II 5-year adjuvant imatinib trial, PERSIST5, has completed its accrual, and still survival data reports are pending. Whether patients who had R1 resection for their GISTs should receive adjuvant imatinib is also not clear as there are no data to support adjuvant imatinib therapy in such cases. Re-excision may be appropriate in these situations.

8.2. Management of metastatic and recurrent GIST

GISTs mostly recur in the first 5 years after surgical resection, while less recurrence is observed after 10 years [92]. A study, with pooled analysis from 10 series and included 1625 patients, reported that 5-year, 10-year, and 15-year RFS were 70.5, 62.9, and 59.9%, respectively [92]. It was observed that the larger the size of the tumor, the higher the risk of recurrence. Compared with tumors of <1.1 cm in size, tumors with sizes of 1.1–2, 2.1–5, 5.1–10.0, 10.1–15.0, and > 15 cm were associated with a hazard ratio (HR) of 2.19, 4.45, 21.56, and 27.98, respectively. There was also a positive correlation between tumor mitosis rates and risk of recurrence. Compared with tumors with a very low mitosis count (<2/50 HPF), tumors with a low count (2–5/50 HPF), a moderate count (6–10/50 HPF), and a high count (>10/50 HPF) were associated with HR of 3.78, 11.1, and 22.09, respectively. Gastric GISTs had better RFS than other types of GISTs. Tumor rupture was associated with a worse prognosis. About two-third and half of patients with recurrence had liver metastasis and peritoneal disease, respectively [93].

Patients with advanced (primary unresectable or metastatic GIST) are treated initially with imatinib rather than surgery.

A phase III randomized trail (EU-AUS trial) [94] included 946 patients randomized to either receive imatinib once or twice daily. At a median follow-up of 760 days, the trial reported that 56% of 473 patients receiving imatinib 400 mg/day had progressed while 50% (235) of 473 patients assigned to imatinib 400 twice/day had progressed. OS was 69 and 74%, respectively. There was no significant difference in response rates between the two groups. The study concluded that, although a daily dose of 400 mg of imatinib is enough, a dose of 400 mg twice daily significantly prolongs PFS.

In a phase II open-label multicentric randomized trial, B2222 study, which included 147 patients with advanced GIST, 73 patients received imatinib 400 mg/day and 74 patients received imatinib 600 mg/day. The study reported equal response rates, median progression-free survival, and median overall survival among both groups with a median survival of 57 months for all patients. No advantage was seen with using a higher dose of imatinib (600 mg/day) in this study. This study was followed by another phase III open-label multicentric randomized trial, S0033 study [95], which compared imatinib dose 400 mg/day to imatinib dose 400/mg twice daily. The study included 746 patients with advanced GIST with a median follow-up of 4.5 years. Similar findings were found with no statistically significant difference in response rates, PFS, or OS between either doses of imatinib. However, after progression on imatinib dose of 400 mg/day, 33% of the patients who were crossed over to receive a higher imatinib dose 400 mg twice daily achieved either an objective response or a stable disease [95].

Further analysis of data from EU-AUS and S0033 trials reported that tumor genotype has a significant prognostic impact on PFS and OS, with tumors with mutation of KIT exon 9 having a worse prognosis when compared to tumors with mutation of KIT exon 11 [96, 97].

A subsequent meta-analysis combining S0033 and EU-AUS trials [98] reported a minor albeit significant PFS advantage for a higher imatinib dose of 400 mg twice daily for patients with advanced GIST. The PFS benefit was only evident in patients with KIT exon 9 mutations treated with a high-dose imatinib without difference in OS between the two groups, while patients with KIT exon 11 had a more favorable prognosis. Thus, genotype is required for the treatment of advanced or metastatic GISTs.

The findings of the results of the previous studies [94, 95, 98] designated imatinib dosage of 400 mg/day to be the standard treatment for patients with advanced GISTs, and patients with advanced GISTs with KIT exon 9 mutations to be started on the higher imatinib dose (400 mg twice daily), keeping in mind that the toxicity of imatinib is dose-dependent [99]. Imatinib treatment should be life long as interruption of treatment has a higher rate of disease progression as proven by the phase III randomized trial [100–102]. Indications of surgery in advanced GISTs are still debatable. Multiple retrospective studies have shown that debulking surgery may be beneficial in patients with a stable disease without generalized progression as surgery may improve the prognosis. However, patients should be treated with imatinib first before attempting surgery [103–108].

8.3. Alternatives of imatinib in case of resistance or progression of disease with imatinib therapy

Most patients with advanced GISTs will show improvement with imatinib therapy, although a subgroup of patients will fail to show a response. Resistance to imatinib may be primary or secondary. Primary resistance is defined as continuous growth or growth within 6 months of therapy, and occurs in 15–20% of patients with advanced GIST [109] and occurs frequently in patients with wild-type (WT) GIST or KIT exon 9 mutations or D842V mutation in PDGFRA exon 18 [110]. Unfortunately, most patients develop secondary resistance, which is defined as patients who received treatment with imatinib for longer than 6 months and had an initial response and then developed progressive disease. Secondary KIT mutations occur frequently in KIT exons 13, 14, and 17 and a D842V mutation in PDGFRA exon 18 [111–113].

If a patient develops resistance, escalating imatinib dosage to 800 mg daily or shifting to a second-line therapy like sunitinib may be recommended.

Sunitinib is considered a second-line therapy for patients with advanced GIST refractory to imatinib therapy. Outcomes of a randomized phase III trial versus placebo reported a prolongation of the time to progression from 1.5 to 6.3 months in patients with GIST who progressed on imatinib treatment [114]. It is approved by the EMA and the FDA for the treatment of patients with GIST resistant to imatinib therapy and for patients who are not tolerant to imatinib therapy.

In case of progression on imatinib and sunitinib, regorafenib is considered a third-line therapy [4]. It was recently approved by EMA and FDA for the treatment of patients with unresectable or metastatic GISTs who are resistant or intolerant to imatinib and sunitinib, and it was tested in a phase III randomized trial which included patients with advanced GIST who progressed after imatinib and sunitinib failed. The study reported that regorafenib, when compared to placebo, has significant improvement in PFS [115]. Inadequate data are available for the efficacy of other tyrosine kinase inhibitors (e.g., sorafenib, pazopanib, and ponatinib) for imatinib and sunitinib refractory GISTs [4].

9. Follow-up

There are no studies assessing the efficacy of different follow-up modules. Nevertheless, follow-up strategies were created based on the fact that most recurrences occur within the first 5 years after surgery.

A follow-up schedule frequency is based on the risk of aggressiveness and recurrence of GISTs [4]. CT is favored over other imagings, such as MRI and FDG-PET scan, because it is more readily obtainable, although other modalities can be used in case CT is inconclusive.

9.1. Follow-up for localized resectable GISTs

Very low-risk patients with surgically removed tumor do not require a follow-up. Low-risk patients require an annual CT. Intermediate- and high-risk patients require CT every 4 months for the first 1–2 years, every 6 months for 3–5 years, and then CT every year thereafter [4].

9.2. Follow-up for unresectable/metastatic GISTs

Follow-up should be done at the start of every 3 months and can be delayed to every 6 months if there is response to the treatment.

10. Conclusion

Surgery is the only curative option for GISTs. The discovery of KIT protein had allowed the development of tyrosine kinase inhibitors which considerably affected the diagnosis and management of GISTs. A multidisciplinary approach is required for optimal management. Neoadjuvant imatinib therapy has produced favorable results so far; however, more studies are needed to define the optimal dose and duration of imatinib therapy. Adjuvant imatinib therapy for 3 years improves outcome in patients with high risk. Mutational analysis has an important role in the management of GISTs. New therapeutic agents have been developed for patients with imatinib resistance.

Author details

Tamer Saafan

Address all correspondence to: tsaafan@gmail.com

General Surgery Department, Hamad General Hospital, Hamad Medical Corporation, Doha, Qatar

References

[1] Eisenberg BL, Harris J, Blanke CD, et al. Phase II trial of neoadjuvant/adjuvant imatinib mesylate (IM) for advanced primary and metastatic/recurrent operable gastrointestinal stromal tumor (GIST): Early results of RTOG 0132/ACRIN 6665. Journal of Surgical Oncology. 2009;**99**(1):42-47. [PubMed: 18942073]

[2] McAuliffe JC, Hunt KK, Lazar AJ, et al. A randomized, phase II study of preoperative plus postoperative imatinib in GIST: Evidence of rapid radiographic response and temporal induction of tumor cell apoptosis. Annals of Surgical Oncology. 2009;**16**(4):910-919 [PubMed: 18953611]

[3] Miettinen M, Killian JK, Wang ZF, et al. Immunohistochemical loss of succinate dehydrogenase subunit A (SDHA) in gastrointestinal stromal tumors (GISTs) signals SDHA germline mutation. The American Journal of Surgical Pathology. 2013;**37**(2):234-240 [PubMed: 23282968]

[4] Poveda A, García Del Muro X, López-Guerrero JA, Cubedo R, Martínez V, Romero I, Serrano C, Valverde C, Martín-Broto J. GEIS (Grupo Español de Investigación en Sarcomas/Spanish Group for Sarcoma Research). GEIS guidelines for gastrointestinal sarcomas (GIST). Cancer Treatment Reviews. 2017 Apr;**55**:107-119. DOI: 10.1016/j.ctrv.2016.11.011. Epub 2017 Mar 2. Review. PubMed PMID: 28351781

[5] Ducimetiere F, Lurkin A, Ranchere-Vince D, et al. Incidence of sarcoma histotypes and molecular subtypes in a prospective epidemiological study with central pathology review and molecular testing. PLoS One. 2011;**6**(8):e20294

[6] Fletcher CD, Berman JJ, Corless C, et al. Diagnosis of gastrointestinal stromal tumors: A consensus approach. Human Pathology. 2002;**33**(5):459, 465. [PubMed: 12094370]

[7] Perez EA, Livingstone AS, Franceschi D, et al. Current incidence and outcomes of gastrointestinal mesenchymal tumors including gastrointestinal stromal tumors. Journal of the American College of Surgeons. 2006;**202**(4):623-629. [PubMed: 16571433]

[8] Miettinen M, Virolainen M, Maarit SR. Gastrointestinal stromal tumors—value of CD34 antigen in their identification and separation from true leiomyomas and schwannomas. The American Journal of Surgical Pathology. 1995;**19**(2):207-216. [PubMed: 7530409]

[9] Hirota S, Isozaki K, Moriyama Y, et al. Gain-of-function mutations of c-kit in human gastrointestinal stromal tumors. Science. 1998;**279**(5350):577-580. [PubMed: 9438854]

[10] Ma GL, Murphy JD, Martinez ME, Sicklick JK. Epidemiology of gastrointestinal stromal tumors in the era of histology codes: Results of a population-based study. Cancer Epidemiology, Biomarkers and Prevention. 2015;**24**:298

[11] Ducimetiere F, Lurkin A, Ranchere-Vince D, et al. Incidence of sarcoma histotypes and molecular subtypes in a prospective epidemiological study with central pathology review and molecular testing. PLoS One. 2011;**6**(8):e20294

[12] Tran T, Davila JA, El-Serag HB. The epidemiology of malignant gastrointestinal stromal tumors: An analysis of 1,458 cases from 1992 to 2000. The American Journal of Gastroenterology. 2005;**100**(1):162-168. [PubMed: 15654796]

[13] DeMatteo RP, Lewis JJ, Leung D, et al. Two hundred gastrointestinal stromal tumors: Recurrence patterns and prognostic factors for survival. Annals of Surgery. 2000;**231**(1):51-58

[14] Cassier PA, Ducimetière F, Lurkin A, et al. A prospective epidemiological study of new incident GISTs during two consecutive years in Rhône Alpes region: Incidence and molecular distribution of GIST in a European region. British Journal of Cancer. 2010;**103**:165

[15] Miettinen M, Lasota J, Sobin LH. Gastrointestinal stromal tumors of the stomach in children and young adults: A clinicopathologic, immunohistochemical, and molecular genetic study of 44 cases with long-term follow-up and review of the literature. The American Journal of Surgical Pathology. 2005;**29**(10):1373-1381. [PubMed: 16160481]

[16] Prakash S, Sarran L, Socci N, et al. Gastrointestinal stromal tumors in children and young adults: A clinicopathologic, molecular, and genomic study of 15 cases and review of the literature. Journal of Pediatric Hematology/Oncology. 2005;**27**(4):179-187. [PubMed: 15838387]

[17] Kaemmer DA, Otto J, Lassay L, et al. The GIST of literature on pediatric GIST: Review of clinical presentation. Journal of Pediatric Hematology/Oncology. 2009;**31**(2):108-112

[18] Agaram NP, Laquaglia MP, Ustun B, et al. Molecular characterization of pediatric gastrointestinal stromal tumors. Clinical Cancer Research. 2008;**14**(10):3204-3215

[19] Maeyama H, Hidaka E, Ota H, et al. Familial gastrointestinal stromal tumor with hyperpigmentation: Association with a germline mutation of the c-kit gene. Gastroenterology. 2001;**120**:210

[20] Nishida T, Hirota S, Taniguchi M, et al. Familial gastrointestinal stromal tumours with germline mutation of the KIT gene. Nature Genetics. 1998;**19**:323

[21] Tarn C, Merkel E, Canutescu AA, Shen W, Skorobogatko Y, Heslin MJ, Eisenberg B, Birbe R, Patchefsky A, Dunbrack R, Arnoletti JP, von Mehren M, Godwin AK. Analysis of KIT mutations in sporadic and familial gastrointestinal stromal tumors: therapeutic implications through protein modeling. Clinical Cancer Research. 2005 May 15;**11**(10):3668-3677

[22] Hirota S, Okazaki T, Kitamura Y, et al. Cause of familial and multiple gastrointestinal autonomic nerve tumors with hyperplasia of interstitial cells of Cajal is germline mutation of the c-kit gene. The American Journal of Surgical Pathology. 2000;**24**:326

[23] Beghini A, Tibiletti MG, Roversi G, et al. Germline mutation in the juxtamembrane domain of the kit gene in a family with gastrointestinal stromal tumors and urticaria pigmentosa. Cancer. 2001;**92**:657

[24] Hirota S, Nishida T, Isozaki K, et al. Familial gastrointestinal stromal tumors associated with dysphagia and novel type germline mutation of KIT gene. Gastroenterology. 2002;**122**:1493

[25] Chompret A, Kannengiesser C, Barrois M, et al. PDGFRA germline mutation in a family with multiple cases of gastrointestinal stromal tumor. Gastroenterology. 2004;**126**:318

[26] de Raedt T, Cools J, Debiec-Rychter M, et al. Intestinal neurofibromatosis is a subtype of familial GIST and results from a dominant activating mutation in PDGFRA. Gastro enterology. 2006;**131**:1907

[27] Pasini B, Matyakhina L, Bei T, et al. Multiple gastrointestinal stromal and other tumors caused by platelet-derived growth factor receptor alpha gene mutations: A case associated with a germline V561D defect. The Journal of Clinical Endocrinology and Metabolism. 2007;**92**:3728

[28] Ricci R, Martini M, Cenci T, et al. PDGFRA-mutant syndrome. Modern Pathology. 2015;**28**:954

[29] Stratakis CA, Carney JA. The triad of paragangliomas, gastric stromal tumours and pulmonary chondromas (Carney triad), and the dyad of paragangliomas and gastric stromal sarcomas (Carney–Stratakis syndrome): Molecular genetics and clinical implications. Journal of Internal Medicine. 2009;**266**(1):43-52. [PubMed: 19522824]

[30] Miettinen M, Killian JK, Wang ZF, et al. Immunohistochemical loss of succinate dehydrogenase subunit A (SDHA) in gastrointestinal stromal tumors (GISTs) signals SDHA germline mutation. The American Journal of Surgical Pathology. 2013;**37**(2):234-240. [PubMed: 23282968]

[31] Andersson J, Sihto H, Meis-Kindblom JM, et al. NF1-associated gastrointestinal stromal tumors have unique clinical, phenotypic, and genotypic characteristics. The American Journal of Surgical Pathology. 2005;**29**(9):1170-1176. [PubMed: 16096406]

[32] Rubin BP. Gastrointestinal stromal tumours: An update. Histopathology. 2006;**48**:83-96. [PubMed PMID: 16359540]

[33] Martin-Broto J, Rubio L, Alemany R, Lopez-Guerrero JA. Clinical implications of KIT and PDGFRA genotyping in GIST. Clinical and Translational Oncology: Official Publication of the Federation of Spanish Oncology Societies and of the National Cancer Institute of Mexico. 2010;**12**:670-676. [PubMed PMID: 20947481]

[34] Lasota J, Dansonka-Mieszkowska A, Sobin LH, et al. A great majority of GISTs with PDGFRA mutations represent gastric tumors of low or no malignant potential. Laboratory Investigation. 2004;**84**(7):874-883. [PubMed: 15146165]

[35] Hostein I, Faur N, Primois C, et al. BRAF mutation status in gastrointestinal stromal tumors. American Journal of Clinical Pathology. 2010;**133**(1):141-148. [PubMed: 20023270]

[36] Agaram NP, Wong GC, Guo T, et al. Novel V600E BRAF mutations in imatinib-naive and imatinib-resistant gastrointestinal stromal tumors. Genes, Chromosomes and Cancer. 2008;**47**(10):853-859. [PubMed: 18615679]

[37] Bamboat ZM, Dematteo RP. Updates on the management of gastrointestinal stromal tumors. Surgical Oncology Clinics of North America. 2012;**21**(2):301-316. [PubMed: 22365521]

[38] Miettinen M, Lasota J. Gastrointestinal stromal tumors–definition, clinical, histological, immunohistochemical, and molecular genetic features and differential diagnosis. Virchows Archiv-An International Journal of Pathology. 2001;**438**:1-12. [PubMed PMID: 11213830]

[39] Novelli M, Rossi S, Rodriguez-Justo M, et al. DOG1 and CD117 are the antibodies of choice in the diagnosis of gastrointestinal stromal tumours. Histopathology. 2010;**57**(2):259-270. [PubMed: 20716168]

[40] Liegl B, Hornick JL, Corless CL, Fletcher CD. Monoclonal antibody DOG1.1 shows higher sensitivity than KIT in the diagnosis of gastrointestinal stromal tumors, including unusual subtypes. The American Journal of Surgical Pathology. 2009 Mar;**33**(3):437-446. DOI: 10.1097/PAS.0b013e318186b158. [PubMed PMID: 19011564]

[41] Nilsson B, Bumming P, Meis-Kindblom JM, et al. Gastrointestinal stromal tumors: the incidence, prevalence, clinical course, and prognostication in the preimatinib mesylate era–a population-based study in western Sweden. Cancer. 2005;**103**(4):821-829. [PubMed: 15648083]

[42] Chaudhry UI, DeMatteo RP. Management of resectable gastrointestinal stromal tumor. Hematology/Oncology Clinics of North America. 2009;**23**(1):79-96. [PubMed: 19248972]

[43] Reith JD, Goldblum JR, Lyles RH, et al. Extragastrointestinal (soft tissue) stromal tumors: An analysis of 48 cases with emphasis on histologic predictors of outcome. Modern Pathology. 2000;**13**(5):577-585. [PubMed: 10824931]

[44] DeMatteo RP, Maki RG, Agulnik M, et al. Gastrointestinal Stromal Tumor. In: Amin MB, editor, AJCC Cancer Staging Manual, 8th, AJCC, Chicago 2017. p. 523. no abstract available

[45] Joensuu H. Risk stratification of patients diagnosed with gastrointestinal stromal tumor. Human Pathology. 2008;**39**(10):1411-1419. [PubMed: 18774375]

[46] Miettinen M, Lasota J. Gastrointestinal stromal tumors: Review on morphology, molec ular pathology, prognosis, and differential diagnosis. Archives of Pathology and Labora tory Medicine. 2006;**130**(10):1466-1478. [PubMed PMID: 17090188]

[47] Takahashi T, Nakajima K, Nishitani A, Souma Y, Hirota S, Sawa Y, Nishida T. An enhanced risk-group stratification system for more practical prognostication of clinically malignant gastrointestinal stromal tumors. International Journal of Clinical Oncology. 2007;**12**:369-374

[48] DeMatteo RP, Maki RG, Agulnik M, et al. Gastrointestinal Stromal Tumor. In: Amin MB, editor. AJCC Cancer Staging Manual, 8th, AJCC, Chicago 2017. p. 523

[49] Gold JS, Gönen M, Gutiérrez A, et al. Development and validation of a prognostic nomogram for recurrence-free survival after complete surgical resection of localised primary gastrointestinal stromal tumour: A retrospective analysis. The Lancet Oncology. 2009;**10**:1045

[50] Bischof DA, Kim Y, Behman R, et al. A nomogram to predict disease-free survival after surgical resection of GIST. Journal of Gastrointestinal Surgery. 2014;**18**:2123

[51] Joensuu H, Vehtari A, Riihimäki J, et al. Risk of recurrence of gastrointestinal stromal tumour after surgery: An analysis of pooled population-based cohorts. The Lancet Oncology. 2012;**13**:265

[52] Orita H, Ito T, Kushida T, et al. Pfetin as a risk factor of recurrence in gastrointestinal stromal tumors. BioMed Research International. 2014;**2014**:651935. DOI: 10.1155/2014/651935

[53] Kim HC, Lee JM, Choi SH, et al. Imaging of gastrointestinal stromal tumors. Journal of Computer Assisted Tomography. 2004;**28**(5):596-604. [PubMed: 15480031]

[54] Jiang ZX, Zhang SJ, Peng WJ, et al. Rectal gastrointestinal stromal tumors: Imaging features with clinical and pathological correlation. World Journal of Gastroenterology. 2013;**19**(20):3108-3116. [PubMed: 23716991]

[55] Gold JS, Dematteo RP. Combined surgical and molecular therapy: The gastrointestinal stromal tumor model. Annals of Surgery. 2006;**244**(2):176-184. [PubMed: 16858179]

[56] Van den Abbeele AD. The lessons of GIST–PET and PET/CT: A new paradigm for imaging. The Oncologist. 2008;**13**(suppl 2):8-13

[57] Watson RR, Binmoeller KF, Hamerski CM, et al. Yield and performance characteristics of endoscopic ultrasound-guided fine needle aspiration for diagnosing upper GI tract stromal tumors. Digestive Diseases and Sciences. 2011;**56**(6):1757-1762. [PubMed: 21360279]

[58] Wang D, Zhang Q, Blanke CD, et al. Phase II trial of neoadjuvant/adjuvant imatinib mesylate for advanced primary and metastatic/recurrent operable gastrointestinal stromal tumors: Long-term follow-up results of radiation therapy oncology group 0132. Annals of Surgical Oncology. 2012;**19**(4):1074-1080

[59] Kurokawa Y, Yang HK, Cho H, Ryu MH, Masuzawa T, Park SR, Matsumoto S, Lee HJ, Honda H, Kwon OK, Ishikawa T, Lee KH, Nabeshima K, Kong SH, Shimokawa T, Yook JH, Doki Y, Im SA, Hirota S, Hahn S, Nishida T, Kang YK. Phase II study of neoadjuvant imatinib in large gastrointestinal stromal tumours of the stomach. British Journal of Cancer. 2017 Jun 27;**117**(1):25-32. DOI: 10.1038/bjc.2017.144 Epub 2017 May 23. PubMed PMID: 28535156; PubMed Central PMCID: PMC5520207

[60] Ng EH, Pollock RE, Munsell MF, et al. Prognostic factors influencing survival in gastrointestinal leiomyosarcomas. Implications for surgical management and staging. Annals of Surgery. 1992;**215**(1):68-77. [PubMed: 1731651]

[61] NCCN 2010 guidelines. NCCN Task Force report: Management of patients with gastrointestinal stromal tumor (GisT)—update of the NCCN clinical practice guidelines. Journal of the National Comprehensive Cancer Network. 2007;**5**(suppl. 2):1-29

[62] Casali PG, Jost L, Reichardt P, et al. Gastrointestinal stromal tumours: ESMO clinical recommendations for diagnosis, treatment and follow-up. Annals of Oncology. 2009;**20**(Suppl 4):64

[63] Blackstein ME, Blay JY, Corless C, et al. Gastrointestinal stromal tumours: Consensus statement on diagnosis and treatment. Canadian Journal of Gastroenterology. 2006;**20**:157

[64] Abraham SC, Krasinskas AM, Hofstetter WL, Swisher SG, Wu TT. Seedling mesenchymal tumors (gastrointestinal stromal tumors and leiomyomas) are common incidental tumors of the esophagogastric junction. The American Journal of Surgical Pathology. 2007;**31**:1629-1635

[65] Agaimy A et al. Microscopic gastrointestinal stromal tumors in esophageal and intestinal surgical resection specimens: A clinicopathologic, immunohistochemical, and molecular study of 19 lesions. The American Journal of Surgical Pathology. 2008;**32**:867-873

[66] Agaimy A et al. Minute gastric sclerosing stromal tumors (GisT tumorlets) are common in adults and frequently show c-KiT mutations. The American Journal of Surgical Pathology. 2007;**31**:113-120

[67] Kawanowa K et al. High incidence of microscopic gastrointestinal stromal tumors in the stomach. Human Pathology. 2006;**37**:1527-1535

[68] Agaimy A, Wunsch PH, Dirnhofer S, et al. Microscopic gastrointestinal stromal tumors in esophageal and intestinal surgical resection specimens: A clinicopathologic, immunohistochemical, and molecular study of 19 lesions. The American Journal of Surgical Pathology. 2008;**32**(6):867-873. [PubMed: 18408593]

[69] Saafan T, Bashah M, El Ansari W, Karam M. Erratum to: Histopathological changes in laparoscopic sleeve Gastrectomy specimens: Prevalence, risk factors, and value of routine Histopathologic examination. Obesity Surgery. 2017 Oct;**27**(10):2778. DOI: 10.1007/s11695-017-2819-y. [PubMed PMID: 28752381]

[70] Salama A, Saafan T, El Ansari W, Karam M, Bashah M. Erratum to: Is routine preoperative esophagogastroduodenoscopy screening necessary prior to laparoscopic sleeve Gastrectomy? Review of 1555 cases and comparison with current literature. Obesity Sur gery. 2017 Nov;**27**(11):3068. DOI: 10.1007/s11695-017-2837-9. [PubMed PMID: 28748357]

[71] Sepe PS, Brugge WR. A guide for the diagnosis and management of gastrointestinal stromal cell tumors. Nature Reviews. Gastroenterology and Hepatology. 2009 Jun;**6**(6): 363-371. DOI: 10.1038/nrgastro.2009.43 Epub 2009 Apr 14. Review. PubMed PMID: 19365407

[72] Demetri GD, von Mehren M, Antonescu CR, et al. Journal of the National Comprehensive Cancer Network. 2010;**8**(suppl 2):S1, S42-S41, S44 [PubMed: 20457867]

[73] Andalib I, Yeoun D, Reddy R, Xie S, Iqbal S. Endoscopic resection of gastric gastrointestinal stromal tumors originating from the muscularis propria layer in North America: Methods and feasibility data. Surgical Endoscopy. 2017 Sep 15. DOI: 10.1007/s00464-017-5862-9. [Epub ahead of print] PubMed PMID: 28916847

[74] Demetri GD, Benjamin RS, Blanke CD, Blay JY, et al. NCCN Task Force report: Management of patients with gastrointestinal stromal tumor (GIST)—update of the NCCN clinical practice guidelines. Journal of the National Comprehensive Cancer Network. 2007;**5**(Suppl 2):S1-S29 quiz S30

[75] Zhou PH, Yao LQ, Qin XY, Cai MY, Xu MD, Zhong YS, Chen WF, Zhang YQ, Qin WZ, Hu JW, Liu JZ. Endoscopic full-thickness resection without laparoscopic assistance for gastric submucosal tumors originated from the muscularis propria. Surgical Endoscopy. 2011 Sep;**25**(9):2926-2931. DOI: 10.1007/s00464-011-1644-y. Epub 2011 Mar 18. PubMed PMID: 21424195

[76] Davila RE, Faigel DO. GI stromal tumors. Gastrointestinal Endoscopy. 2003;**58**:80-88

[77] Raut CP, Ashley SW. How I do it: Surgical management of gastrointestinal stromal tumors. Journal of Gastrointestinal Surgery. 2008 Sep;**12**(9):1592-1599. DOI: 10.1007/s11605-008-0501-3. Epub 2008 Mar 4. Review. PubMed PMID: 18317848

[78] Prakash S, Sarran L, Socci N, et al. Gastrointestinal stromal tumors in children and young adults: A clinicopathologic, molecular, and genomic study of 15 cases and review of the literature. Journal of Pediatric Hematology/Oncology. 2005;**27**:179-187

[79] Kaemmer DA, Otto J, Lassay L, et al. The gist of literature on pediatric GIST: Review of clinical presentation. Journal of Pediatric Hematology/Oncology. 2009;**31**(2):108-112. [PubMed: 19194193]

[80] Agaram NP, Laquaglia MP, Ustun B, et al. Molecular characterization of pediatric gastrointestinal stromal tumors. Clinical Cancer Research. 2008;**14**(10):3204-3215. [PubMed: 18483389]

[81] Kitagawa Y, Dempsey DT. Stomach. In: Brunicardi F, Andersen DK, Billiar TR, Dunn DL, Hunter JG, Matthews JB, Pollock RE, editors. Schwartz's Principles of Surgery, 10eNew. York, NY: McGraw-Hill; 2015. Available from: http://accesssurgery.mhmedical.com/content.aspx?bookid=980&sectionid=59610868. Accessed December 06, 2017

[82] Pelletier JS, Gill RS, Gazala S, Karmali S. A systematic review and meta-analysis of open vs. laparoscopic resection of gastric gastrointestinal stromal tumors. Journal of Clinical Medicine Research. 2015 May;**7**(5):289-296. DOI: 10.14740/jocmr1547w Epub 2015 Mar 1. Review. PubMed PMID: 25780475; PubMed Central PMCID: PMC4356087

[83] Koh YX, Chok AY, Zheng HL, Tan CS, Chow PK, Wong WK, Goh BK. A systematic review and meta-analysis comparing laparoscopic versus open gastric resections for gastrointestinal stromal tumors of the stomach. Annals of Surgical Oncology. 2013 Oct; **20**(11):3549-3560. DOI: 10.1245/s10434-013-3051-1 Epub 2013 Jun 21. Review. PubMed PMID: 23793362

[84] Demetri GD, von Mehren M, Antonescu CR, et al. NCCN Task Force report: Update on the management of patients with gastrointestinal stromal tumors. Journal of the National Comprehensive Cancer Network. 2010;**8**(suppl 2):S1, S42-S41, S44

[85] DeMatteo RP, Ballman KV, Antonescu CR, et al. Long-term results of adjuvant imatinib mesylate in localized, high-risk, primary gastrointestinal stromal tumor: ACOSOG Z9000 (Alliance) Intergroup Phase 2 Trial. Annals of Surgery. 2013;**258**(3):422-429. [PubMed: 23860199]

[86] Dematteo RP, Ballman KV, Antonescu CR, et al. Adjuvant imatinib mesylate after resection of localised, primary gastrointestinal stromal tumour: A randomised, double-blind, placebo-controlled trial. Lancet. 2009;**373**(9669):1097-1104. [PubMed: 19303137]

[87] Joensuu H, Eriksson M, Sundby Hall K, et al. One vs three years of adjuvant imatinib for operable gastrointestinal stromal tumor: A randomized trial. JAMA. 2012;**307**(12): 1265-1272. [PubMed: 22453568]

[88] Casali PG, Cesne AL, Velasco AP, et al. Imatinib failure-free survival (IFS) in patients with localized gastrointestinal stromal tumors (GIST) treated with adjuvant imatinib (IM): The EORTC/AGITG/FSG/GEIS/ISG randomized controlled phase III trial. Journal of Clinical Oncology. 2013;**31**(suppl):abstract 10500

[89] Blanke CD, Demetri GD, von Mehren M, Heinrich MC, Eisenberg B, Fletcher JA, Corless CL, Fletcher CD, Roberts PJ, Heinz D, Wehre E, Nikolova Z, Joensuu H. Long-term results from a randomized phase II trial of standard- versus higher-dose imatinib mesylate for patients with unresectable or metastatic gastrointestinal stromal tumors expressing KIT. Journal of Clinical Oncology. 2008 Feb 1;**26**(4):620-625. DOI: 10.1200/JCO.2007.13.4403. [PubMed PMID: 18235121]

[90] Demetri GD, von Mehren M, Antonescu CR, et al. NCCN Task Force report: Update on the management of patients with gastrointestinal stromal tumors. Journal of the National Comprehensive Cancer Network. 2010;**8**(suppl 2):S1, S42-S41, S44. [PubMed: 20457867]

[91] Joensuu H, Eriksson M, Sundby Hall K, et al. Adjuvant Imatinib for high-risk GI stromal tumor: Analysis of a randomized trial. Journal of Clinical Oncology. 2016;**34**:244

[92] Joensuu H, Vehtari A, Riihimaki J, et al. Risk of recurrence of gastrointestinal stromal tumour after surgery: An analysis of pooled population-based cohorts. The Lancet Oncology. 2012;**13**(3):265-274

[93] Bamboat ZM, Dematteo RP. Updates on the management of gastrointestinal stro mal tumors. Surgical Oncology Clinics of North America. 2012;**21**(2):301-316. [PubMed: 22365521]

[94] Verweij J, Casali PG, Zalcberg J, et al. Progression-free survival in gastrointestinal stromal tumours with high-dose imatinib: Randomised trial. Lancet. 2004;**364**(9440): 1127-1134. [PubMed: 15451219]

[95] Blanke CD, Rankin C, Demetri GD, et al. Phase III randomized, intergroup trial assessing imatinib mesylate at two dose levels in patients with unresectable or metastatic gastrointestinal stromal tumors expressing the kit receptor tyrosine kinase: S0033. Journal of Clinical Oncology. 2008;**26**(4):626-632. [PubMed: 18235122]

[96] Heinrich MC, Owzar K, Corless CL, et al. Correlation of kinase genotype and clinical outcome in the North American Intergroup Phase III Trial of imatinib mesylate for treatment of advanced gastrointestinal stromal tumor: CALGB 150105 Study by Cancer and Leukemia Group B and Southwest Oncology Group. Journal of Clinical Oncology. 2008;**26**(33):5360-5367. [PubMed: 18955451]

[97] Debiec-Rychter M, Sciot R, Le Cesne A, et al. KIT mutations and dose selection for imatinib in patients with advanced gastrointestinal stromal tumours. European Journal of Cancer. 2006;**42**(8):1093-1103. [PubMed: 16624552]

[98] Gastrointestinal Stromal Tumor Meta-Analysis Group (MetaGIST). Comparison of two doses of imatinib for the treatment of unresectable or metastatic gastrointestinal stromal tumors: A meta-analysis of 1,640 patients. Journal of Clinical Oncology. 2010;**28**(7):1247-1253. [PubMed: 20124181]

[99] Van Glabbeke M, Verweij J, Casali PG, et al. Predicting toxicities for patients with advanced gastrointestinal stromal tumours treated with imatinib: A study of the Euro pean Organisation for Research and Treatment of Cancer, the Italian sarcoma group, and the Australasian gastro-intestinal trials group (EORTC-ISG-AGITG). European Journal of Cancer. 2006;**42**:2277-2285

[100] Blay JY, Le Cesne A, Ray-Coquard I, et al. Prospective multicentric randomized phase III study of imatinib in patients with advanced gastrointestinal stromal tumors comparing interruption versus continuation of treatment beyond 1 year: the French Sarcoma Group. Journal of Clinical Oncology. 2007;**25**(9):1107-1113. [PubMed: 17369574]

[101] Le Cesne A, Ray-Coquard I, Bui BN, et al. Discontinuation of imatinib in patients with advanced gastrointestinal stromal tumours after 3 years of treatment: An open-label multicentre randomised phase 3 trial. The Lancet Oncology. 2010;**11**(10):942-949 [PubMed: 20864406]

[102] Ray-Coquard IL, Bin Bui N, Adenis A, et al. Risk of relapse with imatinib (IM) discontinuation at 5 years in advanced GIST patients: Results of the prospective BFR14 randomized phase III study comparing interruption versus continuation of IM at 5 years of treatment: A French Sarcoma Group Study. Journal of Clinical Oncology. 2010;**28**(suppl):15s, abstract 10032

[103] Bonvalot S, Eldweny H, Pechoux CL, et al. Impact of surgery on advanced gastrointestinal stromal tumors (GIST) in the imatinib era. Annals of Surgical Oncology. 2006;**13**(12):1596-1603. [PubMed: 16957966]

[104] Raut CP, Posner M, Desai J, et al. Surgical management of advanced gastrointestinal stromal tumors after treatment with targeted systemic therapy using kinase inhibitors. Journal of Clinical Oncology. 2006;**24**(15):2325-2331. [PubMed: 16710031]

[105] Rutkowski P, Nowecki Z, Nyckowski P, et al. Surgical treatment of patients with initially inoperable and/or metastatic gastrointestinal stromal tumors (GIST) during therapy with imatinib mesylate. Journal of Surgical Oncology. 2006;**93**(4):304-311. [PubMed: 16496358]

[106] Andtbacka RH, Ng CS, Scaife CL, et al. Surgical resection of gastrointestinal stromal tumors after treatment with imatinib. Annals of Surgical Oncology. 2007;**14**(1):14-24. [PubMed: 17072676]

[107] Gronchi A, Fiore M, Miselli F, et al. Surgery of residual disease following molecular-targeted therapy with imatinib mesylate in advanced/metastatic GIST. Annals of Surgery. 2007;**245**(3):341-346. [PubMed: 17435538]

[108] DeMatteo RP, Maki RG, Singer S, et al. Results of tyrosine kinase inhibitor therapy followed by surgical resection for metastatic gastrointestinal stromal tumor. Annals of Surgery. 2007;**245**(3):347-352. [PubMed: 17435539]

[109] Antonescu CR, DeMatteo RP. CCR 20th anniversary commentary: A genetic mechanism of Imatinib resistance in gastrointestinal stromal tumor-where are we a decade later? Clinical Cancer Research. 2015 Aug 1;**21**(15):3363-3365. DOI: 10.1158/1078-0432.CCR-14-3120. [PubMed PMID: 26240289; PubMed Central PMCID: PMC4526110]

[110] Benjamin RS, Debiec-Rychter M, Le Cesne A, et al. Gastrointestinal stromal tumors II: Medical oncology and tumor response assessment. Seminars in Oncology. 2009;**36**(4): 302-311. [PubMed: 19664491]

[111] Debiec-Rychter M, Cools J, Dumez H, et al. Mechanisms of resistance to imatinib mesylate in gastrointestinal stromal tumors and activity of the PKC412 inhibitor against imatinib-resistant mutants. Gastroenterology. 2005;**128**(2):270-279. [PubMed: 15685537]

[112] Heinrich MC, Corless CL, Blanke CD, et al. Molecular correlates of imatinib resistance in gastrointestinal stromal tumors. Journal of Clinical Oncology. 2006;**24**(29):4764-4774. [PubMed: 16954519]

[113] Wardelmann E, Thomas N, Merkelbach-Bruse S, et al. Acquired resistance to imatinib in gastrointestinal stromal tumours caused by multiple KIT mutations. The Lancet Oncology. 2005;**6**(4):249-251. [PubMed: 15811621]

[114] Demetri GD, van Oosterom AT, Garrett CR, et al. Efficacy and safety of sunitinib in patients with advanced gastrointestinal stromal tumour after failure of imatinib: A randomised controlled trial. Lancet. 2006;**368**(9544):1329-1338. [PubMed: 17046465]

[115] Demetri GD, Reichardt P, Kang YK, et al. Efficacy and safety of regorafenib for advanced gastrointestinal stromal tumours after failure of imatinib and sunitinib (GRID): An international, multicentre, randomised, placebo-controlled, phase 3 trial. Lancet. 2013; **381**(9863):295-302. [PubMed: 23177515]

[116] Wang D, Zhang Q, Blanke CD, et al. Phase II trial of neoadjuvant/adjuvant imatinib mesylate for advanced primary and metastatic/recurrent operable gastrointestinal stromal tumors: Long-term follow-up results of Radiation Therapy Oncology Group 0132. Annals of Surgical Oncology. 2012;**19**(4):1074-1080. [PubMed: 22203182]

[117] McAuliffe JC, Hunt KK, Lazar AJ, et al. A randomized, phase II study of preoperative plus postoperative imatinib in GIST: Evidence of rapid radiographic response and temporal induction of tumor cell apoptosis. Annals of Surgical Oncology. 2009;**16**(4): 910-919. [PubMed: 18953611]

[118] Hohenberger P, Langer CM, Wendtner CM, et al. Neoadjuvant treatment of locally advanced GIST: Results of APOLLON, a prospective, open label phase II study in KIT- or PDGFRA-positive tumors. Journal of Clinical Oncology. 2012;**30**(suppl):abstract 10031

12

Radiation Therapy for Esophageal Cancer

Ivan M. Buzurovic, Borbala Daroczi,
Desmond A. O'Farrell, Mandar S. Bhagwat and
Phillip M. Devlin

Abstract

Esophageal cancer develops in the mucosa of the esophagus and spreads toward the muscle layer. The nonsurgical treatment for localized, deeply invasive esophageal cancer has been external beam radiation therapy (EBRT) and concurrent chemotherapy. Recently, intraluminal brachytherapy showed a strong potential for the improvement of the therapeutic ratio. It was found that the fractionated high dose rate (HDR) brachytherapy offered beneficial palliation for a longer period of time with more durable symptom control. A similar was concluded for advanced unresectable esophageal cancer in previously irradiated patients. HDR brachytherapy may be a useful salvage treatment option for inoperable patients diagnosed with local esophageal cancer. Although better local control can be achieved with higher brachytherapy dose, this increases the risk of acute morbidity and late morbidity, especially in the setting of recurrence cancer. It was found that the moderate dose of EBRT and HDR brachytherapy could give a better local response than EBRT alone.

Keywords: esophageal cancer, radiation therapy, brachytherapy

1. Introduction

Esophageal cancer is the eighth most common cancer worldwide, besides being the sixth most common cause of cancer death. There were 456,000 new cases in the world in 2012 [1]. It is four times more common in men than in women; it occurs more frequently among people above 45 years of age and reaches its plateau among people at 65–74 years of age. Its mortality is high; it can be as high as 84%. For the locally advanced disease, the 5-year survival is 15–34%. The cornerstone of treatment remains surgery; however, there is evidence that survival is favorably influenced when additional therapies, such as chemotherapy or radiation therapy or their combination, or targeted therapies are used for lymph node-positive or cT2 or tumors that are larger than cT2. The clinical studies assessing treatment modalities for esophageal cancer are diverse: the modalities (chemotherapy, radiation therapy and surgery) have been evaluated in various orders and combinations. The number of study subjects has rarely been over 100 per study. The study populations have not always been homogeneous; different portions of the esophagus were affected, and the study population is sometimes mixed, regarding staging and histology.

1.1. Histology

Histology is usually based on the histologic analysis of an endoscopic sample. There are two main types of esophageal cancer: squamous cell carcinoma (SCC) and adenocarcinoma. Squamous cell carcinoma mostly occurs in the lining in the upper portion of the esophagus. Adenocarcinoma develops at the junction between the esophagus and the stomach. Most of the tumors are squamous cell carcinoma, but the incidence of adenocarcinoma has been increasing.

1.2. Predisposing factors

Intraepithelial neoplasias, such as epithelial dysplasias and in situ carcinoma, are the most significant precursor lesions for the development of esophageal cancer. Generally, it occurs a decade prior to carcinoma. The classification of dysplasias is based on the extent of the epithelial involvement. Some of the dysplasias show spontaneous regression. Nearly 30% of the severe dysplasias become invasive cancer. Tobacco use and/or consuming alcohol predominantly increase the risk of esophageal squamous cell carcinoma. Being overweight and/or reflux disease can primarily increase the risk of esophageal adenocarcinoma.

The multifocal appearance and intramural spread are common characteristics of esophageal cancer. It often spreads through the lymphatic system. Tumors involving the proximal portion of the esophagus may give metastases to the cervical lymph nodes, and tumors involving the lower portion may also give metastasis to the vicinity of the celiac artery. Cancer can infiltrate its surroundings, the pars membranacea of the trachea and the prevertebral fascia.

2. Treatment options

From a surgical point of view, early cancer means that the lesion only involves the mucosa and/or submucosa. The treatment option remains surgery for very early cancers (up to stage pT1b) while it is palliative in the case of metastatic esophageal cancer. For other cases, additional therapies, such as chemotherapy and/or radiation therapy may result in improved survival.

Regarding epidemiology, tumor biology, pathogenesis, and prognosis, the two main histological types of esophageal cancer, SCC and adenocarcinoma, are different from each other.

The perioperative mortality is higher for squamous cell cancer. It might be due to comorbidities and the localization of cancer since SCC mostly involves the upper third of the esophagus, and the postoperative mortality is significantly higher for esophageal cancer involving the proximal third. Esophageal cancer affecting the upper third and/or middle third of the esophagus recurs in a locoregional manner whereas adenocarcinoma can more often metastasize to distant sites. However, the prognosis of adenocarcinoma in an early stage is more favorable than that of SCC.

2.1. Chemoradiotherapy

The results of several randomized, phase III studies have been reported so far. Practically, a platinum-based medication is used in combination with radiation.

Morbidity and mortality are unclear regarding the use of neoadjuvant chemoradiotherapy. Some authors reported an increase in the anastomosis insufficiency and an increase in mortality, whereas others did not find an increase in mortality. A recent US study analyzed the data obtained from 1939 patients who had undergone esophagectomy. Seven hundred and eight patients received neoadjuvant therapy. They found no differences in mortality or morbidity [2]. The studies are unclear about the stage in which neoadjuvant therapy can be safely omitted. The American recommendation [3] states that neoadjuvant therapy is reasonable in the case of pT1b (>2 cm in size or dedifferentiated) whereas the European recommendation finds it reasonable only in stage T3-4 or lymph node-positive disease [4]. Chemoradiotherapy can be used

- Definitively: in inoperable cases or if the disease involves the upper third portion of the esophagus, with or without preventive, induction chemotherapy;
- In an adjuvant manner; or
- For a neoadjuvant purpose: if the patient is eligible for surgery (chemoradiotherapy, followed by surgery).

In a prospective multicenter study [5] with 186 patients with esophageal squamous cell carcinoma, three-year survival was significantly higher in patients receiving either pre-operative radiation or pre-operative chemotherapy, radiotherapy and surgery. Definitive chemoradiotherapy can be used in patients who are not surgical candidates or if the disease involves the proximal third portion of the esophagus. The main aims of care are to improve the quality of life and to maintain the patient's ability to swallow. The RTOG 8501 [6] study evaluated the benefits of concurrent chemotherapy compared to radiation therapy alone. The randomized portion of the study included 121 patients, and 61 were enrolled in the chemoradiation arm. No one had any distant metastases. Chemotherapy included the combination of continuous 5-fluorouracil (5-FU) and cisplatin. 1000 mg/m^2 of 5-FU was administered daily over 4 days during Week 1 and Week 5 of radiation treatment, as well as cisplatin at 75 mg/m^2 during the first day of Week 1 and Week 5 in combination with 50 Gy irradiation. After completion of radiation therapy, another two cycles were administered at unchanged doses. By contrast, 64 Gy irradiation was delivered as monotherapy in the other arm. Most of the patients (82%) had squamous cell carcinoma. The study proved the superiority of chemoradiotherapy over radiation therapy alone, regarding both median survival (12.5 vs. 8.9 months) and the 5-year survival (26 vs. 0%). A PRODIGE-5/ACCORD-17 study [7] included 267 patients with up to IV/A stage esophageal cancer. Cisplatin and 5-FU used in the RTOG 8501 study were compared with the administration of six cycles of FOLFOX. FOLFOX + radiation yielded results similar to those of the regimen used in the RTOG study (median PFS: 9.7 vs. 9.4 months), but it was significantly less toxic.

Primarily, the combination of taxane and platinum was assessed in the neoadjuvant setup. The most commonly used paclitaxel (50 mg/m^2) and carboplatin (AUC2, weekly over 5 weeks) were at least as efficient as the combination of platinum and 5-FU [8]; therefore, it is accepted as definitive treatment. In general, definitive chemoradiation is a choice of treatment for those patients who are not suitable for surgery or who do not consent to surgery.

Since distant metastases are present nearly in 75% of patients with locally advanced esophageal cancer, induction chemotherapy prior to chemoradiotherapy would be a rational choice. Usually, patients with locally advanced but resectable esophageal cancer were enrolled in the studies. Since there are no phase III study results, these regimens have not become recommendations. Seventy-two patients participated in the phase II, RTOG 0113 study [9]. The induction treatment included 5-FU (5 × 700 mg/m^2), cisplatin (5 × 15 mg/m^2) and paclitaxel (200 mg/m^2) or cisplatin (75 mg/m^2) and paclitaxel (175 mg/m^2), which was followed by a similar combination (5-FU + paclitaxel or cisplatin + paclitaxel) administered simultaneously with a total radiation dose of 50.4 Gy. Median survival showed no significant differences, and the toxicity was similar in both arms.

Neoadjuvant chemoradiotherapy can be used in those patients who are suitable for surgery. The method of treatment is practically identical to that of the definitive chemoradiotherapy. The aim of the treatment of inoperable patients is palliative, and the aim is to improve the proportion of operability or recovery. The studies frequently yielded contradictory results. However, based on several clinical trials and meta-analyses, neoadjuvant chemoradiotherapy proved to be superior to surgery alone in patients with locally advanced esophageal cancer. A significant survival benefit was found in the CROSS study [10] in which 366 patients with potentially resectable esophageal or gastroesophageal junction cancer were randomized to get either preoperative chemoradiotherapy (50 mg/m^2 paclitaxel a week + carboplatin AUC2, concurrent radiotherapy with a total dose of 41.4 Gy over 5 weeks) or surgery alone. Patients tolerated the combined treatment well. There were no significant differences in mortality or morbidity. The complete resection rate was 92 vs. 69% in favor of the combined treatment, and the complete pathological remission (pCR) ratio was 29% in patients receiving chemoradiotherapy. There was a significant difference in median overall survival (preoperative chemoradiotherapy followed by surgery vs. surgery alone: 49.4 vs. 24.0 months).

In the FFCD 9901 study [11], the efficacy of preoperative chemoradiotherapy was evaluated in patients with small-sized, resectable tumors. 195 patients with stage I or II disease were randomized into the preoperative chemoradiation arm (two cycles of 5-FU at 800 m/m^2 daily at Days 1–4 and 29–32, plus cisplatin at 75 mg/m^2 at Day 1 or Day 2 of the cycle, in both cycles, plus a total dose of 45 Gy concurrent radiation) or the surgery alone arm. During this study with a median follow-up of 93.6 months, there were no significant differences in the 3-year survival. No significant survival benefits were noted in any of the subgroups. Based on these data, the combined treatment may not result in any survival benefit.

Numerous meta-analyses have dealt with the comparison of the effects on survival regarding the trimodal treatment or surgery alone. One of the latest studies was published by Sjoquist and his colleagues [12]. It includes the twelve most significant neoadjuvant chemoradiation studies. The reducing effect of neoadjuvant chemoradiotherapy on mortality proved to be significant, which led to an absolute survival benefit of 8.7% after two years. It was independent of the histologic type of the tumor, and it was not associated with increased perioperative mortality, either.

In addition to the conventional cisplatin + 5-FU therapy, adding paclitaxel to platinum has become more popular lately. Results of ten studies were analyzed in another meta-analysis, and a comparison was made between the efficacy of paclitaxel together with platinum and the efficacy of platinum together with 5-FU. The analysis proved the benefit provided by neoadjuvant chemoradiation therapy over both combinations. The risk of mortality was significantly reduced with both chemotherapy combinations, but the benefit was more pronounced in the taxane arm. However, it was only statistically significant in the case of squamous cell cancer [8]. Some small-sized studies have found the combination of docetaxel and platinum effective [13, 14].

Based on the consequent results of several clinical studies, the response to perioperative treatment, especially the pCR, is an important indicator of better overall survival. Thus, intensification of the perioperative treatment could be a potential approach. Based on the results of 22 studies, survival of those patients who achieved pCR as a result of treatment was 2–3 times longer compared to those patients who had residual cancer in the resection specimen obtained via surgery following neoadjuvant chemoradiotherapy. During the intensification of neoadjuvant treatments, the employments of chemotherapy prior to chemoradiation, as well as the increase of the number of the agents have been studied. According to the INT0123 study, radiation dose intensification resulted in no improvement in either the survival or the local control [15].

Some work was conducted in relation to the non-surgical treatment options of patients with squamous cell carcinoma of the esophagus. Trimodal therapy (chemoradiotherapy followed by surgery) was compared with chemoradiotherapy by Stahl et al. and in the FFCD 9102 study. Stahl et al. [16] enrolled 172 patients. Patients received three cycles of bolus 5-FU, leucovorin, etoposide, cisplatin (FLEP) followed by chemoradiotherapy including a total dose of 40 Gy irradiation and cisplatin and etoposide chemotherapy. Patients then underwent either observation or surgery. In the surgery arm, 62 out of 86 patients underwent surgery. However, there were no significant differences in overall survival. The two-year progression-free survival was more beneficial for those patients who had undergone surgery (64.3 vs. 40.7%). Notably, both the radiation dose and the intensity of chemotherapy were lower than those used in conventional treatments. In the FFCD 9102 study [17], 259 patients with locally advanced, resectable SCC were randomized into two arms following low-dose chemoradiotherapy. If a therapeutic response was noted after the induction treatment, surgery was performed or chemoradiotherapy was completed. No significant differences were found in overall survival between the two treatment groups. However, the 3-month mortality was significantly higher ($p = 0.002$) in the surgery arm (9.3 vs. 0.8%).

Little is known about the results of the nonsurgical treatment of patients with adenocarcinoma. Based on a retrospective analysis of the results of 276 patients treated with definitive chemoradiotherapy for esophageal adenocarcinoma at the university of texas MD Anderson cancer center [18]. After a median follow-up of 54.3 months, 33.3% of the patients never had a relapse. Local relapse was present in 51% of the patients, and distant dissemination was detected in 43.5% of the patients.

There are not enough phase III results in relation to adjuvant chemoradiation. In a retrospective study by Bedard et al. [19], data of 38 patients who had undergone surgery for node-positive esophageal cancer, had received postoperative adjuvant chemoradiation (concurrent or sequential radiation therapy plus cisplatin and 5-FU ± epirubicin) were compared with data of patients who had undergone surgery only. Both the local control and median survival proved to be better in patients receiving adjuvant treatment, and so did overall survival. In another retrospective analysis [20], benefits of adjuvant chemoradiation were evaluated in 304 patients who had undergone surgery for node-positive esophageal squamous cell cancer. Based on the data, both the 5-year overall survival and the disease control proved significantly better in patients who had also received chemotherapy in addition to radiotherapy. According to a prospective study [21] that evaluated chemoradiation vs. chemotherapy and included 45 patients, neither survival benefit nor improved locoregional control was shown in the chemoradiation treatment arm relative to chemotherapy alone (cisplatin + 5-FU over 5 weeks plus 50 Gy of irradiation over 5 weeks vs. cisplatin + 5-FU over 5 weeks).

2.1.1. Neoadjuvant chemotherapy

Eight hundred and two patients with either SCC or adenocarcinoma were randomized in the MRC OEO2 study [22]. Patients received either two cycles of cisplatin + 5-FU preoperatively or underwent surgery primarily. The 5-year overall survival was 23 vs. 17% in favor of the neoadjuvant treatment regimen. In Sjoquist's meta-analysis, data of 1981 patients were assessed. Nine neoadjuvant chemotherapies were compared to surgery alone [12]. Chemotherapy reduced mortality in the entire patient population receiving neoadjuvant chemotherapy. It was significant in patients with adenocarcinoma. Based on these, neoadjuvant chemotherapy seems to be superior to surgery alone.

It is unclear whether neoadjuvant chemotherapy can be an alternative to neoadjuvant chemoradiation therapy. Stahl et al. [23] enrolled 119 patients with adenocarcinoma involving the lower third portion of the esophagus or the gastroesophageal junction. In one of the arms, patients received 15 weeks of chemotherapy (cisplatin + leucovorin + continuous 5-FU) followed by surgery. In the other arm, 12 weeks of chemotherapy were followed by concurrent chemoradiation therapy (low-dose radiation therapy and concurrent cisplatin + etoposide) over 3 weeks, and surgery was then performed. The ratio of pCR was significantly higher in the arm that included chemoradiation therapy (2 vs. 15.6%). However, there were no significant differences in median survival and the 3-year overall survival between the two treatment arms. Burmeister et al. [24] received similar results when they evaluated 75 patients with adenocarcinoma. Regarding pCR and R1 resection, chemoradiotherapy was significantly more beneficial, but there were no significant differences in median survival.

Briefly, chemotherapy can be employed as part of chemoradiation, in a neoadjuvant manner, in an adjuvant manner, or as palliation in metastatic disease.

3. Brachytherapy of esophageal cancer

The results in a large cohort of patients indicated that HDR brachytherapy alone was an effective method for the palliation of advanced esophageal cancer [25]. Similar long-term results were reported in favor of treatments involving concurrent chemoradiotherapy followed by HDR brachytherapy [26]. Although brachytherapy was found to be preferable, there are studies (such as Refs. [27, 28]) suggesting the stent placement may play an important role for the palliation of disease. In that case, the prognostic models were used as evidence-based tools in decision making. However, the health-related life quality was reported to be improved in patients treated with the HDR brachytherapy. Recent studies suggested the usage of Californium-252 neutron brachytherapy combined with EBRT for esophageal cancer. The treatment resulted in favorable local control and long-term survival rates with tolerable side effects [29]. Patient selection, timing of brachytherapy and dose specifications were well documented [30–32]. Clinicians continue to urge caution in using brachytherapy treatment techniques since severe toxicity can occur post treatment [15, 26, 30]. Therefore, the addition of brachytherapy, with consequently high surface doses, should be limited to well-selected patients [33].

For that reason, the clinical implementation and accuracy in dose delivery is crucial for favorable treatment outcomes. The radiation dose is delivered using esophageal transoral or transnasal applicators with an external diameter of 0.6–1 cm. Ideally, the single channel applicator needs to be placed centrally in the lumen of the esophagus; however, there exists a possibility that the applicator will be closer to one side of the lumen, delivering a larger dose to the epithelium, lamina propria and muscularis mucosa, resulting in local esophageal complications. In those cases, stricture formation, fistula and esophageal ulceration are the common late toxicities of HDR brachytherapy [34]. A possible difference in the delivered dose is caused by disagreements in the choice of the dose point (i.e. mucosal surface or certain distance from the central line of the applicator) in various institutions, as reported in Ref. [35]. For instance, it was reported in the long-term experience with esophageal brachytherapy treatment [36] that radiation was delivered at a level of 5 mm below the surface of the mucosa. However, no correlation was found between the post-treatment complications and the diameter of the brachytherapy applicator [37]. In most of the HDR brachytherapy treatments, 3D treatment plans were generated using computed tomography (CT) images; however, magnetic resonance imaging (MRI) can be used to assist the localization of the tumor and the applicator [38]. The treatment planning for the esophageal cancer patient is performed using the TG-43 formalism [39], since the dose calculation accuracy of the TPS was confirmed in a homogeneous medium [40].

Overall, this HDR treatment is demonstrated to be well-tolerated and effective for superficial primary and recurrent esophageal cancer in inoperable patients [41, 42]. The authors concluded that dose escalation with larger diameter applicators may allow for improved therapeutic coverage without exceeding the organs ate risk tolerances [43]. The latest research in the combined approach (EBRT and HDR) to palliation in esophageal cancer together with the review of the current techniques is reported in Refs. [44, 45].

3.1. Clinical implementation

To decrease the dose to the organs at risk in the upper gastrointestinal region a novel disposable brachytherapy transoral balloon centering esophageal applicator (BCEA) with five independently inflatable balloons was developed [44]. The complete treatment process for this applicator consisted of three principal steps: pre-treatment preparation, treatment planning and treatment delivery (**Figure 1**). This applicator allows for the central placement of the radioactive source during treatment. The BCEA allows for the treatments outside the balloon region with the constraint where the BCEA becomes similar to the standard esophageal applicator (EA).

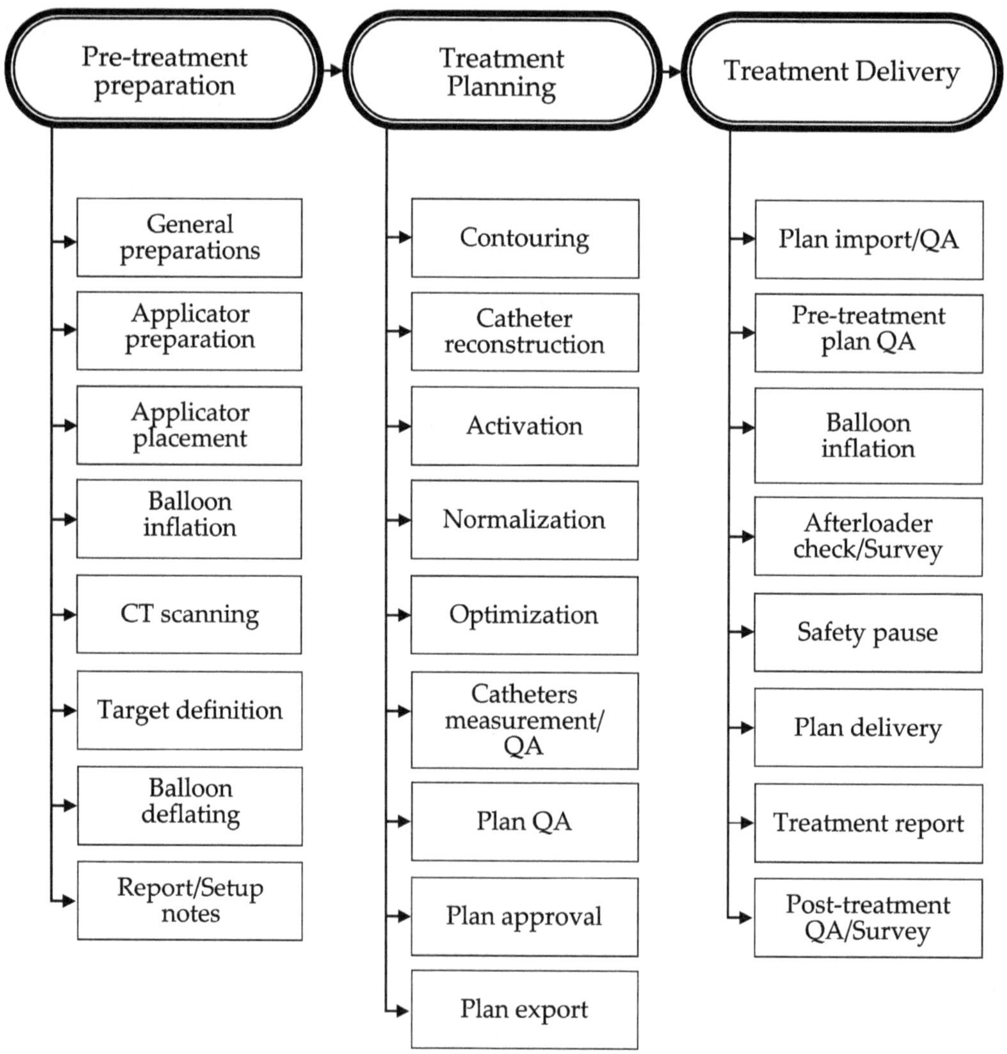

Figure 1. The detailed process map of the treatment was developed for improved treatment plan generation and quality assurance of the process.

The experience in the treatment of esophageal cancer using a standard intraluminal esophageal applicator (EA) was summarized in Ref. [45]. Unlike with the transnasal insertion (EA) where the endoscope would be placed via the anesthetized nose past turbinates and nasopharynx behind the larynx and into the esophagus, the BCEA is placed transorally.

3.2. Treatment planning and delivery

The BCEA positions the catheter centrally when the balloons are inflated. Due to that fact, the treatment plan can be additionally optimized (not the case for the standard EA) for improved dose distribution and conformality. The treatment length was defined as a pretreatment tumor length with 1–2 cm distal and proximal margin determined by pretreatment imaging and confirmed by the CT images.

The prescription dose is usually planned to be delivered to the diameter of 1 cm with respect to the central catheter with an additional optimization to avoid the critical anatomical structures such as the heart, lung, pharyngeal constrictor and spine. The dose calculation is performed using the TG-43 formalism that includes the anisotropy corrections. With the standard EA, the dose point is defined at the mucosal surface or a certain distance from the central line of the applicator with identical dwell times along the treatment length. This was mostly done to minimize the uncertainties in dose delivery related to the positioning of the EA inside the esophagus. In standard approach when EA is used the dose optimization outside the balloon region should be avoided due to the complicated position reproducibility. **Figure 2** shows the differences in the treatment plans between the EA and BCEA.

The centrally placed catheter inside the esophagus lumen resulted in enhanced dose distribution and reproducibility in multi fractional treatment (**Figure 2**). The position of the applicator and the balloon diameters can be verified before the treatments using the planning CT images and the CT images obtained prior to each fraction. Three methods can be used to verify the

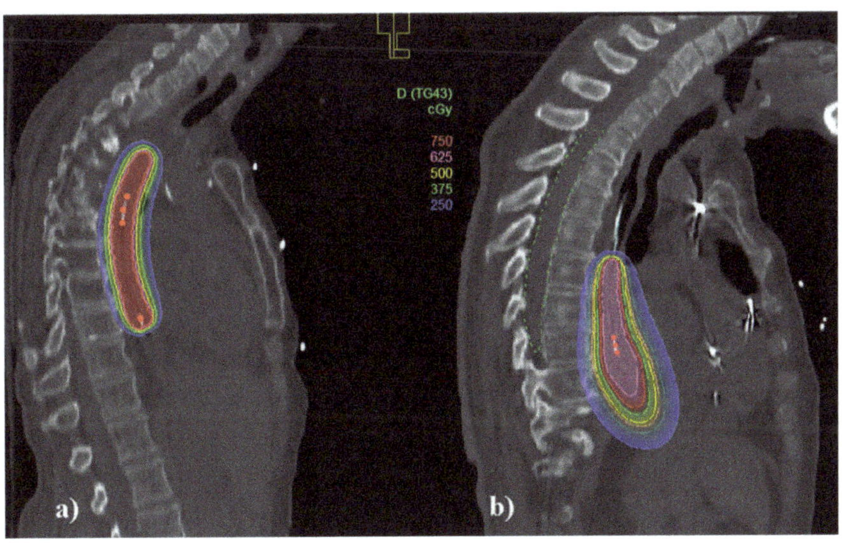

Figure 2. Sagittal images show: (a) the non-optimized plan using the EA and (b) optimized dose distribution achieved with the BCEA.

proper positioning of the BCEA prior to each treatment: (a) using an external marker to verify the length of the catheter in the patient, (b) evaluation of the position of 12 radio-opaque markers on the exterior side of the catheter in the CT images, and (c) measurements of the diameters of the balloons on CT images after inflation to confirm that they were properly inflated.

4. Conclusion

In this chapter, various aspects of esophageal cancers were disused such as histology, predisposing factors and treatment options. It was found that the moderate dose of EBRT and HDR brachytherapy could give a better local response than EBRT alone. Therefore, the brachytherapy of esophageal cancer was elaborated in more detail.

Classically, one of the limitations for the deployment of esophageal brachytherapy has been the difficulties associated with the placement and tolerance of the transnasal applicator [44]. The common adverse effects included significant pain on placement and for the duration of its indwelling. Nasal bleeding, often significant, can be seen from both the scope and catheter placement. There is often the need of significant pain medicine to tolerate this procedure. These effects are pronounced if the applicator is kept in place for an extended period of time.

Long-term toxicities and the correlation between the formation of a fistula or ulceration and the novel design of the BCEA are the topics that can be additionally investigated using the data of more patients treated with the novel BCEA and longer follow-up. Due to the limited number of patients, it is not yet possible to conclude if the patients benefit from the treatment using the centrally placed applicator. Furthermore, due to the provision to additionally optimize the dose, there exists a possibility of dose escalations for certain patients, depending on their anatomy and the spread of disease. The initial implementation of this applicator required strict and careful testing, especially in the determination of the accurate treatment length that would allow the radioactive source to be sent to the most distal position (first dwell position). Multiple tests and an interobserver agreement are required since the inaccurate results of this test can potentially offset the whole treatment, causing adverse events. Therefore, the treatment length and BCEA applicator positioning should be evaluated before each fraction.

Author details

Ivan M. Buzurovic[1*], Borbala Daroczi[2], Desmond A. O'Farrell[1], Mandar S. Bhagwat[1] and Phillip M. Devlin[1]

*Address all correspondence to: ibuzurovic@lroc.harvard.edu

1 Department of Radiation Oncology, Dana-Farber/Brigham and Women's Cancer Center, Harvard Medical School, Boston, MA, USA

2 Department of Radiology, Brigham and Women's Hospital, Harvard Medical School, Boston, MA, USA

References

[1] World Cancer Research Fund International. Oesophageal Cancer Statistics [Internet]. Available from: http://www.wcrf.org/int/cancer-facts-figures/data-specific-cancers/oesophageal-cancer-statistics [Accessed: April 17, 2017]

[2] Mungo B, Molena D, Stem M, Yang SC, Battafarano RJ, Brock MV, Lidor AO. Does neoadjuvant therapy for esophageal cancer increase postoperative morbidity or mortality? Diseases of the Esophagus. 2015;**28**(7):644-651

[3] The National Comprehensive Cancer Network. NCCN Clinical Practice Guidelines in Oncology: Esophageal Cancer [Internet]. Available from: www.nccn.org/professionals/physician_gls/pdf/esophageal.pdf [Accessed: April 17, 2017]

[4] European Society for Medical Oncology. Oesophageal Cancer: ESMO Clinical Practice Guidelines [Internet]. Available from: www.esmo.org/Guidelines/Gastrointestinal-Cancers/Oesophageal-Cancer [Accessed: April 17, 2017]

[5] Nygaard K, Hagen S, Hansen HS, Hatlevoll R, Hultborn, R, Jakobsen A, Mäntyla M, Modig H, Munck-Wikland E, Rosengren B, Tausjø J. Pre-operative radiotherapy prolongs survival in operable esophageal carcinoma: A randomized, multicenter study of pre-operative radiotherapy and chemotherapy. The second Scandinavian trial in esophageal cancer. World Journal of Surgery. 1992;**16**(6):1104-1109

[6] Herskovic A, Martz K, Al-Sarraf M, Leichman L, Brindle J, Vaitkevicius V, Cooper J, Byhardt R, Davis L, Emami B. Combined chemotherapy and radiotherapy compared with radiotherapy alone in patients with cancer of the esophagus. New England Journal of Medicine. 1992;**326**(24):1593-1598

[7] Conroy T, Galais MP, Raoul JL, Bouché O, Gourgou-Bourgade S, Douillard JY, Etienne PL, Boige V, Martel-Lafay I, Michel P, Llacer-Moscardo C. Definitive chemoradiotherapy with FOLFOX versus fluorouracil and cisplatin in patients with oesophageal cancer (PRODIGE5/ACCORD17): Final results of a randomised, phase 2/3 trial. The Lancet Oncology. 2014;**15**(3):305-314

[8] Huang TC, Hsu CH, Lin CC, Tu YK. Systematic review and network meta-analysis: Neoadjuvant chemoradiotherapy for locoregional esophageal cancer. Japanese Journal of Clinical Oncology. 2015;**45**:1023-1028

[9] Ajani A, Winter K, Komaki R, Kelsen DP, Minsky BD, Liao Z, Bradley J, Fromm M, Hornback D, Willett CG. Phase II randomized trial of two nonoperative regimens of induction chemotherapy followed by chemoradiation in patients with localized carcinoma of the esophagus: RTOG 0113. Journal of Clinical Oncology. 2008;**26**(28):4551-4556

[10] van Hagen P, Hulshof MC, Van Lanschot JJB, Steyerberg EW, Henegouwen MVB, Wijnhoven BPL, Richel DJ, Nieuwenhuijzen GAP, Hospers GAP, Bonenkamp JJ, Cuesta MA. Preoperative chemoradiotherapy for esophageal or junctional cancer. New England Journal of Medicine. 2012;**366**(22):2074-2084

[11] Mariette C, Dahan L, Mornex F, Maillard E, Thomas PA, Meunier B, Boige V, Pezet D, Robb WB, Le Brun-Ly V, Bosset JF. Surgery alone versus chemoradiotherapy followed by surgery for stage I and II esophageal cancer: Final analysis of randomized controlled phase III trial FFCD 9901. Journal of Clinical Oncology. 2014;**32**(23):2416-2422

[12] Sjoquist KM, Burmeister BH, Smithers BM, Zalcberg JR, Simes RJ, Barbour A, Gebski V, and Australasian Gastro-Intestinal Trials Group. Survival after neoadjuvant chemotherapy or chemoradiotherapy for resectable oesophageal carcinoma: An updated meta-analysis. The Lancet Oncology. 2011;**12**(7):681-692

[13] Li QQ, Liu MZ, Hu YH, Liu H, He ZY, Lin HX. Definitive concomitant chemoradiotherapy with docetaxel and cisplatin in squamous esophageal carcinoma. Diseases of the Esophagus. 2010;**23**(3):253-259

[14] Ma HB, Di ZL, Wen J, Ke Y, Sun X, Ren J. Prospective, open, multicentre Phase I/II trial to assess safety and efficacy of neoadjuvant radiochemotherapy with docetaxel and cisplatin for esophageal carcinoma. Japanese Journal of Clinical Oncology. 2015;**45**(2):169-175

[15] Minsky BD, Pajak TF, Ginsberg RJ, Pisansky TM, Martenson J, Komaki R, Okawara G, Rosenthal SA, Kelsen DP. INT 0123 (Radiation Therapy Oncology Group 94-05) phase III trial of combined-modality therapy for esophageal cancer: High-dose versus standard-dose radiation therapy. Journal of Clinical Oncology. 2002;**20**(5):1167-1174

[16] Stahl M, Stuschke M, Lehmann N, Meyer HJ, Walz MK, Seeber S, Klump B, Budach W, Teichmann R, Schmitt M, Schmitt G. Chemoradiation with and without surgery in patients with locally advanced squamous cell carcinoma of the esophagus. Journal of Clinical Oncology. 2005;**23**(10):2310-2317

[17] Bedenne L, Michel P, Bouché O, Milan C, Mariette C, Conroy T, Pezet D, Roullet B, Seitz JF, Herr JP, Paillot B. Chemoradiation followed by surgery compared with chemoradiation alone in squamous cancer of the esophagus: FFCD 9102. Journal of Clinical Oncology. 2007;**25**(10):1160-1168

[18] Sudo K, Xiao L, Wadhwa R, Shiozaki H, Elimova E, Taketa T, Blum MA, Lee JH, Bhutani MS, Weston B, Ross WA. Importance of surveillance and success of salvage strategies after definitive chemoradiation in patients with esophageal cancer. Journal of Clinical Oncology. 2014;**32**(30):3400-3405

[19] Bedard EL, Inculet RI, Malthaner RA, Brecevic E, Vincent M, Dar R. The role of surgery and postoperative chemoradiation therapy in patients with lymph node positive esophageal carcinoma. Cancer. 2001;**91**(12):2423-2430

[20] Chen J, Pan J, Liu J, Li J, Zhu K, Zheng X, Chen M, Chen M, Liao Z. Postoperative radiation therapy with or without concurrent chemotherapy for node-positive thoracic esophageal squamous cell carcinoma. International Journal of Radiation Oncology Biology Physics. 2013;**86**(4):671-677

[21] Tachibana M, Yoshimura H, Kinugasa S, Shibakita M, Dhar DK, Ueda S, Fujii T, Nagasue N. Postoperative chemotherapy vs. chemoradiotherapy for thoracic esophageal cancer:

A prospective randomized clinical trial. European Journal of Surgical Oncology. 2003;**29**(7):580-587

[22] Swisher SG, Hofstetter W, Komaki R, Correa AM, Erasmus J, Lee JH, Liao Z, Maru D, Mehran R, Patel S, Rice DC. Improved long-term outcome with chemoradiotherapy strategies in esophageal cancer. The Annals of Thoracic Surgery. 2010;**90**(3):892-899

[23] Stahl M, Walz MK, Stuschke M, Lehmann N, Meyer HJ, Riera-Knorrenschild J, Langer P, Engenhart-Cabillic R, Bitzer M, Königsrainer A, Budach W. Phase III comparison of preoperative chemotherapy compared with chemoradiotherapy in patients with locally advanced adenocarcinoma of the esophagogastric junction. Journal of Clinical Oncology. 2009;**27**(6):851-856

[24] Burmeister BH, Thomas JM, Burmeister EA, Walpole ET, Harvey JA, Thomson DB, Barbour AP, Gotley DC, Smithers BM. Is concurrent radiation therapy required in patients receiving preoperative chemotherapy for adenocarcinoma of the oesophagus? A randomised phase II trial. European Journal of Cancer.2011;**47**(3):354-360

[25] Sur RK, Levin CV, Donde B et al. Prospective randomized trial of HDR brachytherapy as a sole modality in palliation of advanced esophageal carcinoma—An International Atomic Energy Agency study. International Journal of Radiation Oncology Biology Physics. 2002;**53**(1):127-133

[26] Yorozu A, Toya K, Dokiya T. Long-term results of concurrent chemoradiotherapy followed by high dose rate brachytherapy for T2-3 N0-1 M0 esophageal carcinoma. Esophagus. 2006;**3**(1):1-5

[27] Steyerberg EW, Homs MY, Stokvis A et al. SIREC Study Group. Stent placement or brachytherapy for palliation of dysphagia from esophageal cancer: A prognostic model to guide treatment selection. Gastrointestinal endoscopy. 2005;**62**(3):333-340

[28] Bergquist H, Wenger U, Johnsson E et al. Stent insertion or endoluminal brachytherapy as palliation of patients with advanced cancer of the esophagus and gastroesophageal junction. Results of a randomized controlled clinical trial. Diseases of the Esophagus. 2005;**18**(3):131-139

[29] Liu H, Wang Q, Wan X et al. Californium-252 neutron brachytherapy combined with external beam radiotherapy for esophageal cancer: Long-term treatment results. Brachytherapy. 2014;**13**(5):514-521

[30] Gaspar LE, Nag S, Herskovic A et al. Clinical Research Committee. American Brachytherapy Society (ABS) consensus guidelines for brachytherapy of esophageal cancer. International Journal of Radiation Oncology Biology Physics. 1997;**38**(1):127-132

[31] Gaspar LE. Radiation therapy for esophageal cancer: Improving the therapeutic ratio. Seminars in Radiation Oncology. 1994;**4**(1):192-201

[32] Gaspar LE, Winter K, Kocha WI et al. A phase I/II study of external beam radiation, brachytherapy, and concurrent chemotherapy for patients with localized carcinoma of the esophagus (Radiation Therapy Oncology Group Study 9207). Cancer. 2000;**88**(5):988-995

[33] Muijs CT, Beukema JC, Mul VE et al. External beam radiotherapy combined with intraluminal brachytherapy in esophageal carcinoma. Radiotherapy and Oncology. 2012;**102**(2):303-308

[34] Chauhan A, Kaur P, Annex E. Radical external beam radiotherapy with intraluminal high rate dose brachytherapy in patients with carcinoma esophagus. The International Journal of Gastroenterology. 2009;**8**(1):1-7

[35] Okawa T, Dokiya T, Nishio M et al. Multi-institutional randomized trial of external radiotherapy with and without intraluminal brachytherapy for esophageal cancer in Japan. International Journal of Radiation Oncology Biology Physics. 1999;**45**(3):623-628

[36] Gaspar LE, Qian C, Kocha WI et al. A phase III study of external beam radiation, brachytherapy and concurrent chemotherapy in localized cancer of the esophagus (RTOG 92-07): Preliminary toxicity report. International Journal of Radiation Oncology Biology Physics. 1997;**37**(3):593-599

[37] Hishikawa Y, Kurisu K, Taniguchi M et al. High-dose-rate intraluminal brachytherapy for esophageal cancer: 10 years experience in Hyogo College of Medicine. Radiotherapy and Oncology. 1991;**21**(2):107-114

[38] Prott FJ, Pötter R, Kovacs G et al. Magnetic resonance imaging assisted localization of tumor and applicator for brachytherapy of cancer of the esophagus. Tumor Response Monitoring and Treatment Planning. 1992;**1**:607-612

[39] Rivard MJ, Coursey BM, DeWerd LA et al. Update of AAPM Task Group No. 43 Report: A revised AAPM protocol for brachytherapy dose calculations. Medical Physics. 2004;**31**(3):633-674

[40] Uniyal SC, Sharma SD, Naithani UC. Dosimetric verification of a high dose rate brachytherapy treatment planning system in homogeneous and heterogeneous media. Physica Medica. 2013;**29**(2):171-177

[41] Folkert MR, Cohen GM, Wu AJ et al. Endoluminal high-dose-rate brachytherapy for early stage and recurrent esophageal cancer in medically inoperable patients. Brachytherapy. 2013;**12**(5):463-470

[42] Bhatt L, Tirmazy S, Sothi S. Intraluminal high dose rate brachytherapy for palliation of dysphagia in cancer of the esophagus: Initial experience at a single UK center. Diseases of the Esophagus. 2013;**26**(1):57-60

[43] Laskar SG, Lewis S, Agarwal JP, Mishra S, Mehta S, Patil P. Combined brachytherapy and external beam radiation: An effective approach for palliation in esophageal cancer. Journal of Contemporary Brachytherapy. 2015;**6**:453-461

[44] Buzurovic IM, Hansen JL, Bhagwat MS, O'Farrell DA, Friesen S, Harris TC, Damato AL, Cormack RA, Martin NE, Devlin PM. Clinical implementation of a novel applicator in high-dose-rate brachytherapy treatment of esophageal cancer. Journal of Contemporary Brachytherapy. 2016;**8**(4):319-325

[45] Stewart AJ, Tselis N, Albert M et al. Gastrointestinal brachytherapy. In: Brachytherapy: Applications and Techniques. Springer Publishing Company, New York, NY, USA; 2015. pp. 319-354

13

Prevention and Management of Complications from Esophagectomy

Jacqueline Oxenberg

Abstract

While surgery plays a major role in the treatment and potential cure of esophageal cancer, esophagectomy continues to have a significant amount of morbidity compared to other surgical oncology procedures. Efforts to improve morbidity and mortality from esophagectomy include the Consensus Guidelines for Complications from Esophagectomies, Enhanced Recovery after Surgery protocols as well as others. Although we strive to improve morbidity and mortality after these surgeries, adverse events still occur. They affect not only patient quality of life and increase cost of care for esophageal cancer but also have a negative impact on overall cancer survival. This chapter reviews the prevention of adverse outcomes from esophagectomies as well as discusses the management of many complications that may occur more common to the operation.

Keywords: esophagectomy complications, prevention of esophagectomy complications, management of esophagectomy complications

1. Introduction

Adverse events from esophagectomies directly impact patient quality of life, cancer recurrence/survival, hospital costs and resources, as well as require a great deal of energy from those managing them [1, 2]. Prevention of surgical complications is of utmost importance; however, adverse events from this major surgical procedure still occur, even in high-volume centers or experienced hands. Mortality can range from 7 to 9% while morbidity ranges from 17 to 74% [3]. Prevention, early recognition, and adequate management of complications can decrease mortality [4]. While many studies evaluate postoperative morbidity using even randomized methods, randomized studies on the management of postsurgical complications are

2. Selection of the appropriate patient and surgeon

2.1. The optimal patient

Patient optimization and use of appropriate selection criteria are key to minimizing postoperative morbidity. Unfortunately, those risk factors for the development of esophageal cancer may also put patients at an increased risk for postoperative complications. Risk factors include age, elevated BMI, ECOG score/functional status, dyspnea, diabetes, chronic obstructive pulmonary disease, smoking, alkaline phosphatase level elevations, low serum albumin, and increased complexity score [5–11]. However, age and performance status continue to be the most commonly reported. Neoadjuvant treatments have not been consistently proven to be a risk factor. While fibrosis often occurs after chemoradiation, potentially making surgical resection more difficult, data showing optimal timing to surgery after neoadjuvant chemoradiation and its affect on postoperative morbidity are mixed [12].

2.2. How to optimize the patient

Malnutrition has been reported in 57–80% of patients with esophageal cancer [13, 14]. Many factors can be attributed to malnutrition prior to surgery and include patient factors, chemotherapy, radiation therapy, and tumor-related causes [15]. It is important to recognize that even obese patients can suffer from malnutrition. While laboratory values and anthropometric measurements can be useful, their values can vary and therefore may not be clinically relevant. Therefore, a weight loss of greater than 10% for 6 months or 5% for 1 month is considered malnourished [16].

For the malnourished patient, preoperative optimization of nutrition through the advice of a dietician is key, but other measures should be considered as well if a patient is unable to tolerate at least 50–75% of their caloric needs [15]. The preferred intervention should be handled in a multidisciplinary setting and be initiated as early as possible. This decreases the amount of weight loss, increases chances of completion of neoadjuvant therapies, and decreases hospital admissions [17].

Recommendations to maximize oral nutrition intake include dividing daily oral intake into five to six small meals where the patient is given enough time to eat, eating only foods with a high nutritional content, paying attention to presentation and preparation of meals to make food as desirable as possible, enriching meals and drinks and taking advantage of those days where the patient feels like eating, modifying the consistency of foods to ease swallowing, preventing fatigue, decreasing the risk of aspiration, eating non-irritating soft and smooth foods at room temperature and maintaining oral hygiene for those with mucositis [15]. Patients should also be advised to supplement meals with dietary supplements. The preoperative intake of combined "immunonutrition" products consisting of arginine, glutamine, polyunsaturated omega-3 fatty acids, nucleotides, and antioxidant micronutrients has been shown to decrease postoperative infectious complications and length of hospital stay [15, 18, 19].

For those unable to tolerate adequate nutrition, even with optimization and supplementation, other interventions are needed. These include either stent placement or percutaneous, endoscopic, or surgical placement of feeding gastrostomy or jejunostomy tubes. Esophageal stent placement has the benefit of being placed during endoscopic ultrasound, a common staging procedure. While it may improve dysphagia in the neoadjuvant setting, chest pain can occur and stent migration can be seen in up to 46% of patients [20]. although stent migration can be problematic, it is often a sign of tumor response to neoadjuvant therapy, and therefore the stent may not always need to be replaced. Other reported complications of stent placement in the neoadjuvant setting include perforation, mediastinitis, bowel perforation from migration, tracheo-esophageal fistula, and bleeding [21].

Jejunostomy and gastrostomy tube placement have been proven safe and effective for perioperative nutrition. These can be placed in the laparoscopic, open, endoscopic, or even percutaneous settings. Endoscopic placement may be difficult if a patient has a severe malignant stricture/obstruction, which is often the case when a patient is suffering from severe malnutrition and unable to pass food or liquids through the site of tumor. Gastrostomy tubes have the advantage of bolus feeding, which may improve quality of life. While gastrostomy tube placement has been proven to be safe without increasing the risk of postoperative morbidity, jejunostomy tube placement is often preferred given the stomach is the preferred organ for a neo-esophagus. Jejunostomy tubes are often placed at the time of esophagectomy as well for supportive care. However, some data support that the placement of jejunostomy tubes during esophagectomy is not always necessary [22–24]. Unfortunately, tube feeds cannot be given in boluses with jejunostomy tubes, which, if occurs, can lead to diarrhea and further dehydration. Patients therefore require an ongoing pump connection for feedings.

Smoking cessation is crucial to improving morbidity from esophagectomy. This may be most beneficial if performed greater than 90 days before surgery [25]. Active smoking has also been shown to increase recurrence rates of cancer after esophagectomy [26]. Therefore, smoking cessation counseling and supportive programs are necessary when patients are being assessed for esophagectomy.

2.3. The optimal surgeon/hospital

When deciding the optimal surgeon, it is important to understand that outcomes depend on two major factors: experience and resources. It is well known that with increasing numbers of esophagectomies performed, postoperative morbidity and mortality are improved. In addition, long-term survival can also improve [27]. While data show improved outcomes at higher volume centers, this is inconsistent and may depend further on individual surgeon volumes and hospital resources [28]. Begg et al. described low-volume hospitals as 1–5 esophagectomies/year, medium volume 6–11 esophagectomies/year, and high-volume centers as those performing >11 esophagectomies/year, with an improved mortality with increasing hospital volumes [29]. Later, Birkmeyer et al. divided hospital volumes to <2 esophagectomies/year as low-volume and high-volume centers as >19 esophagectomies/year [30]. The 2003 Leapfrog Group recommended 13 esophagectomies/year as a minimum volume standard [31]. However, esophagectomies at mid-volume centers can also be safely performed, especially with a two-surgeon approach [32]. Hospital type may also be important where improved reoperation rates and mortality are seen when surgery is performed at University centers or institutions centralizing esophageal cancer care [33–35].

Early recognition and treatment of complications appears to be just as important as prevention to improve mortality [36]. The recognition of postoperative problems improves with experience, making hospital volumes as well as surgeon volumes important. With morbidity rates being high, early intervention is of utmost importance to prevent further adverse outcomes or even death. In fact, even in low-volume hospitals, mortality may remain low if adequate resources are available [28, 37]. Therefore, these surgeries should only be performed at institutions well equipped to handle the possible complications [38–40]. Ancillary departments that should be available in the postoperative care may include gastroenterology, interventional radiology, cardiology, an astute critical care team, and others. Resources readily available and proven to improve complications also include nurse-to-patient ratios, where the incidence of pulmonary and infectious complications was shown to be increased when nurses had more than two patients [41].

2.4. Optimal surgical approach

Tumor location as well as surgeon experience often dictates the type of surgery performed. Multiple accepted operative approaches to esophageal carcinoma include Ivor Lewis esophagogastrectomy, McKeown esophagogastrectomy, transhiatal esophagogastrectomy, and left transthoracic or thoracoabdominal approaches. Minimally invasive techniques include laparoscopic and robotic esophagectomies. While minimally invasive esophagectomies have been shown to be safe and effective with equivalent oncologic outcomes, robotic, rather than laparoscopic approaches are becoming common [42–44]. However, one should be aware that there is a learning curve when a surgeon is transitioning to minimally invasive esophagectomies [45]. Transthoracic esophagectomies include the Ivor Lewis esophagogastrectomy and the McKeown esophagogastrectomy. Morbidity varies on the location of the anastomosis and if the transthoracic approach was used. While the transthoracic approach may have an increased morbidity, it does allow for extended lymphadenectomies to be performed, possibly increasing long term survival [10, 46] .

3. Prevention and management of complications

The Esophagectomy Complications Consensus Group (ECCG) is a group of 21 high-volume surgeons from 14 countries that compiled a complete list of complications from esophagectomies [3]. These adverse events are separated into pulmonary, cardiac, gastrointestinal, urologic, thromboembolic, neurologic/psychiatric, infectious, wound/diaphragm, and others. They also aimed to standardize the definitions and reporting of complications since reported literature varied depending on adverse reactions and even mortality definitions. These definitions were defined for anastomotic leak, conduit necrosis, chyle leak and vocal cord injury/ palsy. Given the large number of possible complications, this chapter reviews those more common or even specific to esophagectomy.

3.1. Atrial fibrillation

Atrial fibrillation can occur in over 20% of patients undergoing esophagectomy, particularly when the transthoracic approach is used [47, 48]. Its occurrence unfortunately can result in hemodynamic instability as well as put patients at an increased risk for stroke. Atrial Fibrillation may also be an early warning sign for morbidity, especially anastomotic leak [49]. The mechanism and pathophysiology of postoperative atrial fibrillation is incompletely understood, although we know predisposing factors include advanced age, coronary artery disease, heart failure, hypertension, mitral valve disease, and previous history of atrial fibrillation [50]. One randomized, controlled trial showed that the preoperative use of amiodarone via IV infusion significantly reduced the incidence of atrial fibrillation; however, no differences were seen in median hospital stay, ICU stay, or adverse events [51]. In a study evaluating amiodarone administration through the jejunostomy tube postoperatively, there was only a trend towards lower occurrence and a shorter length of stay [52]. Beta-blockers should be continued for the prevention of atrial fibrillation as well if a patient is already taking them, but may require a reduced dose for the prevention of hypotension, especially with epidural anesthesia. Calcium channel blockers, particularly diltiazem, can also be used for the prevention of atrial fibrillation and may have less effect on blood pressure than other calcium channel blockers or beta-blockers [53]. If atrial fibrillation occurs, amiodarone, calcium channel blockers, and beta-blockers are all treatments to be considered, depending on the patient's hemodynamics.

3.2. Respiratory failure/pneumonia/prolonged ventilation

Respiratory complications in patients undergoing esophagectomy can be problematic and are often causes of mortality. When patients need to be reintubated, many require bag ventilation or positive pressure prior to intubation, which may cause insufflation of the esophagus and stomach, placing pressure on the anastomosis or staple lines. For that reason, CPAP is often avoided as well. Direct airway visualization during reintubation is also important to prevent mechanical injury in case the esophagus is intubated rather than the trachea, especially if a cervical anastomosis is performed.

Pneumonia has been shown to significantly increase mortality compared to other complications, even anastomotic leak [6, 8]. Unfortunately, it can also be the most common postoperative complication and cause for respiratory failure and prolonged ventilation [7]. The American Thoracic Society and American Infections Diseases Society define pneumonia into hospital-acquired pneumonia (HAP), ventilator-associated pneumonia (VAP), and health-care-associated pneumonia (HCAP) [54]. The revised Uniform Pneumonia Score aims to define pneumonia occurring after esophagectomies and includes temperature, leukocyte count, and pulmonary radiographic findings [55]. Prevention, early recognition, and treatment as well as correction of causes are key.

Aspiration is a major cause of pneumonia. This occurs more often with a cervical anastomosis, especially with recurrent laryngeal nerve injury. Recurrent laryngeal nerve palsy can occur secondary to stretching, thermal injury, or even compression. If occurs, patients may suffer from hoarseness as well as pulmonary complications such as dyspnea and aspiration, which puts them at an increased risk for pneumonia and reintubation/prolonged ventilation. However, recurrent laryngeal nerve injury may not always present as obvious hoarseness, as we know from thyroid surgery data, and therefore its occurrence may be underreported. The ECCG defines vocal cord injury/palsy as a vocal cord dysfunction postresection where confirmation and assessment are achieved by direct examination [3]. There are three types of injuries/palsies that are each further separated into unilateral (A) and bilateral (B): Type 1 includes a transient injury requiring no therapy, where only dietary modifications are needed; Type 2 is an injury requiring elective surgical procedures such as thyroplasty or medialization procedures; Type 3 is an injury requiring acute surgical intervention due to aspiration or other respiratory issues that include thyroplasty or medialization procedures. Injury to the left recurrent laryngeal nerve is most common and is mainly associated with esophagectomies that include cervical anastomoses or dissections, McKeown-type operations. Therefore, prevention may include performing thoracic anastomoses or careful dissection and prevention of injury from the above causes. The early recognition of injury and treatment (which may include medialization of the vocal fold) may prevent aspiration and pneumonia and therefore may be of benefit early in the postoperative course [56, 57].

Other causes of respiratory failure or shortness of breath can include ARDS, cardiac causes, pleural effusions, pneumothorax, phrenic nerve injury, or fistula. Other infections can put patients at risk for ARDS (acute respiratory distress syndrome), and cardiac causes may also result in respiratory failure and need for reintubation. If ARDS occurs, the cause should be evaluated, including examining for other infections (urine, leak, etc.). If cardiac in nature, most commonly secondary to atrial fibrillation, heart rate control is usually necessary to alleviate symptoms. Pleural effusions and pneumothorax are common and can be managed with chest tube placement or percutaneous radiologic drainage, depending on the size of the effusion or pneumothorax. If effusions occur simultaneously with anastomotic leak, adequate drainage should be performed to prevent empyema and life-threatening mediastinitis. While phrenic nerve injury is rare, immediate surgical intervention is not always needed. However, patients may require tracheostomy placement for pulmonary conditioning. It is also important to remember that patients are at an increased risk for deep vein thrombosis and even pulmonary embolism. This may occur prior to or even after esophagectomy. Perioperative prophylactic anticoagulation should be administered in the perioperative setting to prevent deep vein thrombosis/pulmonary embolism. Tracheoesophageal fistula should also be considered, especially later in the recovery period or in a complicated postoperative recovery setting.

Impaired lung function is a significant risk factor for pulmonary complications [8]. With preoperative chemoradiation, pneumonitis can occur, making patients at an increased risk for postoperative respiratory failure and pneumonia [8]. While some degree of inflammation is often seen in preoperative imaging, assuring patient lung function has not decompensated is prudent. This can often cause delays in surgery; however, allowing the recovery of lung function may improve postoperative pulmonary failure.

Consistent with the recommendations of the Enhanced Recovery After Surgery pathways, intravenous fluid administration should be minimized to improve time to return of bowel function and decrease the length of hospital stay. Excessive fluid administration/fluid overload should also be considered in all patients with acute respiratory failure since the administration of diuretics may quickly improve symptoms.

3.3. *Anastomotic leak/conduit necrosis*

Anastomotic leak after esophagectomy can be difficult to manage and has a major impact on patient quality of life as well as may affect long-term survival [58, 59]. Incidence varies from 5.7 to 14.3% with a higher incidence in cervical anastomoses versus thoracic [60]. The International Study Group for Rectal Cancer proposed the verbiage of anastomotic leak as, "A defect of the integrity in a surgical joint between two hollow viscera with communication between the intraluminal and extraluminal compartments," which was later validated and expanded to the entire gastrointestinal tract [61]. Lerut et al. with the Surgery Infection Study Group defined anastomotic leak severity as Type 1, a radiological leak without any clinical findings; Type 2 with minor clinical findings of local inflammation (cervical wound) or X-ray showed suppressed leak (thoracic anastomosis); Type 3, a major clinical leak with severe disruption and sepsis; Type 4, conduit necrosis seen by endoscopic confirmation [62]. The Early Complications Consensus Group (ECCG) defined anastomotic leak as a full-thickness GI defect involving esophagus, anastomosis, staple line, or conduit, irrespective of the presentation of the method of identification [3]. Type 1 includes a local defect requiring no change in therapy or treated medically or with dietary modification. Type 2 is a localized defect requiring interventional but not surgical therapy (interventional radiology drainage, stent or bedside opening and packing of incision). Type 3 is a localized defect requiring surgical therapy.

Many patient factors as well as peri- and intraoperative factors can contribute to anastomotic leak. Patients at an increased risk for anastomotic leak include those with increased comorbidities, advanced pathologic stage, prior esophagogastric surgeries, and active smoking [63]. Patient factors can include preoperative malnutrition, diabetes, prolonged hospitalization, hypotension, hypoxemia, preoperative chemotherapy, preoperative chemoradiation, and age. Technical factors also impacting the rate of anastomotic leak include the location of the anastomosis, surgery type, tension on the anastomosis, the type of anastomosis (hand sewn vs. stapled), arterial and venous insufficiency, excessive bleeding, and surgeon experience. While leak incidence may be higher in a single-layer anastomosis, the incidence of stricture may be higher in a double-layer anastomosis [64–66]. While data are mixed, the incidence of leak and stricture may also be lower with a stapled anastomosis [67, 68]. Postoperative factors may include gastric distention, external compression, infection, re-exploration for bleeding, prolonged mechanical ventilation, and continued hypoxemia and hypotension [69]. Technical considerations to decrease the rate of anastomotic leak may include anastomotic support with omentum, pleura, pericardium, and fat tissue. Prospective randomized studies have shown that omental wrapping of the anastomosis may decrease the rate of leak or even stricture [70, 71].

Diagnosis can be made by clinical suspicion if a patient presents with fevers, leukocytosis, empyema, pleural effusion, pneumomediastinum, increased drainage from the chest tube (bile or other gastric contents), the presence of enteric bacteria or bacterial culture or tachycardia. The early detection of anastomotic leaks may also include CRP/ESR elevation, an increase in procalcitonin level, and leukocytosis extending past the second and fifth postoperative days, respectively [72, 73]. While contrast esophagogram can be performed to determine subclinical leaks, caution is advised given the risks of aspiration [4, 74]. A barium swallow can be performed to detect an anastomotic leak; however, its sensitivity can be relatively low and may often be performed too early to detect [75, 76]. The oral intake of methylene blue may be used given it is otherwise nontoxic. CT scan with oral contrast may also be helpful and show contrast extravasation as well as concerning areas for infection.

The etiology of the leak is vital to ascertain where patients with conduit tip necrosis or complete conduit ischemia may require different interventions. This often requires direct visualization with EGD for conduit evaluation as well as evaluation of the defect size. The ECCG defines conduit necrosis into three types, with recommendations for specific treatments: Type 1 includes a focal conduit necrosis that is identified endoscopically, requiring only additional monitoring or nonsurgical therapy; Type 2 includes focal conduit necrosis that is identified endoscopically and is not associated with free anastomotic or conduit leak. Surgical therapy not involving esophageal diversion is performed; Type 3 includes extensive conduit necrosis that is treated with conduit resection and diversion [3].

If a leak occurs, source control with drain placement with or without operative intervention remains key to preventing mortality. For this reason, intraoperative drain placement for detection and source control is common. Management often is determined by anastomotic location; however, mediastinitis can occur with both intrathoracic and cervical anastomoses, a possibly fatal diagnosis for which requires close monitoring and rapid evaluation and treatment. Turkyilmaz et al. created algorithms to help guide treatment for anastomotic leak. For cervical anastomoses, a limited leak that is clinically occult may be managed with antibiotics, dressing changes, and cleansing with oral isotonic fluid. If there is a clinically prominent cervical leak, antibiotics, opening of the cervical wound, drain placement, nasogastric decompression, nutritional support, and cleaning are typically needed. For cervical anastomotic leaks that have intrathoracic complications and clinical sepsis failing to improve, drain placement, stent placement, decortication, resection/diversion or resection/colonic interposition may be needed. For thoracic anastomoses, if a contained leak with less than 30% disruption, injection with fibrin glue, endoclips, or stents can be used for management. However, if the defect is larger, drainage and esophageal stent placement can be performed followed by surgery if stent placement and drainage are unsuccessful (can include primary or supporting tissue repair). However, if the anastomosis has a greater than 70% disruption, surgery including drainage and primary repair should be performed first with esophageal diversion with possible colonic interposition if unable to be performed [69].

With the use of self-expanding metal stents, endoscopic management alone has become possible for anastomotic leaks/disruptions. Covered stents can be placed to control the leak, preventing further seeding into the mediastinum for both cervical and thoracic anastomoses. If well controlled, oral intake may also be safe. However, stent migration can occur, requiring retrieval and replacement [77]. Stent use may be limited in large defects (which may occur from conduit necrosis or staple line disruption). It is also important to understand that lumen caliber differences between the esophagus and gastric conduit can result in the reflux of gastric contents around the distal aspect of a stent. This unfortunately may not be seen with an esophagogram, but rather be noticed with other imaging such as CT after the reflux of contrast and gastric contents occur and may be delayed. Therefore, other options for control have emerged including endoscopic vacuum-assisted closure devices and may even be more effective than stent placement [78–81].

3.4. Fistula

In addition to source control, the awareness and prevention of esophago/gastrotracheal fistula is also necessary. This can occur from infection itself or even the erosion of foreign material (stent, staples, etc.) into the trachea. One should be suspicious in patients with frequent uncontrolled coughing, especially after swallowing, or "Ono's sign" [82]. Workup and diagnosis can include an upper gastrointestinal X-ray with oral contrast or even direct visualization with esophagoscopy or bronchoscopy. Prevention may include a pleural wrap around the anastomosis at the time of original operation or even at the time of reoperation if a leak occurs and anastomotic repair is possible. If reoperation is not performed, stent placement may help control symptoms and healing [83]. However, distal feeding tube placement and resection may be needed. Treatment is necessary to prevent recurring pneumonia.

3.5. Delayed gastric emptying

Delayed or inappropriate gastric emptying can occur secondary to the disruption of vagal nerve complexes to the stomach. This can result in delayed emptying of the stomach, which affects not only patient quality of life and inability to obtain oral nutrition but also can put patients at an increased risk for reflux of gastric contents and even aspiration. The most common options for the management of the pylorus include pyloromyotomy, pyloroplasty, intra-pyloric botulinum toxin injection as well as no intervention. While one multicenter study showed no significant difference between pyloroplasty, botulinum toxin-injection, and no pyloric treatment, one study did show that intra-pyloric botulinum toxin can increase the risk of postoperative reflux and increase the use of promotility agents and endoscopic interventions [84, 85]. While delayed gastric emptying can occur anywhere from 10 to 50%, it also can be successfully managed with prokinetic agents (75%) and endoscopic dilation [86].

3.6. Chyle leak/chylothorax

With the thoracic duct being the largest lymphatic vessel in the body as well as being located in the chest, posterior to the esophagus, injury can occur. Its location, however, often varies. The incidence of chyle leak is rather low (1–4%); however, when it occurs, it can be very problematic [87]. Chyle contains triglycerides in the form of chylomicrons as well as lymphocytes. Chyle leaks can result in malnutrition (with continued protein loss), immune compromise, hypovolemia, electrolyte abnormalities, hypoalbuminemia, lymphopenia, and infection [88]. The ECCG defines a chyle leak into three different types, where output <1 L/day is further classified as "A," and "B" is further classified as >1 L/day [3]. Type 1 leaks can be managed with enteric dietary modifications alone. Type 2 can be managed with total parenteral nutrition. Type 3 requires management with interventional or surgical therapy.

Following esophagectomy, drainage from a chest tube of >500 mL/day is suggestive of a chyle leak; however, the measurement of chylomicrons or triglycerides is most commonly utilized [89]. A measurement of >4% chylomicrons or fluid containing >100–110 mg/dL of triglycerides is typically considered indicative of a chyle leak. Since a chyle leak may present with increased serous or even serosanguinous drainage while fasting, a clinical diagnosis can be made by the oral intake of cream followed by milky drainage from the chest tube/drains.

Prevention unfortunately is difficult. Selective en masse ligation has been shown to reduce the rate of chylothorax [90]. Also, the preoperative oral administration of cream may help identify the thoracic duct to aid in the prevention of its injury or to identify the thoracic duct for prophylactic ligation [91]. The initial management of a chyle leak usually includes drainage as well as TPN and bowel rest. Decreasing oral or enteral fat intake decreases the flow of chyle through the leak, possibly allowing spontaneous closure [92]. Long chain fatty acids should be avoided with diets supported by high percentages of medium-chain triglycerides since they are typically absorbed directly into intestinal cells, bypassing the thoracic duct [87]. If conservative management is not successful, surgical intervention may be necessary, especially if the fistula is of high output. Aggressive surgical intervention should be performed if chyle output is >1.5 L/day for >5–7 days [93]. Surgical intervention includes thoracotomy or thoracoscopic thoracic duct ligation on the side of the chylothorax. This is usually assisted by the preoperative administration of cream or lipophilic dye to help identify the thoracic duct. If the leak can be localized, this may be controlled with clips or suture; however, if the leak is unclear, ligation of the thoracic duct just cephalad to the aortic hiatus is recommended [94–96]. Pleurodesis can also be performed at the time of ligation as well.

Radiologic-guided/percutaneous embolization is becoming more popular, especially for patients who are poor operative candidates. This includes lymphangiography followed by transabdominal percutaneous needle cannulation, although a retrograde subclavian vein approach can be used [97, 98]. Once the cisterna chyli is canalized, a catheter is advanced into the thoracic duct and contrast used to identify the leak. Embolization can then be performed. Since surgical intervention to ligate the thoracic duct using thoracoscopy or a thoracotomy can result in increased morbidity and mortality, thoracic duct embolization has become increasingly more popular when conservative management fails.

Author details

Jacqueline Oxenberg

Address all correspondence to: jcoxenberg@geisinger.edu

Geisinger Wyoming Valley, Wilkes-Barre, PA, USA

References

[1] Kataoka K, Takeuchi H, Mizusawa J, et al. Prognostic impact of postoperative morbidity after esophagectomy for esophageal cancer: Exploratory analysis of JCOG9907. Annals of Surgery. 2017;**265**(6):1152-1157. DOI: 10.1097/SLA.0000000000001828

[2] Lerut T, Moons J, Coosemans W, et al. Postoperative complications after transthoracic esophagectomy for cancer of the esophagus and gastroesophageal junction are correlated with early cancer recurrence: Role of systematic grading of complications using the modified clavien classification. Annals of Surgery. 2009;**250**(5):798-806. DOI: 10.1097/SLA.0b013e3181bdd5a8

[3] Low DE, Alderson D, Cecconello I, et al. International consensus on standardization of data collection for complications associated with esophagectomy: Esophagectomy complications consensus group (ECCG). Annals of Surgery. 2015;**262**(2):286-294. DOI: 10.1097/SLA.0000000000001098

[4] Griffin SM, Lamb PJ, Dresner SM, Richardson DL, Hayes N. Diagnosis and management of a mediastinal leak following radical oesophagectomy. The British Journal of Surgery. 2001;**88**(10):1346-1351. DOI: 10.1046/j.0007-1323.2001.01918.x

[5] Law S, Wong K, Kwok K, Chu K, Wong J. Predictive factors for postoperative pulmonary complications and mortality after esophagectomy for cancer. Annals of Surgery. 2004;**240**(5):791-800. DOI: 10.1097/01.sla.0000143123.24556.1c

[6] Atkins BZ, Shah AS, Hutcheson KA, et al. Reducing hospital morbidity and mortality following esophagectomy. The Annals of Thoracic Surgery. 2004;**78**(4):1170-1176. DOI: 10.1016/j.athoracsur.2004.02.034

[7] Bailey SH, Bull DA, Harpole DH, et al. Outcomes after esophagectomy: A ten-year prospective cohort. The Annals of Thoracic Surgery. 2003;**75**(1):217-222. DOI: 10.1016/S0003-4975(02)04368-0

[8] Avendano CE, Flume PA, Silvestri GA, King LB, Reed CE. Pulmonary complications after esophagectomy. The Annals of Thoracic Surgery. 2002;**73**(3):922-926. DOI: 10.1016/S0003-4975(01)03584-6

[9] Kinugasa S, Tachibana M, Yoshimura H, et al. Postoperative pulmonary complications are associated with worse short- and long-term outcomes after extended esophagectomy. Journal of Surgical Oncology. 2004;**88**(2):71-77. DOI: 10.1002/jso.20137

[10] Raymond DP, Seder CW, Wright CD, et al. Predictors of major morbidity or mortality after resection for esophageal cancer: A society of thoracic surgeons general thoracic surgery database risk adjustment model. The Annals of Thoracic Surgery. 2016;**102**(1):207-214. DOI: 10.1016/j.athoracsur.2016.04.055

[11] Ferguson MK, Martin TR, Reeder LB, Olak J. Mortality after esophagectomy: Risk factor analysis. World Journal of Surgery. 1997;**21**(6):599-604. DOI: 10.1007/s002689900279

[12] Kim JY, Correa AM, Vaporciyan AA, et al. Does the timing of esophagectomy after chemoradiation affect outcome? The Annals of Thoracic Surgery. 2012;**93**(1):207-212; discussion 212-3. DOI: 10.1016/j.athoracsur.2011.05.021

[13] Daly JM, Fry WA, Little AG, et al. Esophageal cancer: Results of American college of surgeons patient care evaluation study. Journal of the American College of Surgeons. 2000;**190**(5):562-573

[14] Dewys WD, Begg C, Lavin PT, et al. Prognostic effect of weight loss prior to chemotherapy in cancer patients. Eastern cooperative oncology group. The American Journal of Medicine. 1980;**69**(4):491-497

[15] Mariette C, De Botton M, Piessen G. Surgery in esophageal and gastric cancer patients: What is the role for nutrition support in your daily practice? Annals of Surgical Oncology. 2012;**19**(7):2128-2134. DOI: 10.1245/s10434-012-2225-6

[16] Nitenberg G, Raynard B. Nutritional support of the cancer patient: Issues and dilemmas. Critical Reviews in Oncology/Hematology. 2000;**34**(3):137-168. DOI: 10.1016/S1040-8428(00)00048-2

[17] Odelli C, Burgess D, Bateman L, et al. Nutrition support improves patient outcomes, treatment tolerance and admission characteristics in oesophageal cancer. Clinical Oncology. 2005;**17**(8):639-645. DOI: 10.1016/j.clon.2005.03.015

[18] Beale RJ, Bryg DJ, Bihari DJ. Immunonutrition in the critically ill: A systematic review of clinical outcome. Critical Care Medicine. 1999;**27**(12):2799-2805. DOI: 10.1097/00003246-199912000-00032

[19] Heys SD, Walker LG, Smith I, Eremin O. Enteral nutritional supplementation with key nutrients in patients with critical illness and caner: A meta-analysis of randomized controlled clinical trials. Nutrition Clinique et Metabolisme. 2000;**14**(1):62-63

[20] Adler DG, Fang J, Wong R, Wills J, Hilden K. Placement of polyflex stents in patients with locally advanced esophageal cancer is safe and improves dysphagia during neoadjuvant therapy. Gastrointestinal Endoscopy. 2009;**70**(4):614-619. DOI: 10.1016/j.gie.2009.01.026

[21] Langer FB, Schoppmann SF, Prager G, et al. Temporary placement of self-expanding oesophageal stents as bridging for neo-adjuvant therapy. Annals of Surgical Oncology. 2010;**17**(2):470-475. DOI: 10.1245/s10434-009-0760-6

[22] Srinathan SK, Hamin T, Walter S, Tan AL, Unruh HW, Guyatt G. Jejunostomy tube feeding in patients undergoing esophagectomy. Canadian Journal of Surgery. 2013;**56**(6):409-414. DOI: 10.1503/cjs.008612

[23] Fenton JR, Bergeron EJ, Coello M, Welsh RJ, Chmielewski GW. Feeding jejunostomy tubes placed during esophagectomy: Are they necessary? The Annals of Thoracic Surgery. 2011;**92**(2):504-11; discussion 511-2. DOI: 10.1016/j.athoracsur.2011.03.101

[24] Weijs TJ, van Eden HWJ, Ruurda JP, et al. Routine jejunostomy tube feeding following esophagectomy. Journal of Thoracic Disease. 2017;**9**:S851-S860. DOI: 10.21037/jtd.2017.06.73

[25] Yoshida N, Baba Y, Hiyoshi Y, et al. Duration of smoking cessation and postoperative morbidity after esophagectomy for esophageal cancer: How long should patients stop smoking before surgery? World Journal of Surgery. 2016;**40**(1):142-147. DOI: 10.1007/s00268-015-3236-9

[26] Mantziari S, Allemann P, Winiker M, Demartines N, Schäfer M. Locoregional tumor extension and preoperative smoking are significant risk factors for early recurrence after esophagectomy for cancer. World Journal of Surgery. 2017;**42**(7):2209-2217. DOI: 10.1007/s00268-017-4422-8

[27] Brusselaers N, Mattsson F, Lagergren J. Hospital and surgeon volume in relation to long-term survival after oesophagectomy: Systematic review and meta-analysis. Gut. 2014;**63**(9):1393-1400. DOI: 10.1136/gutjnl-2013-306074

[28] Varghese TK, Wood DE, Farjah F, et al. Variation in esophagectomy outcomes in hospitals meeting leapfrog volume outcome standards. The Annals of Thoracic Surgery. 2011;**91**(4):1003-1009. DOI: 10.1016/j.athoracsur.2010.11.006

[29] Begg CB, Cramer LD, Hoskins WJ, Brennan MF. Impact of hospital volume on operative mortality for major cancer surgery. Journal of the American Medical Association. 1998;**280**(20):1747-1751

[30] Birkmeyer JD, Lucas FL, Wennberg DE. Potential benefits of regionalizing major surgery in medicare patients. Effective Clinical Practice. 1999;**2**(6):277-283

[31] Birkmeyer JD, Dimick JB. Potential benefits of the new leapfrog standards: Effect of process and outcomes measures. Surgery. 2004;**135**(6):569-575. DOI: 10.1016/j.surg.2004.03.004

[32] McCahill LE, May M, Morrow JB, et al. Esophagectomy outcomes at a mid-volume cancer center utilizing prospective multidisciplinary care and a 2-surgeon team approach. American Journal of Surgery. 2014;**207**(3):380-386. DOI: 10.1016/j.amjsurg.2013.09.013

[33] Kauppila JH, Wahlin K, Lagergren P, Lagergren J. University hospital status and surgeon volume and risk of reoperation following surgery for esophageal cancer. European Journal of Surgical Oncology. 2018;**44**(5):632-637. DOI: 10.1016/j.ejso.2018.02.212

[34] Varagunam M, Hardwick R, Riley S, Chadwick G, Cromwell DA, Groene O. Changes in volume, clinical practice and outcome after reorganisation of oesophago-gastric cancer care in England: A longitudinal observational study. European Journal of Surgical Oncology. 2018;**44**(4):524-531. DOI: 10.1016/j.ejso.2018.01.001

[35] Hummel R, Ha NH, Lord A, Trochsler MI, Maddern G, Kanhere H. Centralisation of oesophagectomy in Australia: Is only caseload critical? Australian Health Review. 2017. DOI: 10.1071/AH17095

[36] Michael Griffin S, Shaw IH, Dresner SM. Early complications after ivorlewis subtotal esophagectomy with two-field lymphadenectomy: Risk factors and management. Journal of the American College of Surgeons. 2002;**194**(3):285-297. DOI: 10.1016/S1072-7515(01)01177-2

[37] Funk LM, Gawande AA, Semel ME, et al. Esophagectomy outcomes at low-volume hospitals: The association between systems characteristics and mortality. Annals of Surgery. 2011;**253**(5):912-917. DOI: 10.1097/SLA.0b013e318213862f

[38] Dudley RA, Johansen KL, Brand R, Rennie DJ, Milstein A. Selective referral to high-volume hospitals: Estimating potentially avoidable deaths. Journal of the American Medical Association. 2000;**283**(9):1159-1166

[39] Birkmeyer JD, Siewers AE, Finlayson EVA, et al. Hospital volume and surgical mortality in the United States. New England Journal of Medicine. 2002;**346**(15):1128-1137. DOI: 10.1056/NEJMsa012337

[40] Halm EA, Lee C, Chassin MR. Is volume related to outcome in health care? A systematic review and methodologic critique of the literature. Annals of Internal Medicine. 2002;**137**(6):511-520

[41] Amaravadi RK, Dimick JB, Pronovost PJ, Lipsett PA. ICU nurse-to-patient ratio is associated with complications and resource use after esophagectomy. Intensive Care Medicine. 2000;**26**(12):1857-1862. DOI: 10.1007/s001340000720

[42] Pennathur A, Farkas A, Krasinskas AM, et al. Esophagectomy for T1 esophageal cancer: Outcomes in 100 patients and implications for endoscopic therapy. The Annals of Thoracic Surgery. 2009;**87**(4):1048-1055. DOI: 10.1016/j.athoracsur.2008.12.060

[43] Luketich JD, Pennathur A, Awais O, et al. Outcomes after minimally invasive esophagectomy: Review of over 1000 patients. Annals of Surgery. 2012;**256**(1):95-103. DOI: 10.1097/SLA.0b013e3182590603

[44] Luketich JD, Pennathur A, Franchetti Y, et al. Minimally invasive esophagectomy: Results of a prospective phase II multicenter trial-the eastern cooperative oncology group (E2202) study. Annals of Surgery. 2015;**261**(4):702-707. DOI: 10.1097/SLA.0000000000000993

[45] Sarkaria IS, Rizk NP, Grosser R, et al. Attaining proficiency in robotic-assisted minimally invasive esophagectomy while maximizing safety during procedure development. Innovations Technology and Techniques in Cardiothoracic and Vascular Surgery. 2016; **11**(4):268-273. DOI: 10.1097/IMI.0000000000000297

[46] Junginger T, Gockel I, Heckhoff S. A comparison of transhiatal and transthoracic resections on the prognosis in patients with squamous cell carcinoma of the esophagus. European Journal of Surgical Oncology. 2006;**32**(7):749-755. DOI: 10.1016/j.ejso.2006.03.048

[47] Stawicki SPA, Prosciak MP, Gerlach AT, et al. Atrial fibrillation after esophagectomy: An indicator of postoperative morbidity. General Thoracic and Cardiovascular Surgery. 2011;**59**(6):399-405. DOI: 10.1007/s11748-010-0713-9

[48] Lohani KR, Nandipati KC, Rollins SE, et al. Transthoracic approach is associated with increased incidence of atrial fibrillation after esophageal resection. Surgical Endoscopy. 2015;**29**(7):2039-2045. DOI: 10.1007/s00464-014-3908-9

[49] Seesing MFJ, Scheijmans JCG, Borggreve AS, van Hillegersberg R, Ruurda JP. The predictive value of new-onset atrial fibrillation on postoperative morbidity after esophagectomy. Diseases of the Esophagus. 2018. DOI: 10.1093/dote/doy028

[50] Turagam MK, Downey FX, Kress DC, Sra J, Tajik AJ, Jahangir A. Pharmacological strategies for prevention of postoperative atrial fibrillation. Expert Review of Clinical Pharmacology. 2015;**8**(2):233-250. DOI: 10.1586/17512433.2015.1018182

[51] Tisdale JE, Wroblewski HA, Wall DS, et al. A randomized, controlled study of amiodarone for prevention of atrial fibrillation after transthoracic esophagectomy. The Journal of Thoracic and Cardiovascular Surgery. 2010;**140**(1):45-51. DOI: 10.1016/j.jtcvs.2010.01.026

[52] Fabian T, Rassias DJ, Daneshmand MA, Ilves R. Amiodarone for atrial fibrillation prophylaxis in patients undergoing esophagectomy. Chest. 2004;**126**(4):800S

[53] Fernando HC, Jaklitsch MT, Walsh GL, et al. The society of thoracic surgeons practice guideline on the prophylaxis and management of atrial fibrillation associated with

general thoracic surgery: Executive summary. The Annals of Thoracic Surgery. 2011; **92**(3):1144-1152. DOI: 10.1016/j.athoracsur.2011.06.104

[54] Kalil AC, Metersky ML, Klompas M, et al. Executive summary: Management of adults with hospital-acquired and ventilator-associated pneumonia: 2016 clinical practice guidelines by the infectious diseases society of America and the American thoracic society. Clinical Infectious Diseases. 2016;**63**(5):575-582. DOI: 10.1093/cid/ciw504

[55] Weijs TJ, Seesing MFJ, van Rossum PSN, et al. Internal and external validation of a multivariable model to define hospital-acquired pneumonia after esophagectomy. Journal of Gastrointestinal Surgery. 2016;**20**(4):680-687. DOI: 10.1007/s11605-016-3083-5

[56] Bhattacharyya N, Batirel H, Swanson SJ. Improved outcomes with early vocal fold medialization for vocal fold paralysis after thoracic surgery. Auris, Nasus, Larynx. 2003;**30**(1):71-75. DOI: 10.1016/S0385-8146(02)00114-1

[57] Scholtemeijer MG, Seesing MFJ, Brenkman HJF, Janssen LM, van Hillegersberg R, Ruurda JP. Recurrent laryngeal nerve injury after esophagectomy for esophageal cancer: Incidence, management, and impact on short- and long-term outcomes. Journal of Thoracic Disease. 2017;**9**(Suppl 8):S868-S878. DOI: 10.21037/jtd.2017.06.92 [doi]

[58] Sierzega M, Kolodziejczyk P, Kulig J. Impact of anastomotic leakage on long-term survival after total gastrectomy for carcinoma of the stomach. The British Journal of Surgery. 2010;**97**(7):1035-1042. DOI: 10.1002/bjs.7038

[59] Rizk NP, Ishwaran H, Rice TW, et al. Optimum lymphadenectomy for esophageal cancer. Annals of Surgery. 2010;**251**(1):46-50. DOI: 10.1097/SLA.0b013e3181b2f6ee

[60] Kassis ES, Kosinski AS, Ross P, Koppes KE, Donahue JM, Daniel VC. Predictors of anastomotic leak after esophagectomy: An analysis of the society of thoracic surgeons general thoracic database. The Annals of Thoracic Surgery. 2013;**96**(6):1919-1926. DOI: 10.1016/j.athoracsur.2013.07.119

[61] Chadi SA, Fingerhut A, Berho M, et al. Emerging trends in the etiology, prevention, and treatment of gastrointestinal anastomotic leakage. Journal of Gastrointestinal Surgery. 2016;**20**(12):2035-2051. DOI: 10.1007/s11605-016-3255-3

[62] Lerut T, Coosemans W, Decker G, De Leyn P, Nafteux P, Van Raemdonck D. Anastomotic complications after esophagectomy. Digestive Surgery. 2002;**19**(2):92-98. DOI: 10.1159/000052018

[63] Cooke DT, Lin GC, Lau CL, et al. Analysis of cervical esophagogastric anastomotic leaks after transhiatal esophagectomy: Risk factors, presentation, and detection. The Annals of Thoracic Surgery. 2009;**88**(1):177-185. DOI: 10.1016/j.athoracsur.2009.03.035

[64] Wilson SE, Stone R, Scully M, Ozeran L, Benfield JR. Modern management of anastomotic leak after esophagogastrectomy. American Journal of Surgery. 1982;**144**(1):95-101. DOI: 10.1016/0002-9610(82)90608-0

[65] Mathisen DJ, Grillo HC, Wilkins EW Jr, Moncure AC, Hilgenberg AD. Transthoracic esophagectomy: A safe approach to carcinoma of the esophagus. The Annals of Thoracic Surgery. 1988;**45**(2):137-143

[66] Postlethwait RW. Complications and deaths after operations for esophageal carcinoma. The Journal of Thoracic and Cardiovascular Surgery. 1983;**85**(6):827-831

[67] Okuyama M, Motoyama S, Suzuki H, Saito R, Maruyama K, Ogawa J. Hand-sewn cervical anastomosis versus stapled intrathoracic anastomosis after esophagectomy for middle or lower thoracic esophageal cancer: A prospective randomized controlled study. Surgery Today. 2007;**37**(11):947-952. DOI: 10.1007/s00595-007-3541-5

[68] Orringer MB, Marshall B, Iannettoni MD. Eliminating the cervical esophagogastric anastomotic leak with a side-to-side stapled anastomosis. The Journal of Thoracic and Cardiovascular Surgery. 2000;**119**(2):277-288. DOI: 10.1016/S0022-5223(00)70183-8

[69] Turkyilmaz A, Eroglu A, Aydin Y, Tekinbas C, Muharrem Erol M, Karaoglanoglu N. The management of esophagogastric anastomotic leak after esophagectomy for esophageal-carcinoma. Diseases of the Esophagus. 2009;**22**(2):119-126. DOI: 10.1111/j.1442-2050.2008.00866.x

[70] Dai JG, Zhang ZY, Min JX, Huang XB, Wang JS. Wrapping of the omental pedicle flap around esophagogastric anastomosis after esophagectomy for esophageal cancer. Surgery (USA). 2011;**149**(3):404-410. DOI: 10.1016/j.surg.2010.08.005

[71] Bhat MA, Dar MA, Lone GN, Dar AM. Use of pedicledomentum in esophagogastric anastomosis for prevention of anastomotic leak. The Annals of Thoracic Surgery. 2006;**82**(5):1857-1862. DOI: 10.1016/j.athoracsur.2006.05.101

[72] Deitmar S, Anthoni C, Palmes D, Haier J, Senninger N, Brüwer M. Are leukocytes and CRP early indicators for anastomotic leakage after esophageal resection? Zentralblatt für Chirurgie. 2009;**134**(1):83-89. DOI: 10.1055/s-0028-1098768

[73] Veeramootoo D, Parameswaran R, Krishnadas R, et al. Classification and early recognition of gastric conduit failure after minimally invasive esophagectomy. Surgical Endoscopy. 2009;**23**(9):2110-2116. DOI: 10.1007/s00464-008-0233-1

[74] Sauvanet A, Baltar J, Le Mee J, Belghiti J. Diagnosis and conservative management of intrathoracic leakage after oesophagectomy. The British Journal of Surgery. 1998;**85**(10):1446-1449. DOI: 10.1046/j.1365-2168.1998.00869.x

[75] Roh S, Iannettoni MD, Keech JC, Bashir M, Gruber PJ, Parekh KR. Role of barium swallow in diagnosing clinically significant anastomotic leak following esophagectomy. Korean Journal of Thoracic and Cardiovascular Surgery. 2016;**49**(2):99-106. DOI: 10.5090/kjtcs.2016.49.2.99

[76] Andreou A, Struecker B, Biebl M, Pratschke J. Routine barium swallow may be unnecessary after resection of esophageal cancer. Journal of the American College of Surgeons. 2015;**221**(4):S145. DOI: 10.1016/j.jamcollsurg.2015.07.347

[77] Kauer WKH, Stein HJ, Dittler H, Siewert JR. Stent implantation as a treatment option in patients with thoracic anastomotic leaks after esophagectomy. Surgical Endoscopy. 2008;**22**(1):50-53. DOI: 10.1007/s00464-007-9504-5

[78] Brangewitz M, Voigtländer T, Helfritz FA, et al. Endoscopic closure of esophageal intrathoracic leaks: Stent versus endoscopic vacuum-assisted closure, a retrospective analysis. Endoscopy. 2013;**45**(6):433-438. DOI: 10.1055/s-0032-1326435

[79] Ahrens M, Schulte T, Egberts J, et al. Drainage of esophageal leakage using endoscopic vacuum therapy: A prospective pilot study. Endoscopy. 2010;**42**(9):693-698. DOI: 10.1055/s-0030-1255688

[80] Wedemeyer J, Brangewitz M, Kubicka S, et al. Management of major postsurgical gastroesophageal intrathoracic leaks with an endoscopic vacuum-assisted closure system. Gastrointestinal Endoscopy. 2010;**71**(2):382-386. DOI: 10.1016/j.gie.2009.07.011

[81] Mennigen R, Harting C, Lindner K, et al. Comparison of endoscopic vacuum therapy versus stent for anastomotic leak after esophagectomy. Journal of Gastrointestinal Surgery. 2015;**19**(7):1229-1235. DOI: 10.1007/s11605-015-2847-7

[82] Diddee R, Shaw IH. Acquired tracheo-oesophageal fistula in adults. Continuing Education in Anaesthesia Critical Care & Pain. 2006;**6**(3):105-108. DOI: 10.1093/bjaceaccp/mkl019

[83] Blackmon SH, Santora R, Schwarz P, Barroso A, Dunkin BJ. Utility of removable esophageal covered self-expanding metal stents for leak and fistula management. The Annals of Thoracic Surgery. 2010;**89**(3):931-937. DOI: 10.1016/j.athoracsur.2009.10.061

[84] Marchese S, Qureshi YA, Hafiz SP, et al. Intraoperative pyloric interventions during oesophagectomy: A multicentre study. Journal of Gastrointestinal Surgery. 2018:1-6. DOI: 10.1007/s11605-018-3759-0

[85] Eldaif SM, Lee R, Adams KN, et al. Intrapyloric botulinum injection increases postoperative esophagectomy complications. The Annals of Thoracic Surgery. 2014;**97**(6):1959-1965. DOI: 10.1016/j.athoracsur.2013.11.026

[86] Zhang L, Hou S, Miao J, Lee H. Risk factors for delayed gastric emptying in patients undergoing esophagectomy without pyloric drainage. The Journal of Surgical Research. 2017;**213**:46-50. DOI: 10.1016/j.jss.2017.02.012

[87] Smoke A, Delegge MH. Chyle leaks: Consensus on management? Nutrition in Clinical Practice. 2008;**23**(5):529-532. DOI: 10.1177/0884533608323424

[88] Jensen GL, Mascioli EA, Meyer LP, et al. Dietary modification of chyle composition in chylothorax. Gastroenterology. 1989;**97**(3):761-765. DOI: 10.1016/0016-5085(89)90650-1

[89] Dugue L, Sauvanet A, Farges O, Goharin A, Le Mee J, Belghiti J. Output of chyle as an indicator of treatment for chylothorax complicating oesophagectomy. The British Journal of Surgery. 1998;**85**(8):1147-1149. DOI: 10.1046/j.1365-2168.1998.00819.x

[90] Lin Y, Li Z, Li G, et al. Selective en masse ligation of the thoracic duct to prevent chyle leak after esophagectomy. The Annals of Thoracic Surgery. 2017;**103**(6):1802-1807

[91] Shackcloth MJ, Poullis M, Lu J, Page RD. Preventing of chylothorax after oesophagectomy by routine pre-operative administration of oral cream. European Journal of Cardio-Thoracic Surgery. 2001;**20**(5):1035-1036. DOI: 10.1016/S1010-7940(01)00928-9

[92] Sriram K, Meguid RA, Meguid MM. Nutritional support in adults with chyle leaks. Nutrition. 2016;**32**(2):281-286. DOI: 10.1016/j.nut.2015.08.002

[93] Browse NL, Allen DR, Wilson NM. Management of chylothorax. The British Journal of Surgery. 1997;**84**(12):1711-1716. DOI: 10.1046/j.1365-2168.1997.02858.x

[94] Martucci N, Tracey M, Rocco G. Postoperative chylothorax. Thoracic Surgery Clinics. Nov. 2015;**25**(4):523-528

[95] Zabeck H, Muley TF, Dienemann HF, Hoffmann H. Management of chylothorax in adults: When is surgery indicated? The Thoracic and Cardiovascular Surgeon. 2011;**59**(4): 243-246

[96] Nair SK, Petko M, Hayward MP. Aetiology and management of chylothorax in adults. European Journal of Cardio-Thoracic Surgery. 2007;**32**(2):362-369. DOI: 10.1016/j.ejcts.2007.04.024

[97] Pamarthi V, Stecker MS, Schenker MP, et al. Thoracic duct embolization and disruption for treatment of chylous effusions: Experience with 105 patients. Journal of Vascular and Interventional Radiology. 2014;**25**(9):1398-1404. DOI: 10.1016/j.jvir.2014.03.027

[98] Guevara CJ, Rialon KL, Ramaswamy RS, Kim SK, Darcy MD. US-guided, direct puncture retrograde thoracic duct access, lymphangiography, and embolization: Feasibility and efficacy. Journal of Vascular and Interventional Radiology. Dec. 2016;**27**(12):1890-1896

Permissions

All chapters in this book were first published in ECB, by InTech Open; hereby published with permission under the Creative Commons Attribution License or equivalent. Every chapter published in this book has been scrutinized by our experts. Their significance has been extensively debated. The topics covered herein carry significant findings which will fuel the growth of the discipline. They may even be implemented as practical applications or may be referred to as a beginning point for another development.

The contributors of this book come from diverse backgrounds, making this book a truly international effort. This book will bring forth new frontiers with its revolutionizing research information and detailed analysis of the nascent developments around the world.

We would like to thank all the contributing authors for lending their expertise to make the book truly unique. They have played a crucial role in the development of this book. Without their invaluable contributions this book wouldn't have been possible. They have made vital efforts to compile up to date information on the varied aspects of this subject to make this book a valuable addition to the collection of many professionals and students.

This book was conceptualized with the vision of imparting up-to-date information and advanced data in this field. To ensure the same, a matchless editorial board was set up. Every individual on the board went through rigorous rounds of assessment to prove their worth. After which they invested a large part of their time researching and compiling the most relevant data for our readers.

The editorial board has been involved in producing this book since its inception. They have spent rigorous hours researching and exploring the diverse topics which have resulted in the successful publishing of this book. They have passed on their knowledge of decades through this book. To expedite this challenging task, the publisher supported the team at every step. A small team of assistant editors was also appointed to further simplify the editing procedure and attain best results for the readers.

Apart from the editorial board, the designing team has also invested a significant amount of their time in understanding the subject and creating the most relevant covers. They scrutinized every image to scout for the most suitable representation of the subject and create an appropriate cover for the book.

The publishing team has been an ardent support to the editorial, designing and production team. Their endless efforts to recruit the best for this project, has resulted in the accomplishment of this book. They are a veteran in the field of academics and their pool of knowledge is as vast as their experience in printing. Their expertise and guidance has proved useful at every step. Their uncompromising quality standards have made this book an exceptional effort. Their encouragement from time to time has been an inspiration for everyone.

The publisher and the editorial board hope that this book will prove to be a valuable piece of knowledge for researchers, students, practitioners and scholars across the globe.

List of Contributors

Dimitrios Schizas, Irene Lidoriki and Theodore Liakakos
First Department of Surgery, Laikon General Hospital, National and Kapodistrian University of Athens, Athens, Greece

Demetrios Moris
Department of Surgery, Division of Surgical Oncology, The Ohio State University Wexner Medical Center and James Cancer Hospital and Solove Research Institute, Columbus, OH, USA

Tian Wang and Yi Zhang
Biotherapy Center, The First Affiliated Hospital of Zhengzhou University, Zhengzhou, Henan, China

Talha Sarigoz
Department of General Surgery, Sason State Hospital, Batman, Turkey

Inanc Samil Sarici
Department of General Surgery, Kanuni Sultan Suleyman Training and Research Hospital, Istanbul, Turkey

Ozgul Duzgun
Division of Surgical Oncology, Department of General Surgery, Umraniye Training and Research Hospital, Istanbul, Turkey

Mustafa Uygar Kalayci
Department of General Surgery, Kanuni Sultan Suleyman Training and Research Hospital, Istanbul, Turkey

Shunsuke Sakuraba
Department of Surgery, Juntendo Shizuoka Hospital, Shizuoka, Japan

Ljiljana Širić
Department of Otorhinolaryngology and Head and Neck Surgery, University Hospital Centre Osijek, Osijek, Croatia

Marinela Rosso
Polyclinic Rosso, Osijek, Croatia

Aleksandar Včev
Faculty of Medicine, J. J. Strossmayer University of Osijek, Osijek, Croatia

Byoung Jo Suh
Department of Surgery, Memorial Jin-Pok Kim Gastric Cancer Center, Haeundae Paik Hospital, Inje University College of Medicine, Busan, Korea

Satoshi Kanda and Tetsu Fukunaga
Gastroenterology and Minimally Invasive Surgery, Juntendo University, Tokyo, Japan

Aragona Salvatore Emanuele and Mereghetti Giada
Center of Regenerative Medicine, Humanitas Mater Domini, Castellanza (VA), Italy

Giorgio Ciprandi
Ospedale Policlinico San Martino, Genoa, Italy

Shouji Shimoyama
Gastrointestinal Unit, Settlement Clinic, Towa, Adachi-ku, Tokyo, Japan

Nebojsa S. Ignjatovic, Miroslav P. Stojanovic, Goran Z. Stanojevic and Miodrag N. Djordjevic
Department of Surgery, School of Medicine, University of Nis, Nis, Serbia

Tomislav D. Randjelovic
Department of Surgery, School of Medicine, University of Belgrade, Belgrade, Serbia

Tamer Saafan
General Surgery Department, Hamad General Hospital, Hamad Medical Corporation, Doha, Qatar

Ivan M. Buzurovic, Desmond A. O'Farrell, Mandar S. Bhagwat and Phillip M. Devlin
Department of Radiation Oncology, Dana-Farber/ Brigham and Women's Cancer Center, Harvard Medical School, Boston, MA, USA

Borbala Daroczi
Department of Radiology, Brigham and Women's Hospital, Harvard Medical School, Boston, MA, USA

Jacqueline Oxenberg
Geisinger Wyoming Valley, Wilkes-Barre, PA, USA

Index

www.ingramcontent.com/pod-product-compliance
Lightning Source LLC
LaVergne TN
LVHW060537210926
848485LV00005B/1214

* 9 7 8 1 6 3 9 8 9 0 2 2 4 *